Written by Alastair Gray and Philip Payne, in
collaboration with the U205 Course Team

Contents

About this book

A note for the general reader

World Health and Disease examines contemporary and historical patterns of health and disease in the United Kingdom and the rest of the world. The book draws on epidemiology, history, the social sciences and biology to describe and explain its subject matter.

The book contains eleven chapters which can be grouped around the following broad themes. After an introductory chapter, Chapters 2 to 4 provide an epidemiological and demographic survey of the contemporary world, discussing population trends and structures, birth and mortality rates and causes of death in different parts of the world, and recent trends in life expectancy. Chapter 4 offers a sketch of the way in which these patterns manifest themselves in the life of a Bangladeshi village.

Chapters 5 to 8 are concerned with the links between health, population, and social and economic development. Chapters 5 and 6 examine population history and theories, then examine the impact of the Industrial Revolution on the health and the size and structure of England's population. Chapters 7 and 8 then consider the way in which health and population change are related to the process of development in the Third World. The main theme of these chapters is that world patterns of health and disease can only be understood properly within a social and economic context.

In Chapters 9 and 10 the focus changes to one country—the United Kingdom—in order to examine in more detail the nature and causes of health and disease patterns within a nation. Chapter 11 concludes the book with a case study of food and health. The objective of this case study is to bring together the various perspectives adopted elsewhere in the book, and to show as vividly as possible the many factors that influence what we eat, as well as the complex relationship between diet, nutrition and health.

The book is fully indexed and contains an annotated guide to further reading.

World Health and Disease is the third in a series of eight books on the subject of health and disease specially written for the Open University for the second level course U205 Health and Disease. The book is designed so that it can be read on its own, like any other textbook, or studied as part of this course. General readers need not make use of the study comments, learning objectives and other material inserted for OU students, although they may find these helpful. The text also contains references to a collection of readings[1] prepared for the OU course: it is quite possible to follow the text without reading the articles referred to, although doing so should enhance your understanding of this book's contents.

A guide for OU students

World Health and Disease emphasises that social science, epidemiology, and biology can each contribute to an integrated descriptive and explanatory account of health and disease patterns. It therefore draws on a number of different methods of studying health and disease which were discussed earlier in the course, and provides some empirical foundations for later books. The index includes key words in bold type (also printed in bold in the text) which can be looked up easily as an aid to revision as the course proceeds. There is also a further reading list for those who wish to pursue certain aspects of study beyond the limits of this book.

The time allowed for studying *World Health and Disease* is four weeks or around 40–48 hours. The following table gives a more detailed breakdown to help you to pace your study. You need not follow it slavishly but do not allow yourself to fall behind. If you find a section of the work difficult, do what you can at this stage, and then return to the material when you reach the end of the book.

There is a tutor-marked assignment (TMA) associated with this book; about three hours have been allowed for completing it, *in addition* to the time spent in studying the material that it assesses.

Final note:

Many chapters in this book involve the interpretation of data about populations, their lifestyles and their health status. All this material is discussed in some way in the text, although you may wish to refer back to relevant parts of *Studying Health and Disease* when interpreting the data. However, please do not feel that there is any need to *memorise* them: they have been included primarily to illustrate and to help explain the patterns and relationships that the text is exploring.

[1]*Health and Disease: A Reader* (Open University Press 1984; revised edition 1994).

Study guide for Book 3 (total 40–48 hours, including time for the TMA, spread over 4 weeks). Notice that there are some long chapters at the end of the book; you should allow enough time to read them before completing the TMA.

1st week

Chapter 1   **Introduction**

Chapter 2   **World patterns of mortality**

Chapter 3   **Mortality and morbidity: causes and determinants**, including *Reader* article by Strassburg (1982) and TV programme and audiotape on mortality and morbidity in Zimbabwe

Chapter 4   **Livelihood and survival: a case study of Bangladesh**

Chapter 5   **The world transformed: population and the rise of industrial society**, including Reader article by Engels (1844)

2nd week

Chapter 6   **The decline of infectious diseases: the case of England**, including *Reader* articles by McKeown (1976) and Szreter (1988)

Chapter 7   **Health in a world of wealth and poverty**, including *Reader* article by Drèze and Sen (1989)

Chapter 8   **Population and development prospects**

3rd week

Chapter 9   **Contemporary patterns of disease in the United Kingdom**

Chapter 10   **Explaining inequalities in health in the United Kingdom**, including *Reader* article by the Medical Services Study Group of the Royal College of Physicians (1978) and TV programme and audiotape on inequalities in health in the United Kingdom

---

4th week

Chapter 11   **Food, health and disease: a case study**

TMA completion

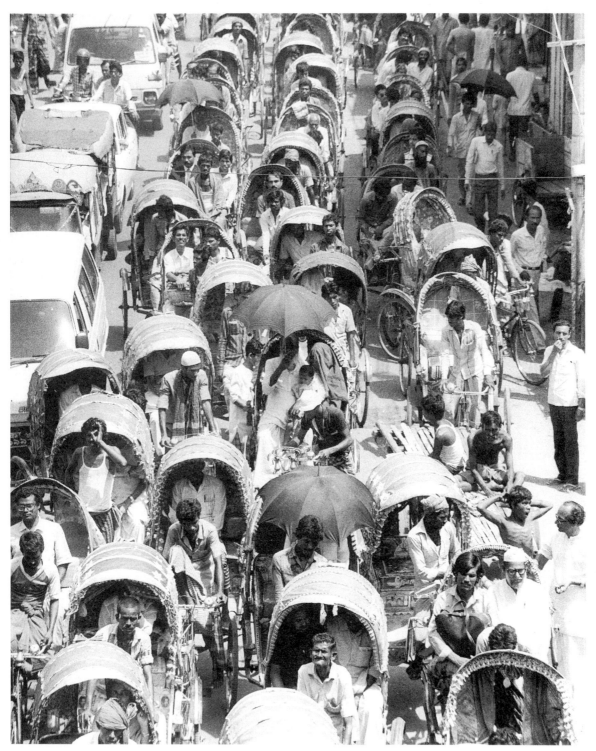

The 'full tide of human existence' on display in this street scene in Dhaka, Bangladesh in 1987.
(Photo: Walter Holt/OXFAM)

1 Introduction

This book is about the patterns of health and disease that exist around the world and in the United Kingdom, how they have changed over time, and the factors that influence them. The first aim of the book is to describe these patterns: for example, the length of life which people in different countries or social groups can expect and what they are likely to die of; or how birth and mortality rates influence population size and structures. The second aim of the book is to consider why these health and disease patterns exist, and what factors can best explain the way they have changed.

Three broad themes run through the book. One is to explore the extent to which world patterns of health and disease have been shaped and continue to be shaped by large-scale social, economic and environmental changes, such as the agricultural and industrial revolutions. A second is to consider whether the countries of the 'Third World' have health and disease patterns similar to those once found in the countries of the world that are now industrialised, and whether they can anticipate the same kinds of epidemiological and demographic changes as those that have accompanied industrialisation elsewhere. The third is to assess the degree to which patterns of health and disease can be related to more detailed aspects of a country's social and economic structure, such as housing, income or occupation.

The broad approach of the book, therefore, emphasises the social, economic and environmental characteristics of societies, and the ways in which these characteristics influence health and disease. This is not a book about the development of medical science, or about the people whose discoveries, skills and work helped to elevate medicine to the position of power and influence it holds today.[1] That approach often teems with the names of outstanding individuals, whereas in this book the 'great names' of history figure hardly at all, and primacy is given to social and economic change and to the natural environment, and the ways in which these interact with human health and population. This approach is not presented as *the* way to understand world health and disease patterns, but it is one powerful way of trying to understand and explain the determinants of these patterns, and how they arose.

The book, therefore, has a number of dimensions: it ranges across different disciplines, drawing on material from epidemiology, history, demography, economics, nutrition, biology, social policy and geography; it seeks both to describe and to explain; and it demonstrates the use of a comparative method. The comparisons made are between nations, between different population groups within nations, and between different historical periods.

These dimensions are complementary, but to present them all simultaneously would be highly confusing. Instead, the book has been designed gradually to build up an integrated view of health and disease patterns through a series of perspective shifts. Thus, Chapters 2 to 4 give an epidemiological survey of world health and disease patterns. Chapter 2 sketches the shape and size of the world's population, then looks at different measures of mortality and how they vary from country to country. Chapter 3 looks more closely at the main causes of death and disease around the world, and at the factors such as environment, demography, and socio-economic circumstances that influence their distribution. Chapter 4 attempts to provide a more human and less statistical account of health in the Third World, by focusing on the changing experience of health of a family in a village in Bangladesh.

Chapters 5 to 8 are concerned to set out and explore the links between health, population, and the social and economic environment. Chapter 5 begins this task by taking a historical look at the relation between health and the process of economic and social development, sketching what little we know about pre-industrial population history and disease patterns, the attempts by theorists such as Thomas Malthus to understand the mechanisms of population change, and the challenge to such theories posed by the Industrial Revolution. Chapter 6 looks in more detail at the way in which the first Industrial Revolution in England affected the health of

[1] This approach is discussed in two other books in this series, *Medical Knowledge: Doubt and Certainty* (Open University Press, 1985; revised edition 1994), and *Caring for Health: History and Diversity* (Open University Press, 1985; revised edition 1993).

the population, and examines the relative contributions of social change and medical intervention to the improved health that eventually resulted. Chapter 7 looks at the initial impact of the Industrial Revolution on the rest of the world, then examines the relation between health and economic and social development in the contemporary world. Chapter 8 examines more closely the ways in which population and development are related.

Following this, Chapters 9 and 10 switch to the epidemiology and social and economic characteristics of the United Kingdom. The contemporary health of people in the United Kingdom is analysed in Chapter 9, which looks at the influence of factors such as gender, social class, ethnicity, marital status and age, and at regional and other variations. Chapter 10 assesses the extent to which these patterns of health and disease can be related to particular social features such as housing, income, and occupation. Finally, Chapter 11 presents a detailed case study of nutrition and health which is intended as an illustration of the ways in which these different perspectives can be combined. In the case study we consider, for example, how our health may be affected by our diet which in turn is affected by the way in which food is produced and distributed.

Because we shall be looking at health patterns across the world we have to use some way of grouping or classifying countries. However, there is no simple or unanimously agreed way of doing this.

◻ Note down some of the ways in which countries can be categorised.

■ You might have thought of some of the following: rich and poor; East and West; developed and developing; North and South; advanced and backward; industrial and non-industrial; modern and traditional; capitalist and socialist; democratic and authoritarian.

All such groupings tend to suffer from two big problems. First, the similarities between countries on which they are supposedly based may be less important than the differences between these same countries. For example, Iceland and Russia are both in the 'North', but their cultures, histories, size, politics and roles in today's world are totally different. Second, the ways in which countries

are grouped and the labels attached to them are not neutral; these choices indicate a particular view of the world with which many might not agree. For example, to talk of the 'developing' countries is to imply that the countries referred to are undergoing progressive changes that in time will make them developed. A quite different view is implied by the word 'underdeveloped', which somehow implies that these countries are not as developed as they should be or could have been, or even that their condition has been imposed on them.

There is no simple solution to these difficulties. Parts of the text that present and discuss official statistics simply make use of the classifications that were used when compiling them. For example, the World Bank, which publishes much useful data on most countries of the world, classifies countries simply according to whether their national income per person is 'low', 'middle' or 'high'. However, in general we have opted to use the terms 'Third World' and 'industrialised' countries, on the grounds that these are the terms often used by countries when classifying themselves, and they avoid the pejorative or value-laden content of terms such as 'backward', 'developing' and 'advanced'. The **Third World** is taken broadly to include the countries of Africa, Central and South America, and most of Asia and the Pacific countries. Clearly, grouping together such a large number of countries is fraught with difficulties: some 'Third World' countries such as India, China or Brazil have substantial industrial sectors and may export aircraft or other advanced technology around the world; others are virtually prostrate economies, without natural resources and heavily dependent on foreign assistance and food aid. The **industrialised countries** are taken to include those in Western and Eastern Europe, North America, the former Soviet Union, and Japan, Australia and New Zealand, and thus include the capitalist industrialised countries (the 'First World'), and the formerly socialist industrialised countries which were until recently considered to be the 'Second World', and arguably have a shared historical experience which continues to set them apart from other industrialised countries in a variety of ways.

We will return to this question of classification at various points, for an important aim of the book is to examine the connection between the economic and social characteristics of countries and their disease burden, mortality rates, and demographic structure. Chapter 2 begins that task by examining world patterns of mortality.

2 *World patterns of mortality*

This chapter builds on some of the basic concepts of demography introduced in Studying Health and Disease[1]*, particularly the age–sex structure of a population, age distribution, age-standardised and age-specific mortality rates, the crude death rate and expectation of life. You may wish to refer to the explanations of these terms, using the index in that book.*

Neither is the population to be reckoned only by numbers. (Francis Bacon, 1561–1626)

In this chapter we shall be looking at the population of the world and how it is distributed: you will see what proportions of the world's population live in the Third World or in industrialised countries, and how these proportions are changing. We will then examine the age- and sex-structure of the populations in different countries, and explore the ways in which birth and death rates influence, and are in turn influenced by, population structure. Finally, you will see whether the mortality differences that separate the Third World and the industrialised world are narrowing.

Measuring health

Before embarking on a comparison of the levels of health of different populations we must be quite clear how we are going to measure health. In its constitution, the World Health Organization (WHO), an agency of the United Nations, has defined health as 'a state of complete physical, mental and social wellbeing' (WHO, 1958, Annex 1). It is easy to see that if we use this famous and frequently quoted definition there are going to be considerable problems in actually measuring the health of a nation or even that of an individual. Using this definition, what proportion of your own life is 'healthy'? Most of us would

have some difficulty in answering this question, even though the state described seems a desirable one to strive towards.

The WHO definition has been criticised on many grounds: for example, because of the difficulty of defining 'complete wellbeing'. So, for practical purposes, we are forced to use other surrogate or 'proxy' measures that are closely correlated with health or its absence, in particular the level of disease and death. (It should be noted, however, that when the WHO defined health, they pointed out that it was 'not merely the absence of disease and infirmity'.) Therefore, instead of looking at world patterns of health we are forced to look at world patterns of disease.

Furthermore, we shall have to use well-defined and perhaps rather rigid and limited definitions of disease— much more restricted than just the absence of health! Some aspects of disease will be neglected almost completely. This is not because they are unimportant but because reliable information is not available from enough places to allow meaningful comparisons. In general, diseases involving major physical sickness with well-defined symptoms and signs are easier to 'count' in different communities than are, for example, mental illness or more minor physiological disturbances.

Even if we select only certain diseases or disease states to study, there are several different measures that we might use to assess the magnitude of the disease problem in a given community. Measures that are commonly used include the disease incidence, prevalence[2], and severity. The last is difficult to measure, sometimes being assessed by the amount of (physical) disability or discomfort caused by the disease, and at other times by the **case-fatality rate**—the proportion of all cases of the disease that result in death. These measures are each useful for different purposes but even these are not generally available for many countries.

The major concern of this chapter is to compare the health of populations in different countries, particularly

---

[1]Another book in this series: *Studying Health and Disease* (Open University Press, 1985; revised edition 1994).

[2]Incidence and prevalence are defined in *Studying Health and Disease* (Open University Press, 1985; revised edition 1994).

in Third World and industrialised countries, a classification which was introduced in Chapter 1. Health data from many Third World countries are very limited and so this chapter concentrates on mortality. You should bear in mind that there are many diseases that kill only a small proportion of the persons they afflict. Chronically disabling diseases such as polio and leprosy in Third World countries or arthritis in industrialised countries are good examples. Nevertheless, it is in general reasonable to assume that communities in which the death rate is high are those in which rates of non-fatal diseases are also high.

Distribution of the world's population

It may be helpful to begin by reviewing how the world's population is distributed over the globe. In 1990, the total population of the world was estimated to be about 5 300 million.

    ☐ Before reading on, write down how you would expect this total to be divided between Africa, North America, Latin America, Asia, Europe, and the USSR.

    ■ Now compare your estimates with Table 2.1, which shows the population estimates for 1990 published by the United Nations.

Asia alone accounts for almost 60 per cent of the world's population. In fact well over a third of all the world's people live in just two countries, China and India. In contrast, less than one in ten of the world's population live in Europe.

    In some of its statistics, the United Nations splits the countries of the world into just two groups: the more developed regions, including North America, Europe (including the former Western and Eastern blocs), Australia, Japan, New Zealand and the (former) USSR, and the less developed regions, including Africa, Latin America, Asia and Oceania other than Australia and New Zealand. Table 2.1 also shows how the world's population was split between these two groups in 1990, and how this is projected to change by the year 2025. Approximately 4 100 million people, or just over three-quarters of the world's population, lived in the less developed countries—that is, the Third World—in 1990. By 2025, the proportion of the world's population living in the Third World will have increased to 84 per cent, although the social and economic structures of some of these countries might well have developed significantly by then.

Table 2.1 World population estimates, 1990 and 2025 (projected), by region

Region	Population in millions		as a percentage of world population	
	1990	2025	1990	2025
Africa	642	1 597	12	19
North/Central America	427	596	8	7
Latin America	297	494	6	6
Asia	3 113	4 913	59	58
(of which): China	1 139	1 513	21	18
India	853	1 442	16	17
Europe	498	515	9	6
Oceania	27	38	0.5	0.4
Former USSR	289	352	5	4
all more developed	1 205	1 353	23	16
all less developed	4 087	7 151	77	84
total	5 292	8 504	100	100

Data from United Nations Population Division, quoted in World Resources Institute (1992), *World Resources 1992–93*, Oxford University Press, Oxford and New York, Table 16.1, p. 246.

The growth of the world's population will be examined in more detail in Chapters 5 and 8. It is a simple arithmetical law that population growth occurs when the birth rate exceeds the death rate. However, both the birth rate and the death rate are influenced by the proportional distribution of the population across different age and sex groupings—the **population's age–sex structure**. And the age–sex structure is in turn influenced by the death rate and the birth rate. So if we wish to examine patterns of health and disease in the world as a whole, we must pay close attention to the age and sex structure of the world's population, and how it varies between countries.

The population pyramid

The **age structure** of a population is entirely defined by the rate at which people enter through birth or immigration from another population, and leave through death or by emigration to another population. To simplify things, we shall not be looking in detail at migration, which in most countries has not had an important influence on the overall population structure in recent decades. It should be noted, however, that migration has often had an important influence on differences in the population structure in different regions within a country. The **sex structure** of a population simply refers to the proportion of males and females. Usually age and sex structures are combined.

A census gives a cross-sectional 'snap-shot' of a population at one point in time. A direct and simple way of presenting this snap-shot of the age–sex structure of a population is by means of a **population pyramid**.

A population pyramid is drawn in much the same way as a histogram. In effect, it consists of two histograms, one for each sex, arranged horizontally (as opposed to the usual vertical orientation), and set back to back. The bar areas are made proportional to the population in each age–sex group.

Figure 2.1 contains population pyramids for four countries, which show strikingly the contrast in population structure between Third World and industrialised countries. The four countries are:

(a)   Sweden: fully industrialised and has been so for a long time.

(b)   Brazil: undergoing rapid industrialisation and urbanisation, but still with a large non-industrialised sector.

(c)   China: a poor country in the process of social and economic change, with a large rural sector and relatively well-developed health and social services.

(d)   Zimbabwe: predominantly rural with only a small industrial/ urban sector.

☐   Describe the pyramids for Zimbabwe (Figure 2.1d) and Brazil (Figure 2.1b), commenting on the distribution by age and sex and noting any obvious differences for males and females.

■   For Zimbabwe and to a slightly lesser extent Brazil, the pyramids are strikingly true to their name, each with a broad base, narrowing upwards so as to give a triangular picture. The most numerous age-groups are the youngest; almost half the population are aged under 15 years in Zimbabwe, and almost two-thirds are aged less than 35 in Brazil. Middle-aged and old people are relatively few in number; the percentage of the population over 64 years is less than 3 per cent in Zimbabwe, and only 5 per cent in Brazil. There is no obvious difference between the pyramids for males and for females.

If mortality rates have been high for all ages, the numbers in each age-group will tend to decrease with advancing age. For example, the broader base of the Zimbabwe pyramid, compared with that of Brazil, suggests a higher mortality under the age of 5 years: because mortality is high, fewer people progress to the next age-band, and so the pyramid narrows.

Another factor leads towards the triangular shape. Throughout most of history, human societies have normally experienced a demographic pattern of high birth rates and high rates of infant and child mortality, and this pattern still prevails in much of the Third World. If these mortality rates fall, then the number of female children who reach childbearing age in each successive generation will increase and the birth rate will rise. This is one of a number of factors that may create an increasing population. Mortality rates are now falling in many Third World countries, and although age-specific fertility rates are also falling in many countries (as you will see in Chapter 8), there are still more births than deaths, over a period of time. This is a major reason for the triangular shape of the population pyramid of a typical Third World country.

Generally, therefore, populations with the triangular shape have high birth rates, high mortality and substantial rates of increase in overall population size.

Now look at the population pyramid in Figure 2.1c for China. It reveals a somewhat different type of demographic structure. The bottom of the pyramid is in fact quite pinched, then there is a bulge in the 10–24 age-groups, and finally a long tapering-off with advancing age with a relatively small proportion of people aged 65 or over. Again, there is no obvious difference between males and females, except in the oldest age-groups.

☐   How might you explain the narrow base of the Chinese pyramid followed by a bulge among young adults?

■   One explanation might be that a 'baby boom' suddenly occurred, creating a large population cohort that is working its way up the pyramid. This phenomenon has been experienced in a number of industrialised countries, creating a bulge in the population structure that is sometimes referred to as the 'pig in the python'. However, in China a much more likely explanation is that the birth rate has been falling substantially in recent decades, thus pinching in the bottom of the pyramid.

The pyramid for China is fairly typical of countries that have experienced a falling death rate and rapidly increasing life expectancy, followed by a falling birth rate. As the generations currently at the bottom of the pyramid get older, so the pyramid will evolve a structure more similar to that in Sweden or other industrialised countries.

If you look more closely at the Chinese pyramid, you can see a number of irregularities. In particular, there is a curious 'waist' caused by the age-group 25–29 being much smaller than the groups on either side of it.

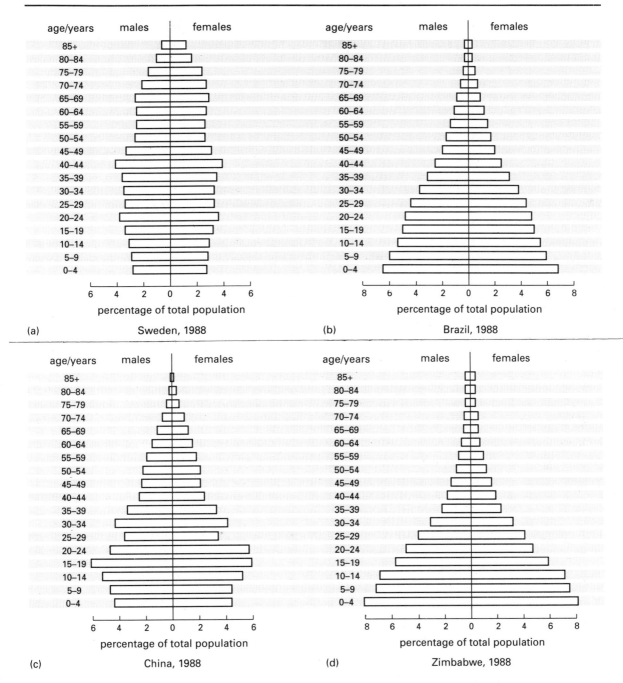

Figure 2.1 *Population pyramids for four countries. (Data from United Nations, 1991,* Demographic Yearbook 1989, *UN, New York, Table 7)*

☐ How might you go about trying to explain this?

■ An obvious starting point would be to look for some event that particularly affected that cohort of the Chinese population, for example when the cohort was born between 1958 and 1963.

In fact, we now know that between 1959 and 1961 parts of China were racked by a famine that may have killed around 15 million people. Famines, and the disproportionate effect that they have on very young children, will be examined in Chapters 7 and 11 of this book, but clearly this particular famine is one very plausible explanation for the irregular shape of China's present demographic structure.

The irregularities in the Chinese pyramid may also reflect the difficulties of conducting censuses of population with limited resources in the world's most populous country, and of determining ages with accuracy. This is a problem in most Third World countries where many people may have little documentary evidence of their date of birth, and are entirely reliant on their own and their parents' memories.

The picture for Sweden (Figure 2.1a) is again quite different. In Sweden, the most numerous age-groups are between 20 years and 44 years. The tapering-off with advancing age, seen so strikingly in the data for Zimbabwe (Figure 2.1d) and other Third World countries such as Brazil (Figure 2.1b), is only evident in the pyramid for Sweden for ages above 65 years. There is a far higher proportion of older people in Sweden and there are rather more elderly females than males. In contrast, the percentage under 15 years of age is well under 20 per cent, much lower than in Zimbabwe.

☐ In the population pyramid of Sweden, there is a low percentage of children under 5 years of age. To what could this be attributed?

■ This low percentage reflects a low birth rate. In fact, the larger percentages in the 5–9 and 10–14

years age-groups compared to the youngest age-group tell us that the numbers of births have declined over the last 10–15 years.

☐ In most Western countries, there was a 'baby boom' immediately after the Second World War. Can you see the effect of this in the Swedish population pyramid?

■ This is reflected by the 'bulge' in the pyramid in the 40–44 years age-group, whose members were born in the period immediately after the war.

You have seen that a triangular pyramid is typical of the population of a Third World country. It was also typical, in the past, of the countries that are now industrialised, such as England and Wales and the USA. Figure 2.2 shows the population of the USA in 1900 and in 1989.

The general resemblance of the American population structure in 1900 to, for example, that of present-day Brazil is quite striking. This has led some people to suggest that as a country undergoes a transition to fully industrialised development, so the population structure also changes, and they refer to this as the **demographic transition.** This is clearly an important concept with wide implications, and we shall return to it in Chapter 6 when we consider the process of industrialisation and development from an historical perspective.

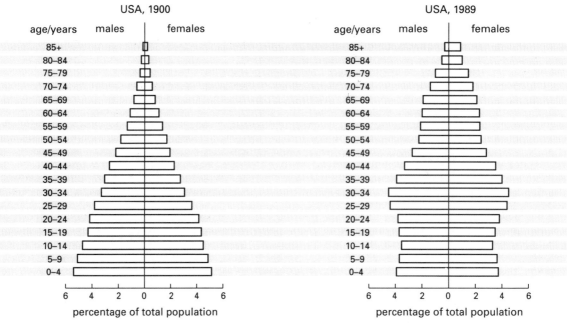

Figure 2.2 *Population pyramids of the USA in 1900 and in 1989. (Data for 1900 from Westoff, C. F., 1974, The populations of the developed countries,* Scientific American, *231 (3), September, p. 114; for 1989 from United Nations, 1991,* Demographic Yearbook 1989, *UN, New York, Table 7)*

Measuring mortality

We have already concluded, from the evidence of population structures, that death rates are in general higher in the countries of the Third World than in the industrialised countries. Let us now look at these variations in more detail.

Various measures are employed to compare mortality in the populations of different countries. The crude death rate, infant mortality rate and expectation of life at birth (defined later in this section) are all widely used for this purpose. Table 2.2 shows estimates of these measures for a sample of countries from each continent. These countries were chosen to illustrate the range of variation in mortality both within and between continents.

Death rates

Consider first the **crude death rates** for a number of selected countries shown in Table 2.2 (the crude death rate is the total number of deaths in a population in a year, expressed as a rate per 1 000 population). Run your eye down the second data column of the table and pick out the highest crude death rates, and the lowest.

Looking at the table, you will see that the highest rates among the countries listed were recorded in the Central African Republic, Mali and Bangladesh, all of which are Third World countries. The rates in these countries ranged from 15 to 20 per 1 000 per year. The rates in the industrialised countries of Europe and North America were lower, generally between 9 and 12 per 1 000. You may have been surprised however, to see that the lowest rates in the table, of 6 or 7 per 1 000, were recorded in Cuba, Jamaica, China, Japan and Sri Lanka. Only one of these—Japan—is a high income country, and Sri Lanka in particular is among the poorest of the world's countries.

In general, there is an inverse relationship between life expectancy in a country and the crude death rate for that country, that is, high life expectancy is associated

Table 2.2 Estimates of crude death rate, infant mortality rate and expectation of life at birth for selected countries, 1990 or nearest date

Country	Population /millions	Crude death rate per 1 000 per year	Infant mortality rate per 1 000 live births	Expectation of life at birth/years Male	Female
Africa					
Central African Republic	3	17	100	44	47
Egypt	52	10	61	59	61
Mali	9	20	164	46	50
Zimbabwe	10	10	61	57	60
Americas					
Brazil	150	8	60	62	68
Cuba	11	7	11	73	76
Jamaica	2	6	16	71	77
USA	249	9	10	71	78
Europe					
Poland	38	10	16	67	76
Portugal	10	10	13	68	75
Sweden	8	12	6	74	80
UK	57	12	9	72	78
Asia					
Bangladesh	116	15	114	57	56
China	1139	7	30	68	71
India	853	11	94	52	52
Japan	124	7	4	75	81
Sri Lanka	17	6	26	68	72
USSR	289	10	25	65	74

Data from United Nations (1991) *United Nations Demographic Yearbook 1989*, UN, New York, Table 4, and United Nations Development Programme (1992) *Human Development Report 1992*, Oxford University Press, Oxford and New York, Tables 22 and 43.

with a low crude death rate. However, this relationship is quite tenuous. For example, Brazil has a lower crude death rate than Sweden, but the life expectancy of both men and women is lower in Brazil. One set of figures appears to indicate that, on average, people live longer in Brazil, the other flatly denies that this is so. How do we reconcile these data? The answer lies in the population pyramids of the two populations. Put simply, Sweden has a higher *crude* death rate than Brazil because it has a higher proportion of old people. If the age distributions of different countries are similar, then crude death rates may be a reasonable basis on which to compare levels of mortality. However, if the age distributions differ (and you have already seen in Figure 2.1 that they do) the use of crude death rates to compare levels of mortality is likely to be misleading. It would be preferable to calculate **age-standardised death rates**, or, if possible, to compare the **age-specific death rates** of the two countries. (Age-specific and sex-specific death rates refer to deaths in a particular age or sex group of a population, expressed as a rate per 1 000 people in that population group.)

A comparison of age-specific death rates for females in Brazil and Sweden is shown in Figure 2.3.

In both countries the mortality rate is higher in the first years of life, then falls to low levels which are maintained from around 5 up to 40 years of age. Mortality then begins to rise steeply, reaching high levels in those aged 70 years and over. For Sweden the result is a 'J'-shaped curve, but for Brazil the curve is a deep 'U'-shape, which is typical of Third World countries, although the actual mortality levels vary considerably between countries, as you have already seen.

□ What are the main differences between the two age-specific mortality curves?

■ Figure 2.3 reveals that in every age-group, the death rate is substantially higher in Brazil than in Sweden. The most important differences are in the first years of life, when death rates are much higher in Brazil than in Sweden. At older ages, the mortality rate is consistently higher in Brazil than in Sweden, but the difference is smaller than it was at young ages.

If the population of Brazil had the same age distribution as that of Sweden, the death rate for all females would be 17 per 1 000 compared with 10 per 1 000 in Sweden: this outcome follows from the fact that the death rates in every age-group are higher in Brazil than in Sweden. However, because Brazil's population has a very different age *distribution*, with a much higher proportion of its population than Sweden in the teen and young adult age-groups that

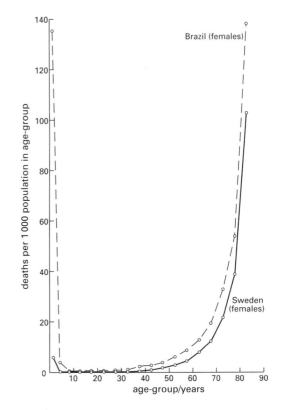

Figure 2.3 *Age-specific mortality rates of females in Brazil and Sweden, 1987. (Data from United Nations, 1991,* United Nations Demographic Yearbook 1989, *UN, New York, Table 20, pp. 418–47)*

tend to experience relatively low mortality, Brazil's crude death rate unadjusted for age is actually lower than Sweden's: among females it is under 5 per 1 000. Taking the very different age structures of Brazil and Sweden into account has reversed the result of the comparison of the unstandardised crude mortality rates in the two countries.

As you saw above, Third World countries are characterised by having populations which are, on average, considerably younger than those of industrialised countries. This very different age structure is the reason why the crude death rate is an unsatisfactory index for comparing mortality in different parts of the world.

The crude death rate is also unsatisfactory for another reason: in many countries it is estimated very inaccurately. In order to calculate the crude death rate, it is necessary to know two things—the number of deaths occurring in a given year and the total population in the middle of that year—and information on both items may be faulty. National censuses are conducted at regular intervals in most countries and often provide a reasonable estimate of the total population, but they can sometimes be misleading. For example, in 1992 a detailed international study of the population of Nigeria, using the most advanced techniques available, concluded that the actual population was up to 20 million less than the official census figure of 110 million. The main reason for this was thought to be a tendency among regions to exaggerate their size, both as a matter of pride and to obtain more national resources. In other countries undercounting is thought to be a problem. Obtaining a reliable estimate of the number of deaths in a given year is even more difficult. In the majority of industrialised countries this is done by means of a national system of death registration, but in most Third World countries either such a system is lacking or else registration is very incomplete. And in such circumstances it is even less likely that accurate breakdowns of the age structure of the population will be available, making age-specific mortality rates even more difficult to estimate reliably.

Infant mortality rates

You have seen that the crude death rate can be an unsatisfactory index for mortality comparisons, because it may be difficult to estimate and is hard to interpret when countries have very different age-structures. Another measure, the **infant mortality rate (IMR)**, is often used as one of the key indicators of socio-economic development. You might think it rather odd to focus on the IMR (the number of deaths in the first year of life per 1 000 live births), when we are really interested in the overall health of a community. It is, however, a very useful index of health for several reasons.

First, the infant mortality rate is relatively easy to measure. In industrialised countries it is calculated by using data on births and infant deaths collected through routine birth and death registration systems. This cannot be done in most Third World countries because of the incompleteness of registration systems, but 'indirect' methods of estimating the IMR have been developed by demographers. These methods generally rely on questioning samples of women of reproductive age about the number of children they have had, and the number that have died. By using this information, obtained either from special surveys or from censuses, demographers have derived fairly reliable estimates of IMR for most countries.

A second strength of the infant mortality measure is that it is quite strongly correlated with adult mortality: if infant mortality is high, then adult mortality is likely to be high.

Third, in countries with high overall mortality, policies to reduce mortality are often directed principally at young children. This is because a high proportion of child deaths in such countries is due to infective and parasitic diseases that could be avoided through simple preventive or curative public health measures. When such measures are implemented, the IMR is likely to change much more dramatically than the crude death rate, making the IMR a useful indicator of the impact of such health measures, and a very sensitive indicator of inequality within a population.

 □ Returning to Table 2.2, identify the three countries with the highest IMR per 1 000 live births and the three countries with the lowest IMR. Guided by this information and by a more general inspection of Table 2.2, identify any consistent pattern in the IMRs across the selected countries.

 ■ The highest IMRs are found in Mali, Bangladesh, the Central African Republic, and India. The lowest IMRs are in Japan, Sweden and the United Kingdom. It is clear that, even allowing for some inaccuracy in the estimates, there are dramatic differences in the IMR between countries. An IMR in Mali of 164 per 1 000 live births means that around one child in six dies before its first birthday, a rate which is over forty times that found in Japan.

Going beyond the sample of countries in Table 2.2, the general pattern is that the IMR is below 10 per 1 000 live births in most of the world's richest countries, but exceeds 100 in many of the poorest countries. However, note that there is also substantial variation within these broad groupings, even between countries in the same region. There are also important exceptions to the general pattern, some of which will be discussed further in Chapter 8: for example Sri Lanka has a reported IMR of 26 per 1 000 live births, which is very low for a poor country.

Expectation of life

Another index of mortality is **the expectation of life at birth**. This can be estimated from a 'life table' of the population. In industrialised countries, life tables are produced using age-specific mortality rates determined through censuses and death registration. Once again this approach is not possible in most Third World countries, and although indirect estimation techniques have been suggested, they are not as reliable as those used to estimate the IMR. Thus, some of the estimates of the expectation of life in Table 2.2 should be regarded as approximations only. We shall return to these expectations of life, and in particular to male/female differences, in the next chapter.

Like the crude death rate, the expectation of life is an index reflecting both childhood and adult mortality. It has the advantage that its interpretation is not complicated by differences in the age structures of populations: an expectation of life must always be related to people at a particular age, usually those who have just been born. However, life expectancy is influenced particularly heavily by childhood mortality, as the following exercise makes clear.

☐ Suppose that 20 per cent of 1 000 newborn children die in the first 5 years of life (near the truth in some countries), and that the rest survive until an average age of 60 years. What is the expectation of life at birth, and at age 5? To keep things simple, assume that the 200 children who die in the first 5 years of life have an average lifetime of 2.5 years.

■ The 800 who do not die in the first 5 years live on average for 60 years. It follows that the total number of years of life lived by the entire 1 000 is (200 × 2.5 years) plus (800 × 60 years) = 48 500. Thus the average—the expectation of life at birth—is 48.5 years per person. At five years of age the expectation is greater—55 more years.

This sharp increase in the expectation of life during early childhood is typical of countries with high childhood mortality. To illustrate this, Table 2.3 shows the expectation of (remaining) life at selected ages, for Bangladesh and the United Kingdom.

Notice first that a boy born in the United Kingdom in 1989 can expect to live on average for 72 years, 15 years

Table 2.3 Expectation of life (years) at various ages, in Bangladesh and the United Kingdom, 1989

Sex	Country	Expectation of life at age/years					
		0	1	5	10	30	50
male	Bangladesh	57	64	63	59	41	23
	UK	72	72	68	63	43	25
female	Bangladesh	56	61	61	57	40	24
	UK	78	77	73	69	49	30

Data from United Nations (1991) *United Nations Demographic Yearbook 1989*, UN, New York, Table 22.

longer than his counterpart in Bangladesh. A girl born in the United Kingdom has a life expectancy of 78 years, which is 22 years longer than her counterpart in Bangladesh. Note also that, whereas in the United Kingdom (and in most other countries in Table 2.2) females have a greater life expectancy than do males, in Bangladesh the opposite is true. As mentioned earlier, we will return to these male/female differences in the next chapter. Next, notice how in Bangladesh the expectation of life increases considerably between birth and the age of one year. Once childhood has been survived, the gap between Bangladesh and the United Kingdom is much narrower. Thus a man aged 30 years in Bangladesh can expect to live to around 71 years of age (30 + 41), whereas a 30-year-old man in the United Kingdom can expect to live to about 73 (30 + 43)—a small difference.

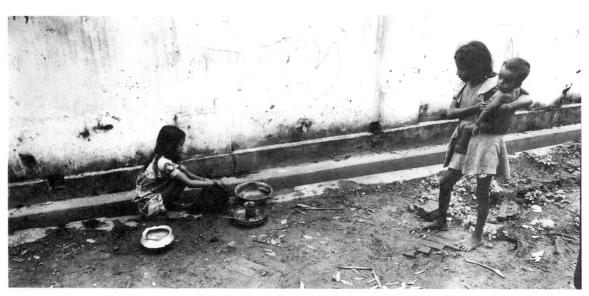

These street-dwelling children in Dhaka, Bangladesh, have survived infancy but live lives of considerable health risk. (Photo: Tom Learmonth)

Turning back to Table 2.2, you can see that expectation of life at birth in the selected countries ranges from 44 to 75 years for men and 47 to 81 years for women: that is, a female born in Japan can now expect on average to live for 81 years. Life expectancy appears to be closely related to the IMR, people in countries with high IMRs tending to have a low expectation of life.

One way of examining the relationship between the IMR and expectation of life, using the information in Table 2.2, is to plot a scatter diagram of IMR and expectation of life.

☐ Figure 2.4 has been designed so that you can create such a scatter diagram from the data in Table 2.2: for each country, plot the IMR along the *x*-axis (horizontal) and the expectation of life for females up the *y*-axis (vertical), then place a dot or cross in the graph. What does the completed scattergram reveal? (A correct version of the graph (Figure 2.8) is given at the end of the chapter.)

■ It reveals a clear negative relationship between the IMR and expectation of life. Of course this is just what would be expected in view of the strong influence of infant mortality on expectation of life that has already been noted.

Height-for-age

Finally, although this chapter is concerned primarily with differences in *mortality* between Third World and industrialised countries, it is important to note that other systematic differences related to health exist. For example, **anthropometric data** (data based on measurement of the human body) reveal large differences between countries in the average height and weight of populations. One of the most commonly used anthropometric measures is **height-for-age**, which is often regarded as a guide to infections in early childhood and past nutritional status. Low height-for-age, referred to as 'stunting', is often taken as an indication that at some point in a person's early life they suffered repeated infections and their food intake may have been chronically inadequate. Figure 2.5 shows height-for-age for females and males in three countries.

The interpretation of such data is complex, and we will return to the whole issue of nutrition and health in Chapter 11. For the moment, however, the key point is that systematic anthropometric differences exist alongside mortality differences.

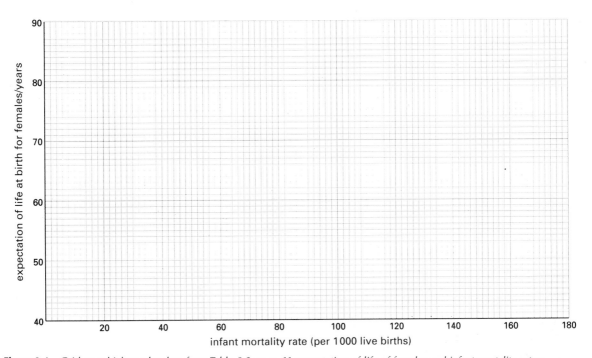

Figure 2.4 *Grid on which to plot data from Table 2.2 on p. 11 expectation of life of females and infant mortality rates: selected countries.*

(a) males

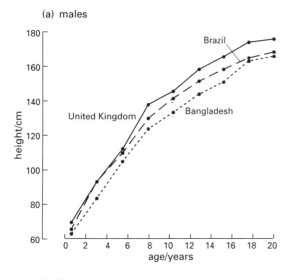

(b) females

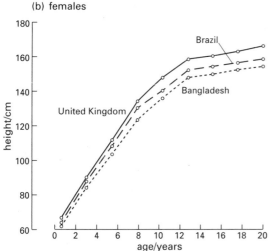

Figure 2.5 *Height-for-age measurements in three countries, 1987. (Data from James, W. P. T. and Schofield, C., 1990,* Human Energy Requirements: a Manual for Planners and Nutritionists, *Oxford Medical Publications, Oxford)*

Recent changes and projected trends in mortality rates

All the evidence considered so far leads to the same conclusion: mortality rates vary greatly between different parts of the world. As noted earlier, however, we are also interested in finding out whether these differences are becoming greater or smaller, and to do this we have to look at trends over time in these mortality rates. For the reasons discussed earlier, the infant mortality rate is a

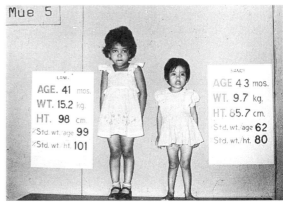

Anthropometric differences in female children in the Philippines. The small-for-age child demonstrates the effects on growth of an adverse early environment, but it is impossible to deduce how much of the 'stunting' has been due to repeated illness and how much to lack of food. (Photo courtesy of Teaching Aids at Low Cost (TALC), P. O. Box 49, St Albans. Details of TALC materials sent free on request.)

particularly useful measure for this purpose. Table 2.4 shows changes in infant mortality rates for selected countries over the period from 1950 to 1990. Note that the IMRs are shown as the average of five-year periods. This removes some of the year-to-year fluctuations which are inevitable in such statistics.

Table 2.4 Infant mortality rates at selected periods from 1950–5 to 1985–90

Country	Infant mortality rate (per 1 000 live births):			
	1950–5	1965–70	1975–80	1985–90
Africa				
Central African Republic	197	160	145	132
Zimbabwe	120	101	86	72
Americas				
Brazil	135	100	79	63
Jamaica	85	45	25	18
Europe				
Sweden	20	13	8	6
UK	24	19	14	9
Asia				
Bangladesh	180	140	137	119
China	195	81	41	32
India	190	145	126	99
more developed world	56	26	19	15
less developed world	180	117	97	79

Data from United Nations (1991) *United Nations Demographic Yearbook 1989,* UN, New York, Table 16, pp.190–7.

□ Describe the main features of the data in Table 2.4, concentrating in particular on similarities and differences between the countries.

■ The countries show a similar pattern in that IMRs have decreased steadily between 1950–5 and 1985–90 for all countries. However, they are different in two main respects: the absolute values of the IMRs vary tremendously in any period, and the rates of decline over time are also very different. To illustrate the last point, the IMRs of Bangladesh and China were similar in 1950–5, but by 1985–90 the Bangladeshi rate was almost four times that of China.

There are two ways of comparing the changes in the infant mortality rates, which will be illustrated by contrasting the IMRs of Zimbabwe and the United Kingdom. One method is to calculate the *absolute difference* in IMRs. In 1950–5 the IMR was 120 in Zimbabwe and 24 in the United Kingdom, an absolute difference of 96 deaths per 1 000 live births. In 1985–90 this difference was 63 (72 – 9), suggesting a narrowing of the difference. However, an alternative, and perhaps more appropriate, measure is to assess the *relative* chance of an infant dying by expressing the two IMRs in the form of a ratio. In 1950–5 the ratio of the IMR in Zimbabwe to that in the United Kingdom was 120 divided by 24, which equals a ratio of 5 : 1. That is, the IMR was 5 times higher in Zimbabwe than in the United Kingdom. This can be compared with 1985–90, when the ratio was 8 : 1 (72/9). So although the IMRs in both countries had dropped considerably between 1950–5 and 1985–90, the relative chance of an infant dying in Zimbabwe had actually increased.

It is possible to generalise the example given above, and consider whether the gap between infant mortality rates in Third World and industrialised countries is closing or widening over time. Figure 2.6 shows the changes in both the absolute difference and the relative difference in IMRs between six countries and the average for the more developed countries.

In absolute terms, the difference between the IMRs for the six selected countries and the average IMR for the more developed countries as a group has in all cases decreased. A different picture emerges, however, from a comparison of the **relative differences in IMR**, with considerable variation from country to country. For example, in 1950–5 a baby born in Jamaica was 1.5 times more likely to die before its first birthday than one born in the more developed world. This difference increased to 1.7 times in 1965–70 but has since been decreasing and in 1985–90 was down to 1.2. Thus in Jamaica there was a period of relative deterioration followed by a relative improvement. In Brazil the IMR in relative terms has

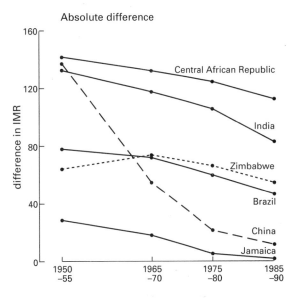

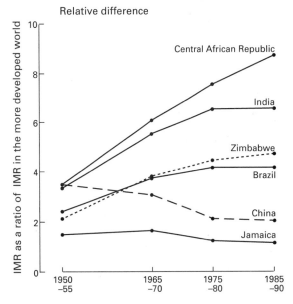

Figure 2.6 *Absolute and relative differences in IMR in selected Third World countries compared with the average IMR for the more developed world, 1950–89. (Data from Table 2.4)*

remained constant since the mid-1960s, while that for China has decreased steadily.

In summary, although the infant mortality rate has been steadily decreasing in almost all Third World countries, in many it has fallen at a much slower rate than in the industrialised countries; thus the relative chance of an infant dying has increased. The lesson is that even when the IMR is falling everywhere, the gap between countries can still be widening. Even in 50 years time the projected rates for Third World countries are predicted to be considerably higher than those currently experienced in industrialised countries.

Another measure of mortality examined earlier was life expectancy at birth, and Figure 2.7 shows how this has changed in major areas of the world, and also how it is predicted to change over the next 20 or so years.

☐ What general trends in life expectancy at birth are shown by Figure 2.7?

■ Figure 2.7 shows some narrowing of differences over time, and a generally increasing life expectancy in every major area of the world, but it also indicates that Latin America, Asia and especially Africa will continue to lag some way behind. By the period 2010–15, average life expectancy at birth in Africa is predicted to have risen to 61 years, still a long way short of the 78 or 79 years that may then be the norm in Europe and North America. The most significant absolute changes are occurring where the IMR is

falling most rapidly. As you have already seen, infant mortality has a profound effect on expectation of life at birth.

In this chapter you have seen that the mortality patterns of people living in Third World countries is systematically different from that of people in industrialised countries. Death rates are higher at all ages, but particularly in the first few years of life, and expectation of life is lower. Moreover, some of these differences do not appear to be decreasing in relative terms, even when they are tracked over several decades or predictions are made well into the twenty-first century.

However, just as average statistics for groups of countries can disguise variations between countries, so mortality statistics for a country as a whole fail to tell us anything about variations that might exist *within* countries. The general patterns established in this chapter are overlaid by variations between and within countries, and these variations raise many intriguing questions about the origins and determinants of such patterns of health and disease. The next step, therefore, is to examine in more detail the main causes of death and types of disease. These are the themes of the next chapter.

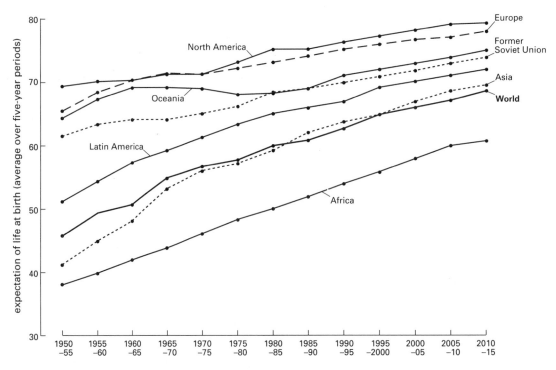

Figure 2.7 *Trends in life expectancy at birth, both sexes, by region, 1950–2015. (Data from United Nations, 1989,* World Population Prospects 1988, *Population Studies No. 106, UN, New York, Table 15, pp. 166–189)*

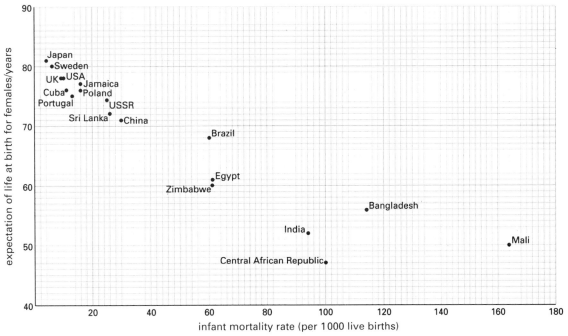

Figure 2.8 *Scatter diagram showing the relationship between infant mortality rate and female expectation of life at birth for selected countries, 1990 or nearest date. (Data from Table 2.2)*

OBJECTIVES FOR CHAPTER 2

When you have studied this chapter you should be able to:

2.1 Demonstrate an understanding of how a population pyramid depicts the age–sex structure of a population, and how population structures tend to differ systematically between industrialised and Third World countries.

2.2 Discuss the advantages and disadvantages of the following three measures of mortality: crude death rate, infant mortality rate, and expectation of life at birth.

2.3 Use different measures of mortality to describe the main differences between industrialised and Third World countries, and give examples of ways in which relative and absolute measures of mortality can suggest different conclusions about changes over time.

QUESTIONS FOR CHAPTER 2

Question 1 (*Objective 2.1*)

(a) Using the data in Figure 2.2, estimate approximately the percentage of the female Brazilian population that, in 1988, was 65 years or older.

(b) Figure 2.9 shows population pyramids for two countries in the late 1980s.

(i) What are their main features and what kind of societies do they suggest to you?

(ii) What difference might you expect to find in comparing crude death rates and age-standardised death rates for these two populations?

(c) Is it possible to predict accurately the life expectancy of a newborn boy or girl from the contemporary population pyramid for the country where he or she was born?

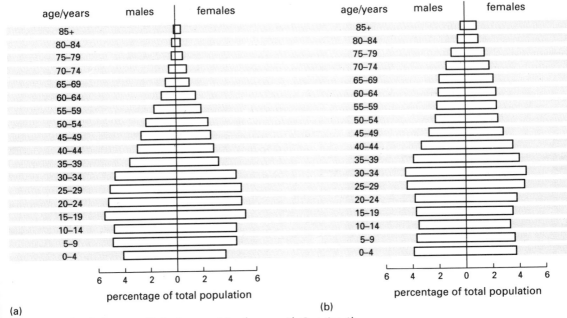

Figure 2.9 *Population pyramids for two countries; for use with Question 1b.*

Question 2 (*Objective 2.2*)

Why is it often more useful to use the infant mortality rate rather than the crude death rate as a measure of the health status of different populations?·

Question 3 (*Objective 2.3*)

Looking at Figure 2.6, what conclusions can you draw about the change in the IMR in India, compared with the average for the more developed world, between 1950–5 and 1985–90?

3
Mortality and morbidity: causes and determinants

There is a television programme and an audio-tape sequence associated with this chapter. They both deal with patterns of health and disease in Zimbabwe. Details can be found in the Broadcast and Audiocassette Notes. During this chapter you will be asked to read an article in **Health and Disease: A Reader**[1]—*'The global eradication of smallpox', by Marc Strassburg.*

In the previous chapter you saw that roughly three-quarters of the world's population live in Third World countries, that their population structure is very different from that of industrialised countries, and that their overall health experience as measured by mortality is generally much poorer than that of the populations of industrialised countries, especially among children. In this chapter we explore further these differences, by considering the main causes of death and morbidity (disease), and then looking for some of the factors influencing these patterns. As a first step, let us have a look at the main causes of death in different parts of the world.

Causes of death

In order to compare patterns of death and disease around the world, we need to have some method of measuring the relative importance of different diseases.

☐ How might the patterns of fatal diseases in different countries be compared?

[1] Another book in this series, *Health and Disease: A Reader* (Open University Press, 1984; revised edition 1994).

■ One method would be to examine the percentages of total deaths that are attributable to different causes, another would be to compare the mortality rates for specific diseases, and a third would be to look at years of life lost from different diseases.

Distribution of deaths by cause

Figure 3.1 (overleaf) illustrates the first of these methods, by comparing the **proportional mortality** (percentage distribution of the main causes of death) in industrial and Third World countries in 1985: the actual numbers of deaths (in millions) are also shown.

The major cause of death in Third World countries, on the evidence of Figure 3.1, is the group of infectious and parasitic diseases. They account for almost half of all deaths. ('Infectious and parasitic diseases' here refers to all diseases caused by micro-organisms — mainly bacteria, viruses and single-celled parasites — or by multicellular parasites such as worms: for every death caused by parasites there are likely to be six or seven caused by bacteria or viruses.)

☐ What proportion of deaths in industrialised and in Third World countries are caused by cancers, circulatory and degenerative diseases?

■ In the industrialised countries, almost three-quarters of all deaths are caused by these diseases. In the Third World, they cause a much smaller proportion of all deaths: about one-quarter.

A look at the actual numbers of deaths by cause reveals something else of interest: because there are far more deaths in total in the Third World, there are actually more deaths there each year from the 'Western' diseases—cancers and circulatory/degenerative diseases—than in the industrialised world.

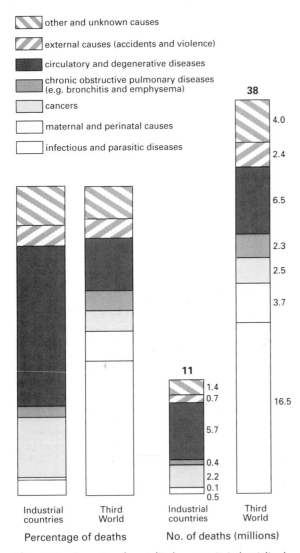

- other and unknown causes
- external causes (accidents and violence)
- circulatory and degenerative diseases
- chronic obstructive pulmonary diseases (e.g. bronchitis and emphysema)
- cancers
- maternal and perinatal causes
- infectious and parasitic diseases

Percentage of deaths   No. of deaths (millions)

Industrial countries   Third World   Industrial countries   Third World

Figure 3.1 *Proportional mortality by cause in industrialised countries and the Third World, around 1985, together with actual numbers of deaths (in millions). (Data from Lopez, A. D., 1993, 'Causes of death in the industrialized and the developing countries: estimates for 1985' in Jamison, D.T. and Mosley, H. (eds) Disease Control Priorities in Developing Countries, Oxford University Press, New York)*

This stark contrast between the Third World and the industrialised countries in the main causes of death exists largely as a consequence of the profound changes that have taken place in industrialised countries over the last century. The most striking change has been the virtual disappearance as major killers of the acute infectious diseases that remain so prevalent in today's Third World.

In their place other diseases, which were relatively unimportant in the past, have become major causes of public health concern in industrialised countries. These changes will be discussed in detail in Chapter 6 in the context of the United Kingdom.

A disease which during the 1980s added itself to the list of major killers in the Third World and the industrialised countries is AIDS (Acquired Immune Deficiency Syndrome), which is caused by infection with the human immunodeficiency virus (HIV). This virus is transmitted primarily via sexual contact or infected blood, and because the period between infection and onset of illness is often very long—as much as eight or more years in many cases—it is extremely hard to know the scale of the epidemic.

By 1991 a cumulative total of around 1 million people had been diagnosed with AIDS world-wide, but during the 1990s it is thought likely that this figure will rise to over 5 million. These will mainly be people who were already infected with HIV by 1990 and therefore a great deal of this increase is beyond the reach of any campaigns to control the epidemic. However, the course of the epidemic into the twenty-first century clearly does depend on the effectiveness of such campaigns.

At first, the country with most reported cases of AIDS was the USA, which contained two-thirds of AIDS patients in 1990. AIDS is now a leading cause of death among young males in the USA. But other countries have increasingly been affected. In 1991 there were an estimated 6–12 million people infected with HIV world-wide, almost half in North America and Europe and most of the remainder in Sub-Saharan Africa, and it has been estimated that by the year 2000 between 35 million and 100 million people world-wide will be infected with HIV. The countries with the highest incidence of AIDS in the world in the early 1990s were in Central Africa—Tanzania, Uganda, Malawi and Burundi. As the epidemic spreads, AIDS will undoubtedly come to figure among the leading causes of death and disease in many regions of the world.

Disease-specific mortality

The differences between Third World and industrialised countries in the causes of mortality which were sketched above can be seen in more detail by examining **disease-specific death rates**. Table 3.1 shows disease-specific death rates for Zimbabwe, Brazil and Sweden, using a classification of diseases very similar to that used in Figure 3.1.

The table bears out strongly the picture provided by Figure 3.1: death rates from infectious and parasitic

Table 3.1 Disease-specific death rates in Zimbabwe, Brazil and Sweden, 1986

Cause	Death rate per 100 000 in		
	Zimbabwe	Brazil	Sweden
infectious and parasitic diseases	32	37	6
maternal and perinatal causes	not known	1 711	255
cancers	23	64	261
chronic obstructive pulmonary diseases (e.g. bronchitis and emphysema)	22	32	72
circulatory and degenerative diseases	36	156	596
external causes (accidents and violence)	41	69	60

Data from United Nations (1991) *Demographic Yearbook 1989*, UN, New York, Table 21, pp. 448–68.

diseases, and from maternal and perinatal causes, are five or six times higher in Zimbabwe and Brazil than in Sweden, while the death rates from cancers, chest diseases and circulatory and degenerative diseases are much higher in Sweden. Finally, and again in line with Figure 3.1, the differences between the countries in the death rates from external causes—injuries, accidents, violence and so on—are less pronounced.

Some of the diseases that predominate in industrialised countries such as Sweden are purely modern epidemics and their emergence has been closely related to changes in patterns of living—the epidemic of lung cancer that has followed the adoption of tobacco smoking on a widespread basis is an example of such a disease. These are the exceptions, however, and other diseases have become important not because the causes of the diseases have become more prevalent, but because the population has 'aged'. Many diseases are more common in elderly people and, as infectious diseases that killed children and young adults in previous centuries have been conquered, increasing numbers of people have survived long enough to be at risk of death from the diseases of older ages, such as cancers and heart disease.[2] Thus, for example, the crude death rate from all cancers, taken together, is much higher now

[2]The biological and sociological dimensions of old age are discussed in two other books in this series: *The Biology of Health and Disease* (Open University Press, 1985; revised as *Human Biology and Health: An Evolutionary Approach*, 1994) and *Birth to Old Age: Health in Transition* (Open University Press, 1985; revised edition 1995).

than it was at the turn of the century but, if we exclude lung cancer and compare age-specific rates of all other cancers combined, the differences in the rates between the two time periods are very small.

Because of the association between degenerative diseases such as cancers and age, it would be preferable to age-standardise death rates when making comparisons between countries. Returning to Table 3.1, you may have noticed that the death rates were *not* age-standardised. If the data existed to do this (unfortunately they do not for all three countries) the differences in death rates would be somewhat reduced, but nevertheless the same broad pattern would remain.

Years of life lost

Comparisons between countries based on the type of mortality data discussed above give only a partial view of the health patterns. Numbers of deaths or crude mortality rates for specific diseases fail to acknowledge that a disease that kills young adults may represent a greater social and economic loss to a country than one that causes the death of elderly people. One modification to mortality rates which attempts to take such problems into account is to calculate the **years of potential life lost** from different diseases due to death from that cause. This helps us to assess the relative importance of each disease.

For example, if a disease kills a person at age 50 years in a country in which they might otherwise have expected to live to 70 years, they have 'lost' 20 years of potential life. Thus, by looking at the ages at which people die of a specific disease and their expectation of life at those ages, it is possible to compute the total years of potential life lost by all persons dying of the disease. Diseases can then be ranked in order of importance according to the years of life that each costs the community.

Tables 3.2 and 3.3 (overleaf) show the results of such an analysis, for the population of the USA and Ghana respectively. Looking at the American data first, you can see that, perhaps surprisingly, accidents come out top, accounting for nearly 19 per cent of the total years of life lost. Cancers are next, followed by heart diseases and then homicide. Infectious diseases do not appear in the top of the list, but years of potential life lost as a result of HIV infection are in sixth place (and rising).

☐ Why do you think accidents have come out first when, in fact, far more people die of cancers than from accidents?

Table 3.2 Leading causes of years of potential life lost by Americans before the age of 65, 1988

Rank order	Cause of death	Percentage of total years of potential life lost
1	accidents	18.9
2	cancers	14.9
3	heart diseases	12.1
4	homicide	5.7
5	suicide	5.5
6	HIV infection	3.6
7	cerebrovascular diseases	2.0
8	chronic liver disease	1.9
9	pneumonia and influenza	1.5
10	chronic obstructive pulmonary diseases	1.1
11	diabetes	1.1
	all causes	**100**

Data from US Department of Health and Human Services (1991) *Health US 1990*, National Center for Health Statistics, Maryland.

■ This method of assessing disease importance gives most weight to diseases that kill at young ages and thus cause a greater loss of years of life. Continuing the assumption suggested above of an average expectation of life at birth of 70 years (a modest assumption for a highly industrialised country such as the USA), a person dying at the age of 1 year loses 69 years of potential life, whereas someone dying at 60 years loses far fewer years. Accident rates are highest in the young and thus are given greater weight than cancer deaths which usually occur at later ages.

Now look at Table 3.3. The methodology used to calculate the Ghanaian table differs slightly from the American data—the American data refer only to years of potential life lost before the age of 65, whereas the Ghanaian data include years lost at all ages. However, these differences had a relatively small effect for all but a few diseases and it is not unreasonable to compare the two tables.

Comparing these tables, the most striking difference is the degree to which infectious diseases, malnutrition and deaths in infancy and childhood dominate the Ghanaian table. Neither cancers nor heart disease appear on the list. At the top of the list it may surprise you to see measles. Measles is certainly not a 'tropical' disease. It is

caused by a virus and is very common in the populations of industrialised countries also, where it is rarely a cause of death. Why it causes so many deaths in Africa (and other areas of the Third World) is not fully understood. Few diseases occur in isolation in children in Third World countries and it is likely that the reason that so many die of measles is that the infection hits hardest those whose defences are already weakened by malnutrition or malaria and other parasitic or infectious diseases.

Another reason why measles may cause so many deaths in the Third World is that it frequently occurs at very young ages, often before the age of one year when the body is less able to cope with such an infection, and often before the age when immunisation would normally be given. In industrialised countries, even before vaccination programmes, measles was predominantly a disease of later childhood, at least in the recent past.

Table 3.3 Leading causes of years of potential life lost in Ghana, mid 1970s

Rank order	Cause of death	Percentage of total years of potential life lost
1	measles	7.9
2	childhood pneumonia	6.5
3	malaria	6.2
4	severe malnutrition	6.1
5	premature birth	5.9
6	sickle-cell disease	5.3
7	birth injury	4.8
8	gastroenteritis	4.7
9	accidents	4.6
10	tuberculosis	3.6
11	adult pneumonia	3.1
12	neonatal tetanus	2.4
13	cerebrovascular disease	2.1
	all causes	**100**

Data recalculated from Ghana Health Assessment Project Team (1981) A quantitative method of assessing the health impact of different diseases in less developed countries, *International Journal of Epidemiology*, **10**, (1), pp. 73–80, Table 1.

To summarise, in contrast to the pattern of diseases in industrialised countries, infectious diseases are the most important category in Third World countries, and the analysis of life-years lost reinforces this fact.

Morbidity

The different methods examined above of assessing the relative importance of different diseases using mortality data each have their merits. However, they share the important limitation that they only provide information about lethal diseases, giving no indication of the **morbidity** (illness) and disability caused by diseases that are seldom lethal.

The measurement of morbidity is fraught with difficulties. Definitions of illness are to some extent subjective, illnesses vary greatly in severity and duration and population surveys are expensive and difficult to conduct, whereas measures based on, for example, visits to hospitals or doctors are likely to be influenced by the numbers of doctors and hospitals and their ease of access. So estimating the number of cases of different types of disease on a world-wide basis is a daunting task and is liable to be error-prone. Nevertheless, one attempt at this ambitious undertaking for the entire Third World is shown in Figure 3.2. The figure shows the main causes of episodes of disease, and the main causes of death.

☐ From Figure 3.2, list three diseases (or groups of diseases) which are important in terms of mortality but less important in terms of disease prevalence.

■ You could have chosen any of: circulatory and degenerative diseases, malaria, measles, injuries, cancers and tetanus and meningitis.

☐ Are there diseases (or groups of diseases) that are more important in terms of disease prevalence than of mortality?

■ Yes: diarrhoeas and respiratory tract infectious diseases.

Respiratory tract infectious diseases together account for 52 per cent of morbidity and 26 per cent of the mortality in the Third World. Viruses such as influenza are mainly responsible for the respiratory infections, and present a severe threat to health and life, especially among infants and young children. Diarrhoeal diseases are caused by a wide variety of different bacteria and parasites, and a few types of virus, which infect the gut and irritate the cells lining its surface. When irritated, these cells secrete large amounts of water and dissolved salts into the gut, which stimulate the muscular gut walls to contract and expel the watery, infected waste. However, if the infection persists and the diarrhoea is prolonged and severe, so much water and essential salts are lost that dehydration and disruption of body chemistry results. At the least, prolonged diarrhoea causes a failure to absorb nutrients effectively and

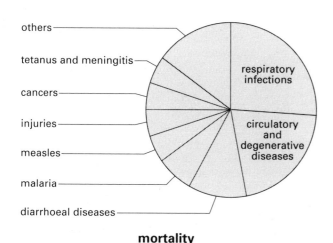

mortality

total 38.4 million deaths

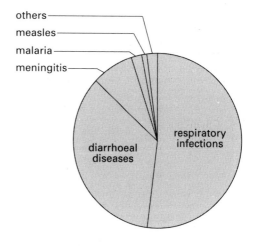

disease prevalence

total 11.4 billion disease episodes

Figure 3.2 *Disease episodes and deaths in the Third World, 1986. (Data derived from Walsh, J. A.,1988,* Establishing Health Priorities in the Developing World, *United Nations Development Programme, New York)*

an increased vulnerability to other infections, which in turn exacerbates the effects of malnutrition. A vicious circle is set up, which acts as a serious check to growth and development among millions of Third World children. Certain diarrhoeal diseases, such as cholera, have high fatality rates because the infectious organism produces a toxin which stimulates the gut wall to secrete exceptionally large amounts of fluid. In as many as 50 per cent of untreated cases of cholera, death occurs within 48 hours.

Treatment of diarrhoeal diseases consists of replenishing the lost water and salts, and giving glucose as an energy source, until the infection subsides. This **oral rehydration therapy (ORT)** is simple, cheap and effective and could save many thousands of lives each year. In 1986 the deaths from diarrhoeas in all age groups were estimated at 4.3 million.

Another aspect of morbidity in the Third World is that it causes a disproportionate amount of economic damage. One study by the World Bank has collated information on the average number of days of sickness and days off work in a variety of countries. Some of the results are shown in Table 3.4.

The countries are ranked in order of their average Gross National Product per person in 1989, with the poorest—Ghana—at the top.

☐ What does the table reveal?

Table 3.4 The economic burden of adult illness, 1989 or nearest year

Country (ranked according to GNP per person 1989)	Average days ill in last month	Work days absent in last month	Percent of normal earnings lost through illness
Ghana (1988)	3.6	1.3	6.4
Mauritania (1988)	2.1	1.6	6.5
Côte d'Ivoire (1988)	2.6	1.3	6.4
Bolivia (1990)	not known	1.2	4.4
Peru (1985)	4.5	0.9	3.1
Jamaica (1989)	1.2	0.5	2.1
USA (1988)	not known	0.3	1.5

Data derived from World Bank (1991) *World Development Report 1991*, Oxford University Press, Oxford and New York, Table 3.1.

■ The poorer the country, the more frequent are days of sickness and days off work, and the greater is the loss of income from illness. Thus workers in the poorest countries listed lose up to one and a half days of work each month through sickness, whereas in the USA barely a third of a day per month is lost. As a result, the proportion of normal earnings lost through sickness is over four times greater in Ghana than in the USA.

In addition to days lost through sickness, the economic burden of morbidity on Third World health-care systems with very limited resources can be overwhelming. For example, even providing basic palliative care to people with AIDS in Africa could absorb one-third or even half of current national health-care budgets.

In summary, therefore, you have seen that infectious diseases are the biggest killers and the biggest cause of ill-health in Third World countries, but that the many exotic sounding 'tropical' diseases do not top the list. In the next section we consider why it is that infectious diseases have such a big impact, by considering some of the main influences on mortality and morbidity in the Third World.

Influences on mortality and morbidity within Third World countries

The occurrence of disease is part of a complex interaction between humans and their social and physical environment. Health is not possible without various prerequisites, such as safe water and sanitation, and at least a basic minimum of nutrition. Human biology exerts its influence in various ways such as via genetic inheritance, which may confer a measure of resistance or susceptibility to a specific disease. Different diseases predominate in different environmental conditions, which include variations in climate, in the prevalence of certain animals and insects, in levels and types of pollution, and in circumstances in the workplace and home. Health care, ranging from immunisation programmes to curative interventions, can affect different aspects of health. And human behaviour and lifestyle, such as drug abuse or smoking, create their own health consequences, as does education via its influence on behaviour and lifestyle. The relationships between these factors are complex; as one set of factors diminishes in importance, others become more pressing.

Here, we will be concerned primarily with environmental factors such as climate, ecological zones, place of residence, and sanitation and clean water; demographic factors such as sex and gender, and intervals between

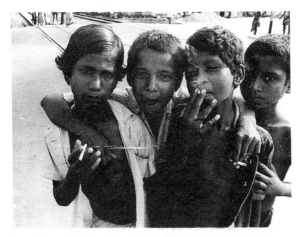

Street boys in Dhaka, Bangladesh. The smoking epidemic, which by the 1990s was in retreat in the developed world, was rapidly spreading in developing countries. (Photo: Tom Learmonth)

births; and a broad group of social and economic factors, including education and social class.[3] Clearly, these are not discrete categories: for example, differences in the mortality of men and women may be partly biological and partly due to different social and economic circumstances; or, the availability of sanitation and safe water supplies could be viewed as an economic issue as much as an environmental one. You should bear these connections in mind at all times when working through the following sections.

Environment and health

As is emphasised elsewhere in this chapter, the Third World is a very heterogeneous group of countries, and this is particularly clear with respect to patterns of disease. Even within the same continent or country, the disease patterns may be very different from one part to another, and this variation is related in part to differences in the natural environment.

The natural environment

The natural environment of a locality can influence human health in a number of ways. First, the chemical make-up of the soil can affect humans through drinking water and food. For example, in mountainous areas such as the Pyrenees, Himalayas and Andes where iodine has been leached from the soil, the iodine-deficiency disease

of goitre has been found to be endemic. Similarly, an absence of fluorine in drinking water can be reflected in high rates of dental caries, whereas an excess of fluorine—as found, for example, in parts of Uttar Pradesh in India—has been associated with severe skeletal abnormalities.

Second, various aspects of climate such as humidity, temperature, and exposure to sunlight can have direct effects on human health. For instance, insufficient sunlight may contribute to diseases associated with a deficiency of vitamin D, whereas excessive sunlight may increase skin cancers.

Next, the physical and climatic conditions together exert a powerful influence over the micro-organisms, plants, and animals and insects that are able to exist in a local environment, and these in turn can have a major impact on human health. A wide range of diseases can be transmitted to humans by organisms that thrive in water contaminated by human faeces; these include typhoid, dysentery, cholera and gastroenteritis. Another group of diseases, called **zoonoses** (or **zoonotic diseases**), are diseases which are shared by humans and other species and can be transmitted to humans from the disease reservoir in these species. Almost 200 such diseases have been identified, including brucellosis, rabies, plague, tuberculosis, gastroenteritis and typhus. Some of these diseases can be transmitted directly: for example, rabies by a dog bite. Others are transmitted by some intermediary insect or animal, called a **disease vector**. For example, yellow fever is found in monkeys and rodents, but is transmitted to humans by certain kinds of mosquito: it is therefore a **vector-borne disease**.

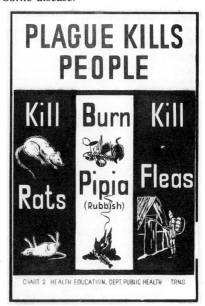

Health education poster from Papua, New Guinea, emphasizing the disease vectors of plague.

[3]For an account of the biological and genetic influences on health and disease, see *The Biology of Health and Disease* (Open University Press, 1985, revised as *Human Biology and Health: An Evoluti*onary Approach, 1994). The impact of health care on health is fully covered in *Caring for Health: History and Diversity*, (Open University Press, 1985, revised edition 1993).

All living things require certain environmental conditions in order to survive, and so all the organisms and zoonotic and vector-borne diseases mentioned above have particular geographic distributions. If the combination of physical and climatic environment is not favourable to the species that harbour a zoonotic disease, or to the disease organism itself, that locality will pose less of a disease threat to humans. Thus people living at low altitude in areas of high relative humidity may be exposed to diseases transmitted by mosquitoes, whereas those at higher altitudes or in areas of low humidity escape because mosquitoes cannot exist there.

The Third World is mostly located in tropical areas whose warmth and humidity do promote the transmission of water-borne and air-borne infectious diseases. However, it would be misleading to explain many of the current differences in mortality and morbidity between industrialised and Third World countries simply in terms of physical or climatic conditions. Many of the water-borne diseases that cause deaths from diarrhoea in the Third World are not due exclusively to 'tropical' environmental conditions, and were prevalent in countries such as the United Kingdom until the late nineteenth century, as you will see in Chapter 6. Similarly, the respiratory diseases that kill in the Third World—including pneumonia, bronchitis, whooping cough, influenza, measles, tuberculosis and diphtheria—can and do occur in industrialised countries. Other diseases such as malaria and cholera have all in the past been prevalent in Europe and North America. So environment is an important factor in human health, but mainly in combination with other factors. This can be illustrated by the examples of malaria and sickle-cell disease.

Malaria —the influence of environment

An example of how the distribution of a disease is affected by a whole range of environmental factors is malaria, which is transmitted by certain kinds of mosquitoes, which in turn require particular conditions for their survival.

There has been a resurgence of malaria around the world since the 1970s. It probably poses the severest health problem in Africa south of the Sahara, in parts of which the majority of the cases reported world-wide occur, but it is also widespread through Asia and Latin America. World-wide about 200 million new cases are thought to occur each year, and there are around 1.5 million deaths, over two-thirds of which occur in Sub-Saharan Africa. Malaria is caused by a single-celled parasite, of which there are four species with different patterns of geographic distribution and severity of symptoms. They all invade red blood cells, causing distortion and malfunction of the cell, anaemia, damage to organs

in which large numbers of infected red blood cells accumulate, and the fevers, nausea, headache and muscle pain associated with the immune response to persistently high levels of infection. The most fatal species, *Plasmodium falciparum*, has a tendency to accumulate in the brain, eventually causing coma and death, but kidney failure and water in the lungs are other common complications.

The parasites are usually transmitted from person to person by a certain species of mosquito (*Anopheles*). In the 1950s and 1960s, mosquito eradication programmes were given priority by the World Health Organisation and malaria was driven out of Europe, North America and parts of Asia. But it remains endemic in the poorer tropical countries, and numbers of cases have risen steadily since the early 1970s.

As Figure 3.3 shows, the life cycle of the malarial parasite is complex, involving passage between humans and mosquitoes.

Among the factors contributing to the transmission of malaria are: the behaviour, species and biology of the mosquito; environmental conditions such as ground water or the design of houses; the temperature and humidity of the climate; and the degree of human immunity including the presence of high-risk groups such

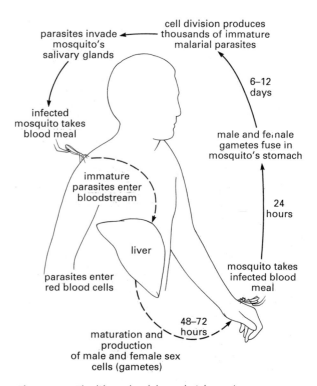

Figure 3.3 *The life cycle of the malarial parasite.*

as recent immigrants or refugees with no immunity. Although malaria used to be endemic to the United States and Europe, it never presented the health problems there that it does in Africa because of less favourable environmental conditions for the transmission of the parasite. Moreover, in much of Africa changing environmental circumstances have encouraged the spread of the disease. Overuse of antimalarial drugs and insecticides has created resistant strains of mosquito; population movements caused by civil wars or growth of human numbers have propelled non-immune people into infected areas and infected people to malaria-free areas; and the spread of irrigation, deforestation and building activity has created many more breeding sites. In consequence, attempts to break the mosquito's life cycle in Africa have been singularly unsuccessful.

Sickle-cell disease: genes and environment

To illustrate further how difficult it is to attribute disease to any single factor, let us now consider the example of sickle-cell disease, which was ranked sixth in Table 3.3 in terms of life years lost in Ghana. Sickle-cell disease is a group of genetically determined conditions (inherited rather than acquired from the environment) in which there is an abnormality in the structure of haemoglobin (the oxygen-carrying molecule in red blood cells). This distorts the cell and makes it fragile and liable to collapse.

Examples of normal and abnormal red cells are shown in Figure 3.4.

When large numbers of red blood cells collapse, in 'sickle-cell crises', huge numbers of damaged red blood cells accumulate in small blood vessels, blocking them and potentially obstructing vital organs. The crisis can subside as new red blood cells replace the collapsing ones, but it can also prove fatal.

About 1 in 400 Africans and people of African descent inherit two sickle-cell genes (one from each parent) and are affected by sickle-cell disease, but about 1 in 10 carry only one sickle-cell gene. These people are said to carry the sickle-cell trait. The single defective gene can only be detected by special blood tests and rarely causes any ill effects. An interesting feature of this trait is that it confers a degree of resistance to malaria, perhaps because the slightly altered haemoglobin in affected people makes their red blood cells less susceptible to infection by malarial parasites. It has been assumed that the high prevalence of sickle-cell disease in African populations has come about because those with the single defective gene (trait) have a survival advantage in terms of resistance to malaria, compared with people with 'normal' genes, which more than compensates for the increased risk of death among those with the two defective genes (sickle-cell disease). Thus environment and genetic inheritance may both be important factors in its distribution.

(a)

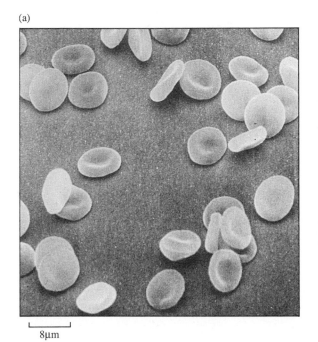

8µm

(b)

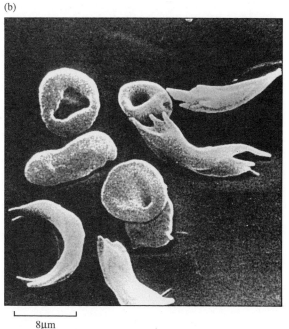

8µm

Figure 3.4 *Normal red blood cells (a) and sickle cells (b). (Source: Science Photo Library, London)*

Water and sanitation

It was noted earlier in this chapter that a wide range of diseases can be transmitted to humans by organisms that thrive in water contaminated by human faeces. The importance of water supplies and sanitation on disease patterns can be illustrated by the example of schistosomiasis (also known as bilharzia), common in many tropical countries. It is a disease caused by a tiny worm (*Schistosoma*) that invades many organs in the body and produces huge numbers of eggs (about 5 million per female worm). The eggs and immature larval stages of the developing worms are particularly damaging as they accumulate in tissues and blood vessels; in 1986, half a million deaths were recorded in Third World countries, but the toll in morbidity is far more extensive. The parasite is transmitted from person to person when the eggs are excreted in the urine or faeces, but first it must pass through an 'intermediate host'—in this instance certain kinds of snails—in which parasites develop and emerge in a form that can reinfect people. Thus there must be faecal or urinary contamination of the water in which people bathe or work (for example on irrigated land), and that water must also contain certain kinds of snail. This cycle is illustrated in Figure 3.5.

If the snails are not present, or if the water ceases to be contaminated, or if people stop bathing or working in contaminated water, then schistosomiasis cannot persist.

Thus the disease is confined to areas in which all elements exist for the life cycle of the parasites to continue. This is true not only of schistosomiasis and malaria, but also of other parasitic diseases. For example, Chagas disease, a serious parasitic infestation which often involves damage to the muscles of the heart, is confined to South America, and sleeping sickness, transmitted by the tsetse fly, does not occur outside Africa.

The impact of the lack of adequate sanitation and clean water can also be seen in the high prevalence of parasitic worm infestations, many of which are waterborne. At least a hundred different species of worm can produce disease in humans and it is estimated that about a billion[4] people are infested with these adaptable parasites. They range from the largest tapeworm, over two metres in length, to worms such as the *Schistosoma* species which are barely visible to the naked eye. Other types of worm that cause significant morbidity in developing countries include the filarial worms, which cause fevers, elephantiasis and river blindness; the hookworms, which suck blood from the gut and cause anaemia and loss of protein; the ascarid worms, which interfere with digestion and stunt the growth of millions of Third World children; and the guinea worms, which erupt

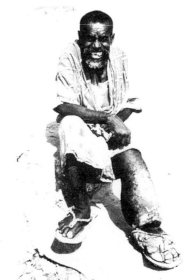

A person infected with a species of filarial worm. The infestation has caused severe tissue damage in the leg, the appearance of which provides the name 'elephantiasis'. (Source: C. J. Webb, London School of Hygiene and Tropical Medicine)

snail, actual size

1 Infected person urinates in water

5 In this way the disease is spread by people washing or swimming in contaminated water

2 Urine contains worm eggs

3 Worm eggs hatch and enter snails

4 Young worms leave snail and enter another person

Figure 3.5 *The life cycle of the worms that cause schistosomiasis (also called bilharzia).*

[4]Throughout this book, 1 billion is taken to equal 1 000 000 000 (one thousand million).

from the skin through disabling and painful swellings, usually on the legs and feet. Studies in Sri Lanka, Bangladesh and Venezuela have found that over 90 per cent of six-year-old children were infested with intestinal parasitic worms, the commonest being hookworm and ascarid worms, which together account for about 60 000 deaths a year.

The prevalence in the Third World of mortality and morbidity associated with water-borne diseases clearly indicate that many people do not have access to safe drinking water or satisfactory sanitation. One World Bank study estimated that in 1990 around two-thirds of urban residents in the Third World had access to satisfactory water, but only one-third to satisfactory sanitation services. In rural areas access was much lower. Another study in 1988 of 20 African countries with a combined population of 325 million found that only 38 per cent had access to safe drinking water and only 21 per cent to satisfactory sanitation. Many Third World countries have been unable to expand their water and sanitation services in line with growing populations, and evidence collected at the beginning of the 1990s by the World Resources Institute suggested that across the Third World as a whole there would be little or no additional resources for water and sanitation during that decade. Safe drinking water and proper sanitation, therefore, are prerequisites for good health, but they are very far from being universally available and it will be a major challenge to expand access to them.

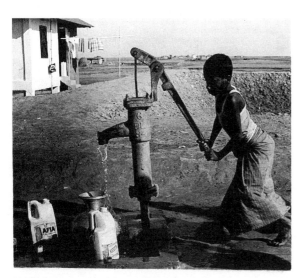

Water being pumped from a shallow tube well, on the island of Uri Char in the Bay of Bengal. (Photo: Tom Learmonth/Christian Aid)

Place of residence

Yet another environmental influence on patterns of mortality and morbidity is **place of residence**. Urban and rural dwellers may be exposed to quite different risks: for example, as you saw above, people in towns generally have more access to safe water and adequate sanitation. Let us now look at the health differences in more detail.

Though few Third World countries publish mortality data classified by place of residence, for a few low-income and middle-income countries there are data available on mortality rates for urban and for rural areas. Table 3.5 contains data for a sample of such countries.

Table 3.5 Mortality rates classified by rural and urban residence for selected countries, 1989 or nearest date

Country	Infant mortality rate (per 1 000 live births)		Crude death rate (per 1 000 population per year)	
	Rural	Urban	Rural	Urban
Bangladesh	112.4	91.3	12.5	8.6
Cuba	11.3	12.1	5.1	7.1
India	104.6	62.0	12.0	7.4
Japan	5.7	5.1	7.9	5.7
USSR	31.6	21.1	11.7	9.0

Data from United Nations (1991) *United Nations Demographic Yearbook 1989*, UN, New York, Tables 15 and 18.

☐ Can you think of any reasons why these data should be interpreted cautiously?

■ There are several reasons.

First, definitions of 'rural' and 'urban' vary from place to place. (You might like to think how you would define them. How large would a town have to be before it would be regarded as urban? What would you do about an area comprising a city surrounded by a large rural area?)

Second, where rates are calculated using a death registration system, registration will often be more complete in urban than in rural areas, so in some instances the rural rates may be artificially low.

Third, in some countries rural dwellers may travel to the nearest urban area to seek hospital treatment for their illness. If any die in hospital, their deaths may artificially inflate the death rate for urban areas. (This would depend on whether care is taken to record the place of usual residence on the death register.)

Finally, it might well be that those people migrating from rural to urban areas, or labour migrants taking jobs far from home, perhaps in another country, tend to be the youngest and healthiest members of the rural population, and those staying behind are the least healthy. In this instance, the death rates for urban areas may be held down and those for rural areas pushed up.

Despite these difficulties, the table shows a clear advantage for urban over rural dwellers in almost every country, and there are many reasons why this might be expected. People in urban areas generally have advantages that include higher incomes, better educational opportunities and greater access to preventive and curative health services. On the other hand, some features of urban living may lead to increased mortality. Accidents and violence are often more common in urban settlements, and overcrowding may enhance the transmission of infectious diseases. In some countries, people living in the slums or shanty towns of the cities may be in a much worse position than peasant farmers in the countryside. Air pollution from traffic, heating fuel or industry can often be worse: in Chinese cities, which are heavily reliant on coal for energy, lung cancer is between 4 and 7 times higher than the national average. And, finally, 'megacities' are growing in the Third World, of a size far beyond all previous human experience: by the year 2000 Mexico City and São Paulo are each expected to contain 24 million inhabitants. The health consequences of such urbanisation can only be guessed.

Demographic influences on mortality

You have already seen that mortality rates vary dramatically with age. This is one reason why crude death rates can be difficult to interpret. But other factors must also be taken into account in trying to explain the variations in mortality within Third World countries, including sex and gender, and family structure. (As Chapter 9 will show, the same factors are also important influences on mortality rates in an industrialised country such as the United Kingdom.) We will look at each of these in turn.

Sex and gender

Health differences between males and females may arise for a variety of reasons, including biological **sex** and culturally-determined **gender**. It is important to keep in mind the distinction between sex and gender as you study the following material.

☐ Look back again at Table 2.2 in the previous chapter, in which the expectation of life is shown separately for men and women in different countries. Do men or women tend to live longer?

■ The expectation of life at birth is greater for females than for males in 16 out of the 18 countries in the table.

☐ However, the difference between the sexes is not uniform. See if you can find any pattern in the figures shown in Table 2.2.

■ In the industrialised countries, the expectation of life is consistently higher for females by between 5 and 10 years. The differences in Third World countries are generally smaller—between 2 and 4 years—and in Bangladesh males actually have a slightly greater expectation of life than females, according to the published data.

The data from industrialised countries have generally been taken to imply that, given favourable living conditions and health care, women have a 'natural' biological advantage in terms of longevity. If this interpretation is correct, the smaller differences between the sexes in some Third World countries suggest that women there are at some special disadvantage. Childbirth is one important factor. In Third World countries, women tend to experience more pregnancies than their counterparts in industrialised countries, and the risk associated with each pregnancy is considerably higher. Many of the deaths of females aged 15–49 in Third World countries are due to complications of pregnancy. This interpretation also fits the information shown in Table 2.3, which shows expectation of life at various ages in Bangladesh for males and females: the female disadvantage persists from birth through childhood and the reproductive years, but by age 50 female life expectancy for the first time is greater than male life expectancy.

However, in addition to the hazards of childbirth, women may be disadvantaged by their position in society. For example, a number of studies have demonstrated that women in Asia and North Africa receive less health care and medical attention in comparison with men. Similar evidence has been compiled in relation to education, nutrition and other factors that may influence health. Cumulatively, such disadvantages can produce startling consequences. For example, Table 3.6 shows the results of an exercise to calculate how many women were 'missing' in a group of Asian and North African countries.

The table first shows the actual ratio of males to females in each country. It can be seen that in each country there is a substantial excess of men over women, ranging from around 4 or 5 per 100 up to almost 11 per 100 in Pakistan. The table then shows the expected ratio if

Table 3.6 The number of 'missing females' in Asia and North Africa

Country	Ratio of males to females		Number of females /millions	Percentage of females missing	Number of missing females/millions
	Actual ratio	Expected ratio			
China, 1990	1.066	1.010	548.7	5.3	29.1
India, 1991	1.077	1.020	406.3	5.6	22.8
Pakistan, 1981	1.105	1.025	40.0	7.8	3.1
Bangladesh, 1981	1.064	1.025	42.2	3.8	1.6
Nepal, 1981	1.050	1.025	7.3	2.4	0.2
West Asia, 1985	1.060	1.030	55.0	3.0	1.7
Egypt, 1986	1.047	1.020	23.5	2.6	0.6

Data from Coale, A. J. (1991) Excess female mortality and the balance of the sexes in the population: an estimate of the number of 'missing females', *Population and Development Review*, **17**, (3), pp. 514–24, Table 1, p. 522.

there were no 'excess' female mortality and if a male : female ratio similar to that in Europe, North America and Japan prevailed. The table then calculates from the actual number of females in the Asian and North African countries the percentage and number of females who are 'missing'. It concludes that there are almost 60 million 'missing females' in the countries studied. Other estimates, for example by the economist Amartya Sen (who focused public attention on this issue through a series of articles), have suggested that the number of missing females in these same countries may be in excess of 100 million.

Of course, gender differences in access to health care, education, occupational stress, nutrition and so on, will vary substantially in different societies and cultures.

Indeed, there is no evidence of excess female mortality in Sub-Saharan Africa, South-East Asia, or other major regions of the Third World: areas where women are more likely to have employment outside the home, and therefore may be more independent and less vulnerable to discrimination. This suggests that gender roles in all societies have an important bearing on health patterns, and require closer examination. Later chapters of this book will return to this issue.

Family structure

Family structure is another factor that appears to be associated with childhood mortality, and the spacing of births seems to be particularly important. Table 3.7 shows the relationship between **birth spacing** and infant mortality in Senegal during the 1970s.

Table 3.7 Relationship between birth spacing and child mortality in Senegal, 1970s

Interval since previous birth/months	Infant mortality rate in that group (per 1 000 live births)
under 11	347
12–23	135
24–35	109
36–47	115
48+	89

Data from United Nations (1986) *Determinants of Mortality Change and Differentials in Developing Countries: a 5-country Case Study Project*, UN Population Studies No. 94, UN, New York, Table 80.

□ Was there any relationship between birth spacing and infant mortality in the data from Senegal?

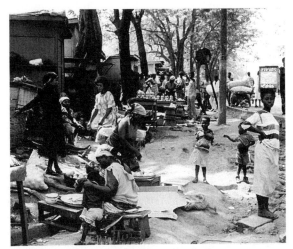

Women running a street market in Ghana, West Africa. In this region, women dominate market selling and trading, and therefore have some economic autonomy. (Photo: Hutchison/Crispin Hughes)

■ Short intervals between births were associated with higher infant mortality.

Short intervals between births can lead to increased infant and childhood mortality for several reasons. First, a rapid succession of pregnancies puts pressure on the mother's health. This can lead to babies with low birth weights, and these are known to be at higher risk of infant death. Second, when the new baby is born, the previous child will no longer be breast-fed, and this may lead to under-nutrition, especially in countries where supplementary foods may be contaminated or inadequate. Third, where there are several young children, the caring resources of the mother are more likely to be stretched.

Socio-economic influences on mortality

A basic difficulty in studying the many socio-economic factors associated with mortality in Third World countries—such as education, social class, housing, income and access to health care—is that they may all be closely associated. Here, we focus on two factors in particular: education and social class.

Education

Numerous studies have shown that childhood mortality is associated with the education of the mother and/or father. Table 3.8, based on research on a sample of women in Zimbabwe, shows that childhood mortality is strongly associated with the level of education of the mother: the risk of dying during early childhood is six times higher for children whose mothers have no formal education than for children whose mothers have a secondary education. There is a weaker but still quite clear association between maternal education and mortality during the first year of a child's life. Research elsewhere shows that the father's level of education is similarly related to childhood and infant mortality.

Table 3.8 Relationship between mother's education and child mortality, Zimbabwe, for period 1978–88

Level of education of mother:	Infant mortality rate (per 1 000 live births)	Childhood mortality rate (per 1 000 aged 1–4)
no education	77	52
primary	55	29
secondary or higher	40	8

Data from Central Statistical Office, Zimbabwe (1990) *Zimbabwe Demographic and Health Survey Report*, CSO, Harare, Table 6.2, p. 79.

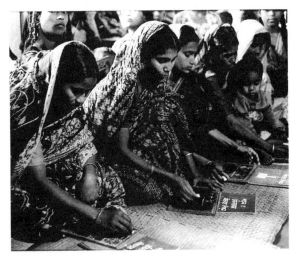

Women's literacy group in Tumulia village, Bangladesh. The female literacy rate in Bangladesh in 1990 was 22 per cent compared with 47 per cent for men. (Photo: Tom Learmonth/Christian Aid])

What factors explain these associations? First, higher levels of parental education are likely to be linked to occupations with higher incomes and hence better social conditions and better access to health care, making it difficult to assess the separate contribution of each of these factors to childhood mortality. Nevertheless, some Latin American studies have shown that the relationship between mortality and parents' education remains strong, even after allowing for the effect of income, suggesting that more education creates a better awareness and use of appropriate health practices.

Social class

Social class, defined by occupation, also has an important influence on patterns of health and disease, but again there are many problems involved in defining, measuring and using occupational class when analysing data, and these are compounded in Third World countries.[5] First, there is the general problem of the availability of data that has been raised several times already in this chapter. There may be no reliable death registration system, and incomplete coverage of the population by censuses. A more fundamental problem, however, is that the whole concept of occupational class measurement has been devised to suit industrialised countries; that is, most of the

[5]See *Studying Health and Disease* (Open University Press, 1985, revised edition 1994).

occupations and work patterns used to assign people to a particular class do not exist in most Third World countries. In consequence, caution is required in transferring occupational class measures to Third World countries. In fact, the emergence of particular forms of social class stratification is an important characteristic of societies at different stages of development, and will be discussed in more detail in Chapter 5.

Bearing this in mind, what can nevertheless be said about variations in mortality rates according to socioeconomic status in the Third World? The most reliable data relate to infant and child mortality rates. Table 3.9 presents data on child mortality rates in Costa Rica, classified by the father's occupation. Such data are not easy to obtain, and this example is now some years out of date, but the picture it reveals remains valid.

Table 3.9 Child mortality rates in Costa Rica, classified by the father's occupation, 1968–9

'Social class'	Number of deaths between birth and age 2 per 1 000 births
high and middle bourgeoisie	20
middle class	39
proletariat	80
agricultural workers	99
average	**80**

Data from Behm, H. (1979) Socioeconomic determinants of mortality in Latin America, *Proceedings of the Meeting on Socioeconomic Determinants and the Consequences of Mortality*, UN/WHO, Mexico, Table 13.

The social class groups used by the researcher may not be familiar to you. Broadly, 'high and middle bourgeoisie' includes farm owners, industrial proprietors, higher executives and managers. 'Middle class' includes other salaried employees, technicians, teachers, and so on. The distinction between the 'proletariat' and 'agricultural workers' is that the former mainly includes wage-earning workers and labourers in manufacturing and service industries, whereas the latter are mainly small farmers and farmworkers.

☐ In Table 3.9, how does the risk of death in Costa Rica vary with social class?

■ There is a dramatic relationship between mortality and social class. The risk of death in the first two years of life increased steeply from 20 per 1 000 births (one child in 50) among the 'bourgeoisie', to almost 100 per 1 000 (one child in 10) among

'agricultural workers'. Mortality rates in the 'middle class' were approximately twice as high as among the 'bourgeoisie', and among the 'proletariat' they were four times as high.

However, these differences could also be related to place of residence, as discussed earlier in the chapter, as farmworkers will be in rural areas and the groups associated with commercial and manufacturing activity are likely to be concentrated in towns. This demonstrates once again that the factors that influence patterns of health and disease are usually intertwined.

Prospects for the control of disease

Despite the high mortality rates experienced by Third World countries, there have been improvements in the health of the people of those countries, and some further improvement is expected, as you saw in Chapter 2. Around one-half of the fall in mortality rates that has occurred over the last few decades has been due to a decline in the number of deaths from malaria, smallpox, tuberculosis and measles. A further one-third of the fall in mortality in Third World countries since 1930 is thought to have resulted from a decline in deaths from the respiratory diseases—influenza, pneumonia, and bronchitis. A smaller fall was due to a reduction in deaths from diarrhoeal diseases. In other words, the commonest cause of illness and death in Third World countries remains one of the most intractable.

The decline in deaths from smallpox was the consequence of a campaign led by the World Health Organisation which succeeded in eradicating this disease globally. This campaign is described in an article in *Health and Disease: A Reader*[6] by Marc Strassburg entitled 'The global eradication of smallpox', which you should now read.

☐ It took almost 200 years from the discovery of an effective vaccine to the eradication of smallpox. What reasons does Strassburg offer for this long delay?

■ First, to be usable in hot climates, the vaccine had to be heat-stable: this was not achieved until the 1950s. Second, the design of needles used in vaccination was greatly improved in the 1960s. And finally, many Third World countries had too few resources to run effective vaccination campaigns without assistance.

[6]*Health and Disease: A Reader* (Open University Press, 1984; revised edition 1994).

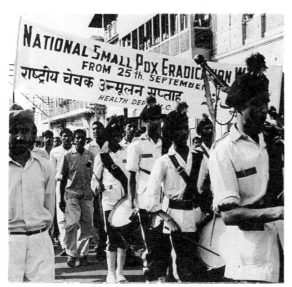

A parade in New Delhi, India, in the 1960s, urges people to get smallpox vaccination. (Source: Popperfoto)

The campaign began in 1967, at which point it was estimated that there were around 10 million cases concentrated in 30 countries. Using an eradication strategy based on surveillance and containment rather than relying solely on mass vaccination, the disease was gradually eliminated from country after country, until the last naturally occurring case was diagnosed in Somalia in 1977.

☐ In what ways did the natural history of smallpox facilitate this eradication strategy?

■ Smallpox spread fairly slowly, tended to cluster, and had no reservoir other than humans; there was no carrier state in which humans could pass on the disease without displaying symptoms; and vaccination conferred long-lasting immunity. Thus case-finding, source-tracing and containment were effective.

☐ What does this article conclude about the likelihood of eradicating other infectious diseases, and why?

■ That many other major infectious diseases would be much more difficult to eradicate, either because not enough is known of their natural history, or because they are zoonotic diseases and the reservoirs of infection are difficult to control, or because the costs of eradication would be so high. However, measles shares certain characteristics with smallpox and might be susceptible to a similar eradication campaign.

There have been attempts to eradicate a number of other diseases prevalent in the Third World, including hookworm, yellow fever and malaria. However, these all failed, and it was partly a disillusionment with this approach that led the World Health Organisation in 1978 to turn to a much broader strategy of comprehensive primary health care, including

> ...education concerning prevailing health problems and the methods of preventing and controlling them; promotion of food supply and proper nutrition; an adequate supply of safe water and basic sanitation; maternal and child health care, including family planning; immunisation against the major infectious diseases; prevention and control of locally endemic diseases; appropriate treatment of common diseases and injuries; and provision of essential drugs. (The Declaration of Alma Ata, World Health Organisation, 1978)

This WHO strategy of 'Health for All by the Year 2000' identifies many of the factors already discussed in this chapter, and has had great influence.[7] However, it has in turn been criticised. One line of argument is that it is too diffuse, too ambitious and too costly to succeed, that all health problems cannot be tackled at the same time, and that a better strategy would be to set realistic and attainable priorities based on the mortality and morbidity caused by particular diseases, and the feasibility and cost of controlling them. During the 1980s this approach led to a massive effort by a group of international agencies to immunise children against a group of immunisable diseases including diphtheria, polio, tetanus, whooping cough and measles, and this did succeed in increasing the proportion of the world's children who were immunised from around 20 per cent in 1984 to around 75 per cent by 1990. This strategy based on specific priorities has also fostered a programme to encourage the use of oral rehydration therapy for acute diarrhoeal diseases.

Another approach to the health problems of the Third World is to argue that the root cause of infectious disease is poverty, which manifests itself in unsatisfactory water supplies and sanitation, insufficient food, poor education and inadequate health care. From this perspective, the industrialised world has largely rid itself of infectious diseases through social and economic development, and therefore some have argued that the

[7]The programme of 'Health for All by the Year 2000' is discussed in more detail in *Caring for Health: History and Diversity* (Open University Press, 1993).

over-riding priority in the Third World is to follow the same path and industrialise. However, the precise ways in which the infectious diseases receded in the industrialised world, the extent to which the present Third World can learn from this historical experience, and indeed the implications of global industrialisation for the future health of humanity, are all fiercely contested

questions to which much of the remainder of this book is devoted. Before turning to some of these issues, the next chapter concludes this initial survey of world health and disease with a case study in which we aim to give you some sense of the experience of health and disease in the Third World, not at the level of national or regional statistics, but by individuals and localities.

OBJECTIVES FOR CHAPTER 3

When you have studied this chapter, you should be able to:

3.1   Compare the important causes of death in Third World and industrialised countries, and the main characteristics of these diseases.

3.2   Describe the use and advantages of the 'years of potential life lost' calculation as a means of comparing the relative importance of different causes of death in a country.

3.3   Compare the main causes of morbidity and mortality in Third World countries.

3.4   Set out the main ways in which environment may influence health, using examples of specific diseases to illustrate the interaction between factors.

3.5   Describe how mortality rates differ between males and females, and offer possible explanations for these patterns.

3.6   Discuss the association between socio-economic status and mortality.

QUESTIONS FOR CHAPTER 3

Question 1 (*Objective 3.1*)

To what extent are the patterns of mortality in Third World countries a result of diseases peculiar to these countries?

Question 2 (*Objective 3.2*)

Given what has been said about causes of death in Third World and industrialised countries, why

might the 'years of potential life lost' measure be a good way of emphasising differences in these patterns?

Question 3 (*Objective 3.3*)

Which diseases (or groups of diseases) are important in terms of mortality in the Third World but *less* important in terms of disease prevalence; and are any diseases (or groups of diseases) more important in terms of disease prevalence than of mortality?

Question 4 (*Objective 3.4*)

Explain, giving examples, what is meant by zoonotic diseases, and why they may be difficult to control.

Question 5 (*Objective 3.5*)

Making use of material from this and the previous chapter, answer the following:

(a)   What is the gender difference in expectation of life at birth in Bangladesh and in the United Kingdom?

(b)   Does the advantage of one sex over the other persist in both countries?

(c)   What is one consequence of these gender differences in Bangladesh on the country's population structure?

Question 6 (*Objective 3.6*)

'Education is bound to be associated with childhood mortality, because it is associated with so many other factors such as income and access to health care'. Discuss.

4
Livelihood and survival: a case study of Bangladesh

We saw why early travellers to the region spoke of its fertility in glowing terms. From the windows of buses and the decks of ferry boats, we looked over a lush green landscape. Rice paddies carpeted the earth and gigantic squash vines climbed over the roofs of the village houses.

The rich alluvial soil, the plentiful water and the hot humid climate made us feel as if we had entered a natural greenhouse. In autumn, as the ripening rice turned gold, we understood why in song and verse the Bengalis call their land 'sonar bangla', 'golden Bengal'…As we travelled through the countryside, trying at once to comprehend the lush beauty of the land and the destitution of so many people, we sensed that we had entered a strange battleground. All around us, beneath the surface calm, silent struggles were being waged, struggles in which the losers met slow bloodless deaths. We began to learn about the quiet violence which rages in Bangladesh, a violence of which the famine victims were only the most visible casualties. (Hartmann and Boyce, 1983, pp. 11 and 17)

This is how the anthropologists Betsy Hartmann and James Boyce, in their book *A Quiet Violence*, tell of their first impressions of rural Bangladesh (see Figure 4.1).

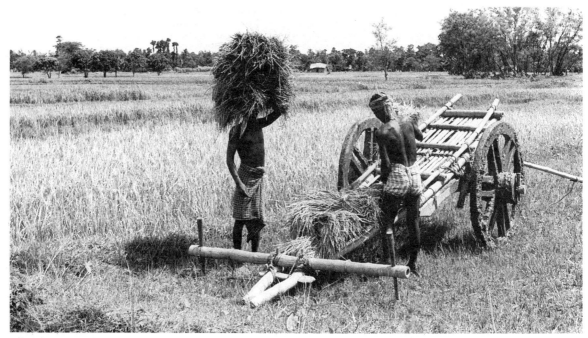

Figure 4.1 *Rural life in Bangladesh. (Source: OXFAM: Philip Jackson)*

We have reproduced this quotation here to set the scene for a different way of looking at and understanding how illness still dominates and shapes the lives of many people living today. Up to this point, we have been making broad general comparisons between the populations of industrialised and Third World countries. For the most part, these have used *quantitative* measures, such as the rates at which disease or death strike in a population and the numbers and ages of the survivors. Now we shall develop a **case study approach** to health and disease by looking in more depth at the lives of people living in a specific Third World country, namely Bangladesh. As well as using numerical data to describe the average levels of health and disease and the social and economic conditions of the population as a whole, we shall show how an account of the life of a single family can typify the conditions of people living in that predominantly rural country. Descriptive accounts such as these are collected quite literally by asking people to tell the stories of their lives.

But, before we begin, we need to discuss the advantages of using case studies which contain descriptive profiles of this kind and point out some of the dangers. We may know from objectively verifiable sources, such as records of hospital admissions, or land sales, that people frequently suffer from a particular infectious disease, that children die of malnutrition, or that small farming families often have to sell up. We may also know in general terms *why* this is so: specific organisms cause the diseases; people live in poverty; sometimes the food supply collapses. But that is not the whole story—case studies can fill in some of the blanks.

☐ What do you think is the main advantage of case studies as a method of researching health problems?

■ The great strength of the case study approach is that it allows us to gain insights into the *processes* by which people's health or even their lives are threatened. It can help us to explain (for example) why certain diseases occur so often in a particular location, or in people dependent on a particular means of livelihood. It may reveal common sequences of events that culminate in the break-up of a family following the death of a productive member. It might identify what the people in villages of type 'A' do for each other to sustain themselves through famines, while the poorest members of villages of type 'B' die.

Potentially offsetting these advantages is the temptation to generalise on the basis of too few examples, or even of a single case description, which might turn out either to be unique (i.e. to be the only member of a class of one), or not be sufficiently typical to justify drawing general conclusions about the nature of the causal processes involved.

Clearly, it is important to develop a case study (such as the one that follows) in a systematic way, which combines descriptive information with statistical sources of data so that one illuminates the other. The systematic approach to developing a case study starts from an investigation of the *general* situation, then focuses down on a *particular* group, individual or situation as a source of ideas about what processes are taking place, and goes back again to the general picture to see if those ideas are consistent with it. If so, the number of specific cases can be extended and their content broadened and so on, in a repeating cycle: the general–to the particular–to the general.

Case studies, therefore, use descriptive, qualitative data to enrich and inform the available quantitative data, which in turn suggests new areas on which to focus.

But the use of descriptive material raises another problem. If we were just interested in getting valid quantitative measurements of average income, or family size, then the statisticians have rules that can be used to estimate the smallest number of cases that would justify the use of an average to extrapolate to the larger population at a given degree of accuracy. If our purpose however, is not just to derive quantitative estimates of some variable, but to use qualitative information, to gain insights into *processes,* then these statistical rules are inadequate. But there are no mathematical rules that will decide how many similar narrative descriptions have to be collected and how these should be combined, in order to be confident that a 'typical' pattern has been established. This means that if they are to be reliable, case studies must be the result of the exercise of judgement. Furthermore, that judgement must be formed not only from a knowledge of the numerical data, but by a combination of the information contained in both observation and measurement. In general, this requires the skills and concepts of anthropology and sociology, together with those of the quantitative life sciences.

Good case studies have practical applications. They can be used to inform planners and politicians about the circumstances and processes in the lives of individuals, families and communities which place them at risk of illness. Such profiles can then provide the basis for the selection and design of programmes and policies which might be effective in reducing those risks.

Against this background, we turn now to Bangladesh.

A case study of rural life in Bangladesh

The following case study begins with a review of the current situation of Bangladesh and of its people as a whole. It then continues with a narrative description of the condition and life experiences of a single family. This is not the story of an actual family, but combines features which have been taken from the life histories of several families and of many individuals. The case study draws upon many different sources of numerical data, surveys and measurements on samples of the population, to give body sizes, ages, food consumption, farm size, etc., which are representative of a particular class of peasants, and it uses the accounts of anthropologists and social scientists who have investigated people's daily lives.

Food, health and survival

Bangladesh is one of the most densely populated countries in the world, and also one of the least industrialised and least urbanised in Asia. Eighty per cent of its people (some 88 million), live in rural or semi-rural areas. More than half of these are either landless, or own such small plots of land that they cannot achieve self sufficiency for food and are wholly or partly dependent on wages earned by working for richer peasants, or in activities related to agriculture or rural commerce. Although the rate of growth of population is now beginning to decline, in 1989 it was still running at 2.6 per cent per year and numbers are expected almost to double by 2025.

Agricultural production has been growing at a rate below that of the natural increase of rural population for some decades. Before the twentieth century, if such a rapid growth of numbers had ever begun, it would have soon have been choked off by a 'positive check', in the form of uncontrolled deaths from famine (as you will learn in Chapter 5). Since Bangladesh gained independence from British colonial rule along with the rest of the Indian sub-continent in 1947, the impact of such disasters has been contained only because of the increasing availability of surplus food grain provided by the industrial countries. In this respect, freedom from colonialism has been counterbalanced by increased economic and political dependence. For example, in 1974 the USA abruptly suspended food aid shipments to Bangladesh in annoyance over Bangladeshi jute exports to Cuba.

The effect of food aid has been to maintain the average food supply per head at a more or less constant level (but a quite low level in comparison with India, for example) and to avoid the mass deaths that were a normal feature of famines before the Second World War. However, stagnation of domestic food production has resulted

in low wage rates, a continuous rise in rural unemployment and hence worsening poverty. Landlessness is increasing, not only because of sub-division of land among the growing numbers of people, but also due to forced sales following indebtedness.

The rate at which families fall into destitution is regularly accelerated by disasters. There was a major famine in 1974–5; a 'near famine' in 1979; flooding and heavy loss of rice crops in 1981; a drought and rural unemployment in 1982; floods leading to the loss of 1.5 million tons of rice in 1984; similar flooding in 1986; even worse floods in 1988; and cyclonic flooding of off-shore islands and coastal land in 1990 and 1991 (see Figure 4.2).

The numbers of deaths resulting from these events seem huge by comparison with those caused by natural disasters in the industrialised countries. But they are much smaller than they would have been before independence, because of better preparedness and much prompter and more extensive relief services, both national and international. The numbers involved are

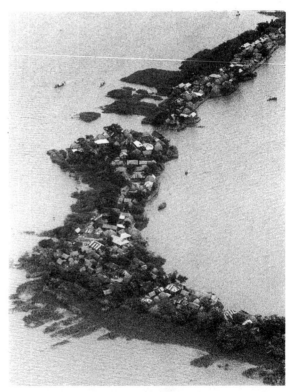

Figure 4.2 *During floods, sea-water covers the rice paddies; aerial view near Dhaka, 1972. (Source: OXFAM: Philip Jackson)*

small, relative to the rate of population growth. The floods of 1990 were said to have killed in excess of 100 000 people: the current rate of natural increase is about 60 000 per week.

However, very much greater numbers than these have their livelihoods destroyed. This happens partly through permanent loss of productive land: low-lying fields are washed away, or salinated (impregnated with salt water). Even temporary displacement, or the loss of part of a crop, can spell disaster for people with no reserves to fall back on. Such crises commonly lead to loss of jobs and possessions and the break-up of families. Men and, increasingly, single women or women supporting children, migrate to the urban slums in search of work (see Figure 4.3). A survey of such migrants by the nutritionist Jane Pryer in 1986 found that nearly 50 per cent gave poverty and lack of employment as the reason for leaving their villages. Another 16 per cent gave loss of land due either to flooding, or to legal problems following a death, disputes over title deeds, or family quarrels. This steady process of impoverishment, followed by the 'squeezing out' of people from their traditional livelihoods, has now brought to Bangladesh one of the fastest rates of urban growth in the world: from 5.2 million living in major cities in 1961 to 22 million in 1989.

In many ways, health has its own balance sheet of good and bad for the first generations since Bangladesh gained independence. In 1950, endemic malaria meant that people were only able to work at limited efficiency. In addition, malaria caused many deaths in infants, children and adults. Two species of parasites are responsible, *Plasmodium falciparum* and the somewhat less virulent *Plasmodium vivax*, both transmitted by mosquitoes.

The introduction of the insecticides DDT and Dieldrin led first to control and then the virtual eradication of the malaria-carrying mosquitoes by about the early 1960s. Like some other infections, malaria is believed to increase the rate of spontaneous abortion. Where it is **endemic** (i.e. numerous small outbreaks occur every year), it certainly contributes to deaths in early childhood. One immediate and dramatic effect of the malaria control programme was an increase in live births and in the rate of population growth. In Bangladesh, as in many other countries, malaria has increased in recent years and has again become a significant threat. Parasites are being carried across the borders of neighbouring countries like Burma, not only by mosquitoes, but by humans. Air travel is an increasing mode of re-infection involving both infected people and mosquitoes taken onto planes in clothing and luggage. In addition, growing insecticide resistance of mosquitoes and drug resistance in the parasites themselves threaten to make the re-emerging disease more difficult to control.

Even more serious is that the type of parasite *Plasmodium falciparum*, which is associated with more

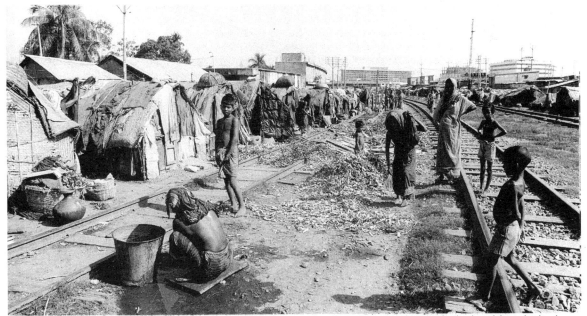

Figure 4.3 *Railway tracks become the focus for squatter camps and makeshift housing for people displaced from the land. (Source: OXFAM: Walter Holt)*

violent symptoms (including cerebral malaria), has increased in proportion to the milder *Plasmodium vivax,* which was the formerly dominant type. This means that if the disease does once again become endemic, more people will die before they acquire any natural immunity.

Diarrhoeal diseases are still a considerable burden, in terms of illness and suffering, loss of production, bereavement and orphaning. One quarter of all children born die before the age of 5 years. This remains true despite improvements in the delivery of technical health interventions such as immunisation, essential drug supplies, and the increasing use of inexpensive techniques for better treatment of diarrhoea such as oral rehydration therapy using home-made solutions of sugar and salt, to prevent deaths from dehydration.

Tetanus remains an important cause of death, especially in children. Outbreaks of typhoid frequently occur. Although water supplies have improved in some areas because of increasing numbers of boreholes, the fields, open wells and water-courses are still massively polluted by human excrement. Measles and influenza are still serious public health problems, with pneumonia often supervening, causing many deaths. Of the 'great' epidemic diseases—smallpox, plague and cholera—smallpox has been eradicated, and plague has almost disappeared, but outbreaks of cholera still occur.

Despite all these problems, the balance so far seems to be slightly on the positive side. Health statistics show overall improvements in life chances. Infant mortality has declined from 144 per 1 000 live births in 1965, to 106 in 1989. As far as adult health is concerned, the picture is of increasing life expectancy once early childhood has been survived. In Matlab, a rural district intensively studied for many years by the International Centre for Diarrhoeal Disease Research, average life expectancy is about 50 years, very similar to the national average, but much of this low figure is the result of high mortality in early life. The 75 per cent of those born who survive the hazards of their first 5 years, can expect to live for about 62 more years. An equivalent figure for the United Kingdom population at age 5 would be about 70 further years of life expectancy.

Surveys of food consumption have been made at regular intervals over the past two or three decades, using samples of households and of individuals living in them. Some of these surveys have included comparisons of food energy intakes at different times of the year, by the same families. These show a slow decline in average energy consumption of about 10 per cent per decade, paralleling the decline in the purchasing power of the average wage. During the 'hungry' period, just before the main harvest, consumption is about 12 per cent lower than just afterwards. Contrary to popular belief, people do not seem to discriminate against small children in terms of food, in Bangladesh at any rate. The nutritionists M. Abdullah and Erica Wheeler found that all the individuals within families—men, women, girls and boys—had energy intakes which were in the same proportion to their estimated energy requirements. This remained true, even in the 'hungry' season.

The proportion of rural Bangladeshi children under 5 years old who are short for their age declined from 72 per cent in 1975 to 57 per cent in 1986. The proportion who were 'thin' (i.e. low in weight for their height) also declined over the same period from 22 per cent to 7 per cent. These improvements, which are probably due to better control of endemic disease and better access to primary health care services rather than to improvements in nutrition, seems to have benefited boys more than girls. A survey in 1981 showed that girls were between two and three times more likely to suffer acute episodes of severe weight loss than boys.

Such differences between the sexes in levels of care, and hence of health and survival, persist at all ages with the result that, over the population as a whole, the ratio of living males to females is 1.064 (as you can see from Table 3.6 in Chapter 3). The equivalent figure for Europe leads demographers to estimate that, in Bangladesh, 1.6 million women are 'missing' (i.e. have died from preventable causes) as a result of discrimination against females in the provision of care.

Against this general background of the national picture, what can we learn from focusing on specific families in Bangladesh? At this point in the case study, we introduce a fictional family constructed from many descriptive accounts, which represents some of the important recurring themes of rural life.

Profile of a typical Bangladeshi peasant family

A typical poor peasant family consists of a husband Abu, a wife whose maiden name was Sofi but who is now known as 'mother of Anis', and four children: Sharifa, a girl of 10, Anis, a boy of 7, Naila, a girl of 5, and a boy of 2, named Hali. They own their house, which is built entirely of palm thatch and has mud floors (see Figure 4.4).

Their water comes from a well which is shared with 30 other households. There is no means of disposal of excreta or refuse, except for the fields and open rubbish heaps. All the members of this family are shorter and lighter than average European or North American people of the same age and sex. The wife weighs 40 kg and the husband 46 kg, 18 per cent and 25 per cent less than their

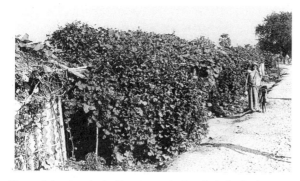

Figure 4.4 *A typical village street in Bangladesh: the houses are covered with squash vines which provide additional shade and food. (Source: OXFAM: Sheena Grossett)*

United Kingdom counterparts. The two older children are about 20 cm shorter than the average for United Kingdom children, whereas the two younger ones are not only short, but are about 10 per cent lighter than Western children, even taking account of their height.

Several times during her life Naila has been severely ill, losing at the time an additional 30 per cent of body weight, relative to a healthy European child of the same age. During the past year, she has had an episode of diarrhoea with fever, scabies and an ear infection with bad fever. Because of her worsening condition, Naila was taken first to a paramedic in the nearest town, who gave her one dose of penicillin. Although trained in the Western tradition, he is well aware that he can care for only

perhaps a fifth of the village population and he encourages respect for traditional Ayurvedic (Hindu) and Unani (Islamic) systems of medicine. When the single injection did no good, Naila was taken to a Hindu herbal doctor, who sold the family pills over which he had chanted mantras. Two other children had been born to this family, both of whom died before reaching their second birthdays.

The family's ability to obtain food is derived in part from a quarter of an acre of land which was left to Abu on the death of Sofi's father. From this, in an average year, they get two crops of rice, enough to provide them with one-fifth of their food energy requirements. The rest of their food procurement relies on payment 'in kind' or from cash, earned by working for richer farmers. In past years, the family 'share-cropped' an additional acre, but the owner now finds it more profitable to farm it himself and to hire their labour when he needs it. Husband and wife both work for wages, as do the two older children: father and son at farm work; mother and daughter chopping and carrying firewood, washing clothes and parboiling rice (a hot soaking of un-milled grain preliminary to re-drying and husking).

Their own piece of land is an essential part of their food procurement and they try to make up for its smallness by the intensity of their labour (see Figure 4.5). They plough with a hired ox and meticulously weed and harvest by hand, although this has to be done just at the time when the best wage rates are on offer by the richer peasants.

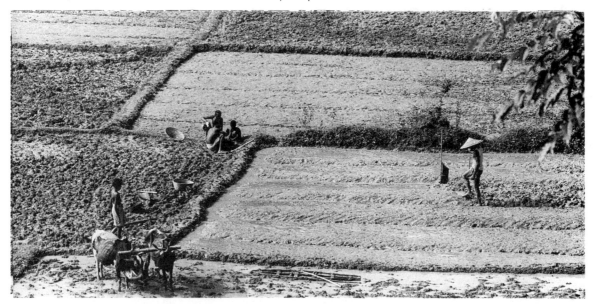

Figure 4.5 *Preparing the fields for rice planting. Notice the small size of the plots. (Source: OXFAM: Philip Jackson)*

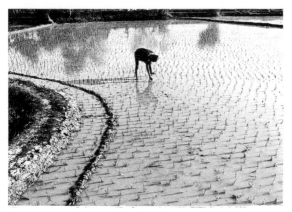

Figure 4.6 *Transplanting rice in the paddy fields. (Source: OXFAM)*

Rice dominates their landscape, their diet and often their thoughts (see Figure 4.6). As the Innuit have many words for snow, so the Bengalis have many words for rice—each of the dozens of varieties has its name and each of these can be eaten in several different ways: parboiled, double parboiled, puffed, flaked, fried, etc. Although their waking hours are devoted to this work, no one takes a daily meal for granted—neighbours greet each other with the simple question 'have you eaten'?

Of the family earnings, 90 per cent is spent on food: the rest goes on clothing, medicines and other essentials. Husband and wife are both illiterate; Anis attends primary school, but only intermittently.

The average year-round food energy consumption of the family is 10 200 kcal[1] per day, or 1 700 kcal per head. Ninety per cent of this comes from rice —2.9 kg a day, the rest from vegetables, occasionally fish.

Even if they did no productive work and only rested quietly all day, the family would still need 7 800 kcal per day, just to stay alive and maintain their present body weights. The 2 400 kcal the family consume over and above this is what is available to them to support their physical activity. This amount of energy has to cover not only what they expend in working their own land and in paid employment, so as to secure their food, but also the energy cost of essential domestic work, carrying water and fuel, cooking and cleaning.

The energy budget for the year includes a peak of food availability after the *aman*, the larger of the two rice

harvests, and a trough or 'hungry' period just before. The difference between this peak and trough in daily consumption for the whole family is 1 200 kcal, equivalent to about 400 grams of rice per day. They 'share' this seasonal hunger among themselves, roughly in proportion to their individual energy needs. That is to say, they each go short by amounts which depend on their body weights and on the amounts of physical work they do: no one makes extra sacrifices and no one is deprived of food by reason of their sex or age.

The struggle to make do is gradually getting worse with each decade that passes. Although, to the casual observer, the intensively cultivated landscape presents an appearance of pastoral harmony, beneath the surface there is an increasingly desperate competition for land and employment.

Abu's greatest worry is that Sofi's brothers have never fully accepted his right to the inherited land from their father. Forgery of land title deeds has become commonplace and people as poor as he is cannot afford legal defence.

For families in this situation, the continuous grind of poverty is both a background and an underlying cause of more dramatic and usually tragic events—a child dies, a wage-earner gets sick, there are droughts and, more commonly, floods.

The initial response to such a crisis is to borrow money and sell household goods and ornaments; later, land and tools have to be sold and finally people themselves, into bonded labour for men and prostitution for women and children.

Of course people do survive. There is food aid relief; crises pass, sometimes just through a better than average harvest. But a number of studies of the rural poor have shown that for many people things are never the same again: those who managed to keep their land have an extra burden of debts to bear; those who sold join the ranks of the landless whose numbers are increasing faster than the rate of growth of the population as a whole. Physical oppression and murder are increasingly evident in the cities to which the landless migrate and, for women especially, suicide has become a relatively common means of escape from the 'quiet violence' of hopeless destitution.

It seems that in Bangladesh, as in most countries, the retreat of the major endemic diseases has had a profound effect upon survival and vitality of the whole population, of all ages, extending even to the rural poor. Similarly, the control of infectious diseases of childhood, together with the adoption of better child-care methods by those who have access, education and the financial means to do so, has begun to reduce the problem of early child deaths.

☐ What do you see as the remaining outstanding health problems facing Bangladesh? Will these be resolved by delivering more technical health services? Better education of the population about health and nutrition? Improved living standards? All of these?

■ From now on it will become increasingly hard to sustain further improvements unless something is done at least to halt the growth of the numbers in absolute destitution. There is little to be gained by 'educating' people in the use of resources they do not possess or of facilities which are out of their reach.

Conclusion

This chapter has served two purposes. First, it has described and demonstrated the way in which the proper use of case study material leads to better interpretation of *measurements* as well as to a deeper understanding of *processes*. Second, the case study of Bangladesh shows vividly how totally interdependent the problems generated by disease and by poor social conditions have now become, for people in some countries. In particular, it is now quite difficult to argue, for countries such as Bangladesh, that they can hope to complete the demographic and health transition achieved in the past by the industrialised countries (which will be introduced in Chapter 5), without at the same time finding an effective way of dealing with the problem of the continuing growth of poverty and destitution. However much financial and human resources, whether from the state, from outside assistance, or from communities themselves, are devoted to delivering health services and to sustaining past efforts to control endemic diseases such as malaria, the potential benefits of these to the quality of people's lives increasingly risk being negated by the combined effects of economic stagnation, population growth and the increasing numbers of people exposed to life-threatening natural crises.

OBJECTIVES FOR CHAPTER 4

When you have studied this chapter, you should be able to:

4.1 Describe the essential features of the case study approach to researching health problems and explain the main advantages and limitations of this method.

4.2 Describe the impact that methods for the control of endemic and epidemic diseases have had in the past on the health of the population of Bangladesh, and the new problems that have arisen with sustaining those interventions.

4.3 Give an account of the way in which the pattern of economic, social and demographic changes, since independence from British colonial rule in 1947, has affected the health of the poor in Bangladesh.

QUESTIONS FOR CHAPTER 4

Question 1 (*Objective 4.1*)

What are the reasons for using case studies and what are their main problems and limitations?

Question 2 (*Objective 4.2*)

What are the problems that face Bangladesh in its efforts to maintain and extend control over infectious diseases?

Question 3 (*Objective 4.3*)

Compare and contrast the benefits that a small farming family might experience from: (a) improved access to basic health services, and (b) improved security of food procurement.

5 The world transformed: population and the rise of industrial society

The interaction of human cultural and biological evolution is introduced here, and discussed at length in another book in this series.[1] During this chapter you will be asked to read an extract contained in Health and Disease: A Reader[2]—*'Health: 1844' by Frederick Engels.*

Amid all the various patterns of health and disease that we examined in Chapters 2 to 4 of this book, probably the most obvious fact to emerge was the degree to which good health is not simply something enjoyed by some individuals and not by others, a biological roulette game where everyone starts more or less equal. In fact, health varies enormously from one society, nation or part of the world to another, such that it is possible to talk about the collective health of different populations: health seems to be a state that is socially shared as much as individually experienced.

Another important element of the material contained in Chapters 2 to 4 is that it questions the widespread assumption that the differences in health that now exist between different parts of the world are narrowing. Of course, it is difficult to generalise over long historical periods, because the further back in time we go the less reliable sources of information become. Nevertheless some of the available measures of health, such as infant mortality rates, indicate a relative widening of differences between a number of Third World countries and the industrialised countries.

How did these differences come about? The period in which these health differences started to become more pronounced—the eighteenth and nineteenth centuries—was also the period when the Industrial Revolution began to transform a small but expanding group of countries. Thus these contemporary international differences in health and disease, and the way in which they have evolved historically, seem to be related to patterns of social and economic development. Broadly, societies that are rich and industrialised also have comparatively high levels of health and relatively stable populations, and societies that are poor have a much poorer health experience and rapidly growing populations. So this and the following three chapters explore some of the reasons for the differences in health between the Third World and industrialised countries, by looking more systematically at the links between health and disease, social and economic development, and population change.

Figure 5.1 charts these links in a simplified way. The figure indicates that each corner of the triangle is linked in both directions to the other corners, suggesting that there is no single direction of causality. In addition, the triangle is placed within an oval representing the environment,

[1] *Human Biology and Health: An Evolutionary Approach* (Open University Press, 1994).

[2] *Health and Disease: a Reader* (Open University Press, 1984; revised edition 1994).

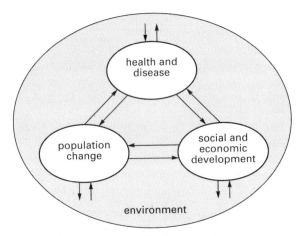

Figure 5.1 *A model of health and disease linkages.*

with each part of the triangle again linked to the environment both directly and via the other corners of the triangle.

Some of these links have already been discussed. For example, in Chapter 2 you saw how death rates affect population structure and how population structure influences death rates, and in Chapter 3 how the natural environment influences the prevalence of specific diseases. Sometimes these links are very direct, but often they are more complex, indirect and subtle. For example, the following three extracts have been selected in order to illustrate different ways in which health and disease are related to social and economic factors and the wider environment. As you read them, make a note of the sequence of events in each extract. Try to define ways in which the sequences differ.

1 From *Mirage of Health*, by R. Dubos

The main reservoirs of the plague bacilli [bacteria] in nature are wild rodents which are infected but sufficiently resistant not to suffer from their infection under normal circumstances. They carry the plague bacilli throughout their life, just as so many healthy men and women are infected with tubercle bacilli or with viruses without showing signs of disease. Among the naturally infected animals are the tarabazan (Manchurian marmot), which has long been hunted for its fur. The professional Manchurian hunters carefully avoid any tarabazan which appears to be sick and in fact a religious taboo specifically instructs them in this regard. This taboo is probably related to the fact that the plague bacilli become active in sick tarabazans and therefore can more readily be transmitted to man. Around 1900 there occurred a change in women's fashion in Europe which increased the demand of the fur trade for the pelt of the tarabazan. Attracted by the high prices of the fur, inexperienced Chinese took to tarabazan hunting. Being ignorant of the ancient taboo, they did not hesitate to catch sick animals which proved the easiest prey. Several of the hunters caught plague from the tarabazans and transmitted it to the population of the inns of Manchuria. Thus began the great epidemic of pneumonic plague in Manchuria. (Dubos, 1979, pp. 187–8)

2 From *Plagues and People*, by W. McNeill

Nearly twenty years ago…I was reading about the Spanish conquest of Mexico. As everyone knows, Hernando Cortez, starting off with fewer than six hundred men, conquered the Aztec empire, whose subjects numbered millions. How could such a tiny handful prevail…?

A casual remark in one of the accounts of Cortez's conquest…suggested an answer to such questions…. For on the night when the Aztecs drove Cortez and his men out of Mexico City, killing many of them, an epidemic of smallpox was raging in the city. The man who had organized the assault on the Spaniards was among those who died on the *nocha triste*, as the Spanish later called it. The paralysing effect of a lethal epidemic goes far to explain why the Aztecs did not pursue the defeated and demoralized Spaniards, giving them time and opportunity to rest and regroup, gather Indian allies and set siege to the city, and so achieve their eventual victory.

Moreover, it is worth considering the psychological impact of a disease that killed only Indians and left Spaniards unharmed. Such partiality could only be explained supernaturally, and there could be no doubt about which side of the struggle enjoyed divine favour…little wonder, then, that the Indians accepted Christianity and submitted to Spanish control so meekly. God had shown himself on their side, and each new outbreak of infectious disease imported from E. Europe (and soon from Africa as well) renewed the lesson. (McNeill, 1976, pp. 1–2)

3 From *Inside the Third World*, by P. Harrison

In a World Bank study in Indonesia, agricultural labourers and rubber tappers with hookworm-induced anaemia were found to be around twenty per cent less productive than their non-anaemic colleagues. Their foreman's views of which workers were 'lazy' or 'weak' were found to correspond closely to the incidence of anaemia. Workers with higher levels of anaemia earned less in incentive payments than their colleagues, and as a result of their lower income they consumed less calories, protein, vitamins, and iron than non-anaemic workers. This poorer nutrition contributed to their poor productivity and lowered their resistance to disease, hence they were more likely to lose time off work.

…Disease may also close up many areas that could be productive: river-blindness and sleeping sickness have emptied the river valleys in West Africa's Sahel region, while the tsetse fly has prevented the development of mixed agriculture in much of Africa. So disease creates poverty, while poverty, continuing the cycle, maintains the conditions that foster disease. (Harrison, 1979, pp. 288–9)

☐ In the first extract, Dubos mentioned a social/economic event, and a change in the pattern of health. What were they, and how were they related?

■ The event Dubos mentions was a change in fashion in Europe; the health change was an outbreak of pneumonic plague in Asia. Dubos is arguing that the change in fashion set off the change in health.

Even in quite unexpected or indirect ways, social or economic factors can have repercussions on health. In this first extract, the 'cause' of the pneumonic plague epidemic to which Dubos refers seems to have been these social and economic influences as much as the plague bacilli.

☐ Now consider the second extract. In what way does the sequence of events described by McNeill differ from that outlined by Dubos?

■ One way of interpreting McNeill's argument is as follows; if it had not been for the debilitating effects of disease on the Aztecs, it would have been much more difficult for the Spaniards to impose their cultural and economic domination. In other words, a change in disease pattern strongly influenced the social and economic history, and the population history, of the Americas.

In fact, the sequence of events described by McNeill seems in some way to be in the opposite direction to that in the first extract.

☐ Finally, how does Harrison's account construct a sequence of events?

■ In the extract from Harrison, the emphasis seems to be placed on interaction and interdependence between health and socio-economic factors. Health conditions are influenced by social and economic factors and the environment, which in turn are influenced by the prevailing pattern of health and disease.

In practice, it is this more complex kind of relationship that is most frequently encountered. To return to the extract from McNeill, for example: the spread of disease assisted the Spanish conquest, but it could be argued that it was the overseas expansion of the Spanish that triggered the spread of disease. It could further be argued that the overseas expansion of Spain would not have been possible without the help of navigational discoveries and new shipbuilding techniques, and so on. In one sense all of these factors caused a change in disease patterns in America, but none was *the* cause.[3]

With this lesson about the complexity of causal relationships in mind, let us now examine in more detail some of the complex ways in which population change is

related to changes in health and to economic and social change.

Population change

The explosive growth in the human population of the world during the period we live in, shown in Figure 5.2, is one of the most dramatic facts of human existence.

Humans and their immediate ancestors have been on Earth for only about 2 million years. It took almost this long for humankind to reach its first billion, around the year 1800. It took just 130 more years to add another billion, 30 years to add a third, and 15 years to add a fourth. By 1990 the world's population was well past 5 billion, by 2000 will be over 6 billion, and by 2025 is very likely to have reached 8 or 9 billion. Clearly such a radically unstable situation cannot continue for very long, but before looking to the future we must try to understand the past. As a starting point, let us look at population and disease in the pre-industrial world, and try to sketch briefly both the kinds of diseases that are likely to have afflicted our early ancestors, and how these might have changed as human society evolved through different stages of development.

Population and disease in the pre-industrial world

40 000 years ago, our human species had colonised most of the inhabitable area of the world. They were food-collectors rather than food-producers, who lived by hunting other animals and gathering foodstuffs such as fruit, seeds, nuts, roots and honey. The only way we can estimate the numbers of these **hunter-gatherers** is by calculating their food-collecting efficiency in relation to the maximum population sustainable by the environments in which they lived (sometimes referred to as the **carrying capacity** of the environment). On this basis, it is unlikely that there were more than two million of our human ancestors at this time.

The causes of illness and rates of death among these human ancestors are largely a matter of speculation. They would have been subject to mites, fleas, ticks and worms, and invaded by viruses, bacteria, fungi and parasites, although the practice of cooking meat (developed early in human evolution) gave humans a unique degree of protection from food-borne diseases. Through their development and mastery of hunting skills, hunter-gatherers dominated the food chain, and this largely removed the threat of being preyed on by other species. However, it posed a new survival risk: slaughter by other humans. Additional stresses would have arisen regularly

[3]Very similar issues are raised in the discussion of scurvy in *Studying Health and Disease*, (Open University Press, 1985, revised edition 1994).

Population (millions)   **Year**

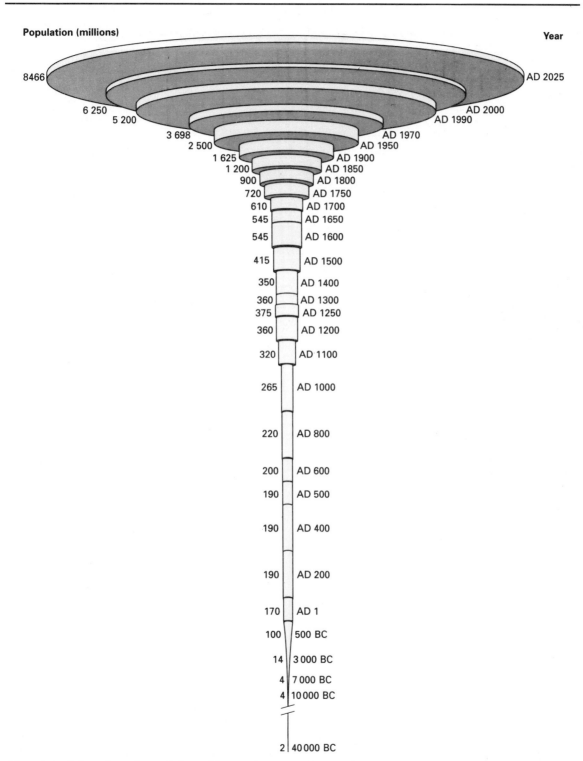

Figure 5.2 *Estimated population of the world. (Data from McEvedy, C. and Jones, R.,1978,* Atlas of World Population History, *Penguin, London, and United Nations, 1989,* World Population Prospects 1988, *Population Studies No. 106, UN, New York)*

from food shortages and from changes in climatic conditions, such as the advance and retreat of successive Ice Ages.

In so far as any species can be said to be in equilibrium with its environment, these human societies were close to stability, both in numbers and in age structure. An An important element in this stability was likely to have been population control, probably by means of infanticide, abortion, sexual abstinence and protracted breast-feeding (which suppresses ovulation). This would have ensured that these societies did not press too hard against the carrying capacity of their environment, but had some safety margin which allowed them to cope with periods of scarcity, and to recover from periodic disease epidemics or famines.

However, underlying this apparent stability it appears that there was a very slow growth in total population size—perhaps 2 per cent per 1 000 years. By approximately 10 000 BC, human numbers may have doubled to around 4 or 5 million. Over the same period a number of major meat sources, such as mammoths and mastodons, were hunted to extinction. Perhaps both the rising human population and its impact on other species are evidence of a kind of human adaptability and skill. But as the last Ice Age retreated around this time, it seems that growing human numbers, the disappearance of some food sources, and unusually large climatic variations may well have combined to create a slow collision between human populations and their resource base. These were the conditions in which an entirely new phase of human history unfolded, as humanity switched from food collecting to food production, and hunting and gathering gave way to the cultivation of crops and the domestication of animals: the first Agricultural Revolution.

The first Agricultural Revolution

The switch from food collecting to food production surged forward from around 8000 BC. This is sometimes referred to as the **Neolithic** period, the last phase of the Stone Age. It was based on the domestication and cultivation of a wide range of plants—cereals such as maize, rice, millet and wheat; roots and tubers such as potatoes and yams; pulses and fruits—and the parallel domestication of many animal species, including sheep, cattle, goats, pigs, camels and chickens. This process was remarkably widespread, and may have commenced independently in a number of regions: the prevailing view at present is that it centred on China, India, the Near East and Central America, from where it advanced into most other regions of the world. As it spread, hunting and gathering was displaced.

This **first Agricultural Revolution** transformed the social organisation of humans. Small, wandering groups who rarely came into contact with one another were replaced by much larger, settled communities in most (though not all) parts of the world. There was a greatly increased division of labour and specialisation of tasks. This has been regarded by some commentators as the most significant change humans have ever experienced:

> Of the 50,000 odd generations in the last million years of history, only about 400 have occurred since agriculture was first adopted by one part of the human population. With agriculture came dramatic changes in diet, population density and patterns of daily life, and the human organism was exposed to stresses that were, in evolutionary terms, novel. It is unlikely that there has been major biological change in man since the Neolithic revolution. Such change is highly improbable with respect to the more recent adoption of urban and advanced industrial patterns of life. (Powles, 1973, p. 4)

The Agricultural Revolution made it possible to produce more food, which in turn allowed a substantial increase in population. From an estimated 4–5 million humans in the world at the beginning of the Agricultural Revolution, numbers increased to perhaps 170 million by the birth of Christ. As regards human disease, the Agricultural Revolution is likely to have led to the rise of infectious diseases as the main cause of illness and death.

☐ Why should infections have assumed such importance as a consequence of the social changes of the Agricultural Revolution?

■ The most important effect was the increase in both the total population size and the size of local groups living in close personal contact.

Many infections require a minimum size of human population if they are to be maintained. Whereas some diseases depend on an animal host (e.g. rats in the case of plague), others, such as measles, are specific to humans. It has been suggested that measles requires a population of about one million to be maintained as an endemic (always present) infection.

Other less important reasons include more numerous intruders such as rats and mice into human habitations, attracted by the stored food that food production necessarily entails. In addition, the switch from the often highly varied diet of the hunter-gatherers to the mono-diets of the early agriculturalists may have had severe health consequences. The American physiologist Jared Diamond, summarising the recent research findings of paleopathology (the science of identifying disease in remains of ancient peoples), has noted that in Greece and Turkey 'the average height of hunter-gatherers...towards the end of the Ice Age was a generous 5 foot 10 inches for men, 5 foot 6 inches for women. With the adoption of agriculture, height crashed, reaching by 4000 BC a low value of only 5 foot 3 inches for men, 5 foot 1 inch for women. By classical times, heights were very slowly on the rise again, but modern Greeks and Turks have still not regained the heights of their healthy hunter-gatherer ancestors.' (Diamond, 1991, p. 168)

Thus, though the Agricultural Revolution may have diminished the risk of death from starvation, predation and possibly violence, it led to an increased risk of infections and other diseases. Infections were to remain the predominant threat to human survival for almost 10 000 years (and in many parts of the world are still the leading cause of death and disease). It is impossible to know what the mortality would have been during this period: life expectancy at birth may have been barely 25 years, but may have been substantially greater for those who survived infancy.

Scarcity or plenty

These stages of development in human society—from hunter-gatherers to agriculturalists—are of course crude approximations to what was a long, complex and still poorly understood series of changes. However, it seems clear beyond reasonable doubt that major shifts in the experience of health and disease attended these changes. A second point to note is less obvious but equally important: each stage of development was characterised by a particular way of obtaining the means of subsistence, and it was the *balance* between that means of subsistence and the number of people it had to sustain which dictated whether there would be scarcity or plenty. To illustrate the relative nature of these concepts, let us examine the traditional view anthropologists once took of hunter-gatherer societies: that they were characterised by permanent scarcity, meagre resources, hand-to-mouth subsistence, and a life of continual struggle for survival. This seems to be remarkably similar to the famous description of life without social organisation suggested by Thomas Hobbes, the seventeenth-century social theorist, as 'solitary, poor, nasty, brutish and short'.

However, as evidence has accumulated on surviving hunter-gatherer societies, it has become increasingly difficult to reconcile these views with their irregular and not prolonged hours of labour, the amount of time spent dozing, chatting, playing games or engaged in ceremonies, and the generally low esteem in which many material possessions were held. Among the !Kung Bush-people of the Kalahari, for example, researchers found that there seemed to be little or no material pressure in life, and possession of objects conferred no status on individuals. Similarly, among Australian natives in Arnhem Land, work was intermittent and averaged around four hours a day, and dietary intake was more than adequate.

One possible explanation for this anomaly is that anthropologists began with inappropriate assumptions. Their point of reference was their own industrial societies, where material wants and desires are great. But supposing human material wants were limited, and the technical means to meet them were unchanging but broadly adequate: in these circumstances, it would be possible to have a 'low' standard of living but enjoy material plenty.

This hypothesis, and evidence to support it, come from the work of the American anthropologist Marshall Sahlins, who has gathered together a great deal of information on hunter-gatherer societies and economies. The emergence of modern societies, he argues, has created new relationships between members of society, one feature of which is the existence of poverty:

> One third to one half of humanity are said to go to bed hungry every night. In the Old Stone Age the fraction must have been much smaller. This is the era of hunger unprecedented. Now, in the time of the greatest technical power, starvation is an institution.... This paradox is my whole point. Hunters and gatherers have by force of circumstances an objectively low standard of living. But...all the people's material wants usually can be easily satisfied. The world's most primitive people have few possessions, but they are not poor. Poverty is not a certain small amount of goods, nor is it just a relation between means and ends; above all, it is a relation between people. Poverty is a social status. As such it is the invention of civilisation. (Sahlins, 1974, pp. 36–7)

On this view, the Agricultural Revolution depended on a much higher degree of social order than previously existed, and the emergence of social hierarchies or strata inevitably produced inequality, wealth and poverty. The existence of social class, or stratification, or hierarchy, is one of the most important aspects of health and disease patterns. But the essential point here is that this is not unique to industrialised societies. In fact, it seems that every society that produces more than is immediately consumed, that can accumulate a surplus of food or other wealth, inevitably confronts the question of how that surplus should be used. Out of this develops conflict, and such conflicts are resolved within a hierarchical structure in which power is exercised. The emergence of poverty as an 'invention of civilisation' is therefore one feature of the power relationships between different groups in a hierarchical structure.

Returning briefly to the human population of the world, it seems that growth slowed down during the early Christian era, as the Agricultural Revolution reached the limits of easily cultivable land. From AD 200 to 500, population may have been virtually static. Then another cycle of growth commenced, as a medieval economy emerged bringing new technologies of farming, new towns and settlements, and the clearance of large areas of forest. By 1200 world population may have reached 360 million. But again growth faltered as medieval society appeared to reach some limit of expansion and was stricken in Europe by plague and in Asia by Mongol attack. Not until 1500 did the upward path of population resume, accelerating after 1800 as the Industrial Revolution took hold.

Over this great sweep of time, therefore, we can see in faint outline the links between population size, disease, and the food supply or more generally the economic base. Historians and paleo-anthropologists face great difficulties in attempting to assess the degree to which food supplies may have affected the health of populations in the past. No one questions that there must be some connection: if a population is constant in size, or nearly so over a long period, there must be sufficient food to sustain it at that level. Equally, if numbers are continuously growing, food supply must be continuously expanding. The controversy is about the nature of the mechanism that holds the balance between the two.

Balancing population and resources

Many people have tried to understand and explain the nature of the links between population and resources, but one of the most influential was Thomas Malthus. Let us now see what light his work casts on the pre-industrial world.

The Malthusian model

The Reverend Thomas Malthus was born near Dorking in Surrey in 1766 and died in 1834. As you will see, the lifetime of 'Population Malthus' (as he was caricatured) covered a key period of history. Like that of Machiavelli, the first great modern political theorist, the name of Malthus has acquired a patina of unpleasantness. It is not always clear whether this is because he has been regarded as having made observations which were

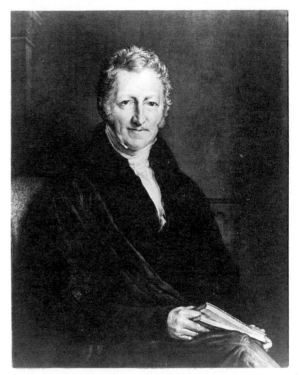

Thomas Malthus, 1766–1834, painted by J. Linnel. (Source: The Mansell Collection)

untrue, or simply unpleasant; certainly his work has at times been enlisted in unpleasant and repressive ideologies. In 1798 Malthus published the first edition of *An Essay on the Principles of Population*, which put forward the following views, which we can call the **Malthusian model**.

1   The survival and increase of a population is completely dependent upon the means of subsistence.

2   The 'passion between the sexes' is so strong and unalterable 'that population, when unchecked, goes on doubling itself every twenty-five years, or increases in a geometrical ratio'.

3   As a general rule, it is simply not possible for the means of subsistence to grow in the same geometrical ratio as population: 'Taking the population of the world at any number, a thousand millions, for instance, the human species would increase in a ratio of: 1, 2, 4, 8, 16, 32, 64, 128, 256, 512, etc., and subsistence as: 1, 2, 3, 4, 5, 6, 7, 8, 9, 10, etc. In two centuries and a quarter, the population would be to the means of subsistence as 512 to 10.' (Malthus, 1970 edition, pp. 25–26)

4   This disequilibrium is prevented from arising by a set of checks, producing 'misery or vice', which are unfortunately to be found 'in ample portion' in 'the cup of human life'. The main checks which he identified were starvation and the outbreak of epidemics of infectious diseases.

☐ What strikes you about the kind of checks on population increase that Malthus identified?

■ In this first essay on population Malthus concentrated on checks which increased *mortality* among the existing population, rather than checks on the number of births.

Malthus labelled these checks on the existing population as **positive checks on population growth**. At this stage, he barely considered the possibility of checks such as *coitus interruptus* and other forms of contraceptive practice which were known and practised, such as abortion, infanticide and—perhaps most important of all—the pattern of marriage. He later styled these as **preventive checks on population growth**.

How can **marriage patterns** influence the birth rate? In most societies childrearing outside marriage carries certain moral, social, legal or economic penalties, which are often strong enough to deter people from having children until they are married. It follows that (a) the proportion of the population who enter into marriage— referred to by demographers as **nuptiality**—and (b) the average age of marriage (which influences the potential childbearing years of women) are two key features of marriage patterns which can affect the birth rate. The importance of marriage patterns in the demographic history of England will be examined in Chapter 6.

Malthus initially failed to understand the importance of marriage patterns: he took a view similar to that of Dr Johnson: 'It is not from reason and prudence that people marry, but from inclination. A man is poor; he thinks, "I cannot be worse, and so I'll e'en take Peggy".' Later, however, Malthus grasped more fully the importance of marriage patterns and other preventive checks, which he put under the heading of 'moral restraint'.

The overall scheme of Malthus' ideas is shown in Figure 5.3.

Looking at this figure, you will see that there are two loops: the upper one deals with the positive checks on populations, and the lower one with the preventive checks.

The upper loop begins by showing a positive association between population size and food prices; that is, a rise in population size leads to a rise in food prices, a fall in population size to a fall in food prices.

The next part of the figure connects food prices and real wages. Rising food prices mean that the same amount of money buys less food, and so real wages fall. Conversely, if prices were to fall, real wages would rise; in other words, there is an *inverse* relationship between them.

As real wages fall so mortality starts to increase through starvation, malnutrition and disease. The rise in mortality is the final positive check on population size, cutting it back as 'nature wields her red pencil', and as the population size comes down so food prices start to fall, and so on.

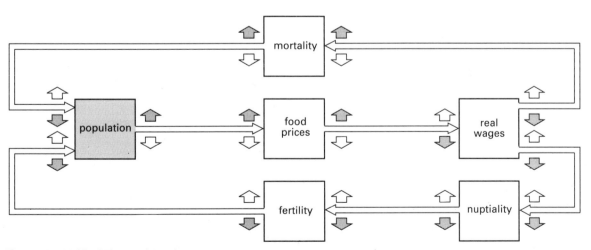

Figure 5.3 *Malthus' Theory of Population.*

Following the lower loop, the effect of a fall in real wages brought about by population increase is to lower the nuptiality rate and increase the average age of marriage: to paraphrase Dr Johnson, a man becomes poorer, realises things are worse, and postpones taking Peggy. As nuptiality falls, so fertility falls, and thus the population increase is thrown into reverse.

Inventiveness and self-regulation

Malthus was one of the first to suggest that 'positive checks' to the size of human populations might be imposed at some point by an upper limit to food production. In part, his argument was an attempt to counter contemporaries such as the anarchist philosopher William Godwin, who believed in the possibility of constant social progress and improvement. 'Man is perfectible, or in other words susceptible of perpetual improvement', Godwin asserted. Godwin railed against Malthus' insistence that the earth imposed limits on social development, stressing instead the almost boundless inventiveness and creativity of humans: in time, he contended, mankind would have the ability to produce its entire food supply from a solitary flowerpot.

More recently, ecologists and evolutionary biologists have developed another position, which modifies Malthus' view that the 'natural' sizes of populations are determined by the capacity of their environments to support them, and introduces the idea of **self-regulation**. The numbers of many small-bodied species such as insects and some small mammals and birds fluctuate continuously through phases of 'boom and bust', and the kind of 'positive checks' Malthus identified are strongly in evidence. However, ecologists have now identified many examples of physiological and/or behavioural mechanisms which provide a 'feedback' link, whereby the *current* density of a population influences the *subsequent* reproductive performance of individual members (**density-dependent reproduction**). The most common way this kind of **spacing behaviour** happens is through territoriality. Each individual or kinship-related group such as a troop of animals dominates a fixed area. Those unable to find and defend territory of their own are denied access to mates or to breeding sites, and are more vulnerable to predators. This results in populations that regulate themselves at levels which are always somewhat below the maximum that existing food supplies could sustain. Such populations tend to vary in size, more or less in parallel with food supplies, by adjusting the number of offspring in *anticipation* of future resources.

Whether humans have self-regulating characteristics which might have operated in the distant past is of course impossible to prove, since it would require detailed long-term studies of human groups living in an environment unmodified by the activities of modern people. However, as you saw earlier in this chapter, evidence collected from surviving groups of hunter-gatherers, and everything that is known about the way such groups lived in the past, suggests that they almost certainly exercised population control to keep their numbers somewhat below the carrying capacity of their environment and provide some safety margin for times of scarcity. Moreover, as ecologists Robert Moss and Adam Watson and zoologist John Ollason suggest in their book *Animal Population Dynamics* (1982), most larger-bodied animals—particularly those, like humans, with slow rates of reproduction and systems of co-operative social group organisation—have been shown either to self-regulate their numbers, or at least display characteristics which would produce density-dependent reproduction or other kinds of 'spacing' behaviour.

Stable characteristics such as these must have evolved over a long time-span, appearing first in one individual and, over many generations, spreading through the whole population. According to modern evolutionary theory, characteristics that become shared by every member of the population did so because they conferred some survival advantage on those individuals in which the characteristics had evolved. When there is competition for resources, **natural selection** of the best adapted individuals ensures that their genes (and hence their characteristics) are passed on to succeeding generations. A characteristic that increases the chance of an individual surviving long enough to reproduce, and for its offspring to reproduce in their turn, is said to increase the individual's reproductive success or **fitness**. But, to return to the theme of biological checks on population growth, spacing behaviour is a characteristic that *reduces* the chance of reproduction.

At first sight it is difficult to understand how evolution could result in characteristics that cause an individual animal to forgo (either consciously, or involuntarily) some part of its own reproductive success in order to promote the fitness of others. This looks like an example of purely altruistic behaviour which (other than that between parents and offspring) could not be expected to evolve, if the only thing which counts is competition for survival and transmission to future generations of sets of genes which are carried by individuals. But many species do display individual behaviour which, translated into human terms, would be described as apparently self-sacrificing. This either involves exposure to immediate risk from predators, or the acceptance of a seemingly reduced chance of procreation.

The clue to understanding this apparent paradox lies in the concept of **inclusive fitness.** In brief, our modern understanding of evolutionary processes suggests that the competition for survival and propagation of genes operates *between groups* of related individuals, as well as between the individuals who belong to these groups. Because, through kinship, they share among them some identical pieces of genetic information, individuals will display characteristics which promote the survival of that common information set, even at the cost of a threat to their own survival: hence inclusive fitness. As the animal behaviourist Richard Dawkins points out in his book *The Selfish Gene* (1976), what looks like a choice of altruistic behaviour by an animal, at the same time looks like an act of pure self-interest on the part of the genes which the animal carries in its cells.

On balance, it seems unlikely that humans would have been such a successful species in biological terms, unless they also displayed a capacity for self-regulation of numbers. As both human history and the study of other species shows, this strategy does not prevent the kind of famines which are the result of external or perhaps random processes, such as shifts of climatic zones, unusual sequences of bad weather, warfare with other groups of humans or invasions of territory by other species such as locusts. It does however prevent famines being repeatedly and regularly caused by population outstripping food supply. What is significant for this discussion of the general relationship between food and health is that it suggests that the prehistoric condition of humanity, although far from paradisiacal, should not be thought of as a more or less permanent state of near starvation. This is the point Sahlins also made in the discussion earlier in this chapter.

Evidence for the Malthusian model

How do these different views of Malthus, Godwinian optimists and evolutionary biologists compare with what we now know of population history around the time that Malthus was alive? In fact, there is evidence in support of all three positions but, putting qualifications temporarily to one side, it is Malthus' harsh picture of human existence in the centuries preceding 1800 that seems to be closest to the mark. Summarising the available evidence, the economic historian Carlo Cipolla gives the following assessment:

…any agricultural society…tends to adhere to a definite set of patterns in the structure and movements of birth- and death-rates. Crude birth-rates are very high throughout, ranging between 35 and 55 per thousand…. Death-rates are also very high, but normally lower than the birth-rates—ranging generally between 30 and 40 per thousand…. [But] death-rates show a remarkable tendency to recurrent, sudden dramatic peaks that reach levels as high as 150 or 300 or even 500 per thousand. On a few occasions these peaks coincided with wars. But much more frequently they were the result of epidemics and famines that wiped out a good part of the existing population…. The intensity and frequency of the peaks controlled the size of agricultural societies. (Cipolla, 1974 edn, pp. 85–7)

A more detailed picture is provided by the French historian, Fernand Braudel, in *The Structures of Everyday Life* (1981), which is the first volume of a monumental and richly referenced history of civilisation and capitalism from the fifteenth to the eighteenth century.

What characterised this period, writes Braudel, was 'a number of deaths roughly equivalent to the number of births; very high infant mortality; famine; chronic undernourishment; and formidable epidemics' (p. 91). It was a precarious battle for existence 'waged on at least two fronts; against the scarcity and inadequacy of the food supply…and against the many and insidious forms of disease that lay in wait' (p. 90). Famine was ever-present: in France, for example, there were '10 general famines during the tenth century; 26 in the eleventh; 2 in the twelfth; 4 in the fourteenth; 7 in the fifteenth; 13 in the sixteenth; 11 in the seventeenth and 16 in the eighteenth' (p. 74). In the 1696–7 famine in Finland a quarter or a third of the population perished. 'Things were far worse in Asia, China and India. Famines there seemed like the end of the world…. In 1555 and again in 1596, violent famine throughout north-west India resulted in scenes of cannibalism…' (p. 76), and on and on.

Moreover, 'famine was never an isolated event. Sooner or later it opened the door to epidemics'. Each fresh disaster, however, was followed by a reassertion of life, as the population bounced back: for example, when plague mowed down the population of Verona in 1637, '…the soldiers of the garrison, almost all French—many of whom had escaped the plague—married the widows and life gained the upper hand again' (p. 71). Rise and fall is the rhythm of population history and of 'standard of living', each cycle permeating the whole fabric of life: 'trees and wild animals overran fields that had once flourished. But soon the population again increased and had to win back the land taken over by animals and wild plants, clear the stones from the fields and pull up trees and shrubs' (p. 33). What evidence we have suggests that this rhythm stretched across the inhabited world, a procession of 'social massacres' and revivals that seems to confirm the Malthusian model.

However, underlying the increases and decreases was a faint but perceptible longer-term trend, where 'revival ultimately had the last word. The ebb never entirely removed what the preceding tide had brought in' (p. 92), and the population of the world slowly increased, as you saw earlier in this chapter. Second, although famines were widespread and sometimes frequent, they were none the less periodic events with some respite allowed in between. The fact that specific dates of violent famines in north-west India are recorded, for instance, could be interpreted as implying that chronic malnutrition and widespread starvation was not the continual norm there. Third, we know from the monuments and relics of the past, that, whatever relationship existed between the mass of population and the means of subsistence, sufficient surplus was provided by the economic system to invest in mammoth schemes of building, often on a scale that might impose severe strains on not only the Third World countries of today, but also on some industrialised countries.

There are so many gaps in our knowledge of the pre-industrial world that there is ample room for disagreement. We have seen one picture of the world as essentially a procession of 'social massacres', of sweeping epidemics, famines, and 'die-offs' as the population seemed to collide with the subsistence barrier in the way Malthus expected. On the other hand there is evidence, at least in parts of the world, that to be poor did not imply

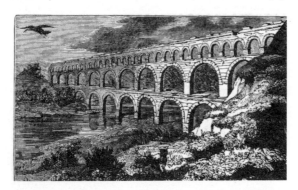

Subsistence or surplus? The Roman Pont du Gard aqueduct, Nimes, is typical of the massive building works that pre-industrial societies could produce. (Source: The Mansell Collection)

continual misery and uncertainty about where the next meal was to come from. What is certain is that, even as Malthus was writing, a decisive break with his scheme of things was about to occur, caused by the sequence of events and changes known as the 'Industrial Revolution'.

The Industrial Revolution

It is paradoxical that the first country in the world for which there is evidence that the Malthusian theory no longer applied was the same country in which the theory was formulated: eighteenth-century England. Here it seems that the population was not pressed hard against the basic means of subsistence, that bad harvests could be overcome without too much hardship or hunger, and that the population could slowly grow without causing real wages to slump. For example, one French traveller, the Abbé le Blanc, making his way from the south coast to London in 1747, was 'struck with the beauties of the country, the care taken to improve lands, the richness of the pastures, the numerous flocks that cover them, and the air of plenty and cleanliness that reigns in the smallest villages' (quoted in Hobsbawm, 1969, p. 11).

Figure 5.4 shows changes in the population of England from the sixteenth to the eighteenth century, and changes in real wages over the same period. Some of the problems involved in estimating population size have already been discussed. The problems of estimating the average value of wages over such a long period are in many ways even more difficult to solve. The real wage index for England from 1550 to 1900 shown in Figure 5.4 is based on the work of two researchers who, remarkably, managed to trace the wage rates of builders and the price of various foodstuffs back to the twelfth century! (Phelps Brown and Hopkins, 1956, reworked by Wrigley and Schofield, 1989).

☐ Look carefully at Figure 5.4. What are the main features of it that strike you as important? Does the figure fit the Malthusian model?

■ In the years up to 1600 we can see population increasing and real wages falling, a pattern that broadly fits in with the Malthusian theory. Around 1650 population growth is checked, while real wages are rising. Then from about 1700 to 1750 population starts rising again (and this growth accelerates after 1800). Meanwhile, real wages decline very slowly, but around 1800 they start rising also: a sustained and rapid increase in the population has not set off the system of checks Malthus predicted.

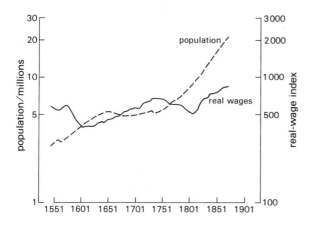

Figure 5.4 *Changes in population and real wages, England, 1550–1900. (Data from Wrigley, E. A. and Schofield, R. S., 1989,* The Population History of England 1541–1871: a Reconstruction, *Cambridge University Press, Cambridge, p. 408)*

England was the first country in the world to experience this pattern of development. This is why it is important to look closely at what happened in England before returning to a world view. The problem in explaining what happened is that it was a unique event, and cannot be repeated experimentally to increase knowledge of why— or even precisely how—it happened. The first key to understanding what was happening takes us back to Malthus and his geometrical versus arithmetical rates of growth of population and agriculture.

In eighteenth-century England agriculture was undergoing a whole series of changes which allowed it to expand at a rate that at least kept up with the increasing population. This expansion was made possible in part by new techniques such as crop rotation, stock-breeding, the famous seed-drilling machine invented by Jethro Tull, and improved drainage and fertilisers. New crops were also introduced: clover and hays (which provided winter feeds so that livestock could be fed over the winter months); root crops (such as carrots and parsnips from the Low Countries); and the potato, introduced in the sixteenth century from America by Walter Raleigh (and first domesticated in Andean America during the first Agricultural Revolution many thousands of years previously). There seems little doubt that the potato was the predominant influence on the growth of population in Ireland, and had a significant effect in Britain from about 1750. Finally, in the eighteenth century, the construction of canals in Britain is thought to have made a major contribution to improving the distribution of the increased amounts of food being produced, as did improvements in coast, river, and road transport.

But these changes in technique and technology were encouraged and widely adopted largely because of other social and economic upheavals which were also taking place. For example, common land was taken over and enclosed by a new class of private landowners and, although this resulted in the size of fields and of farms being rapidly expanded, it also meant that the peasant subsistence farming, which had been based on small plots of land, was completely disrupted and then painfully eliminated.

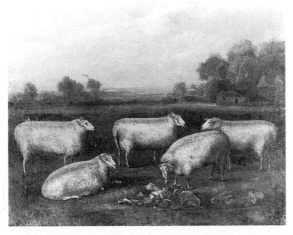
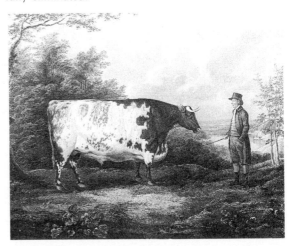

Eighteenth-century agricultural change in England: careful breeding produced improved farm livestock, such as these proudly displayed Leicester sheep and Durham shorthorn cattle. (Source: Institute of Agricultural History, Reading)

Thus Malthus' view that agricultural production could not increase at more than a slow, 'arithmetical' ratio of growth was made obsolete at the very time that he was developing his theory. Agricultural growth was fast enough to lift the check on population growth by facilitating both a reduction in mortality and allowing the birth rate to increase.

As we noted already, there is no agreement over why the Industrial Revolution commenced in the way, the place and the time that it did. Some theories have laid stress on factors such as climate. For example, it has been suggested that weather conditions in the eighteenth century provided a long series of good harvests in England, and that the surplus produced triggered off wider changes. This argument, however, does not explain why previous runs of good harvests did not produce similar changes. Other theories have focused on the values of the Protestant Reformation, arguing that Protestantism was ideally matched to the innovative and individualistic forces required to alter England's economic and social system. But again, this argument does not explain why Catholic Belgium was quicker to follow England's lead than Protestant Holland. The break-down of the Malthusian model, coupled with major agricultural and demographic changes, were simply part of a much bigger set of changes occurring in England at that time, and attributing such changes to a single factor such as climate or religion ignores the many circumstances and combinations of factors that were undoubtedly present.

So what do we mean by the **Industrial Revolution**? We commonly think of it in terms of a sudden increase in economic activity, and this is certainly part of it. The last quarter of the eighteenth century in England witnessed a boom in the construction of canals and roads, a flourishing of the cotton and textiles industries, a doubling of imports and exports, and a sudden increase in the size of towns such as Manchester.

However, to reach a definition of the Industrial Revolution that will help us to understand what was happening we must think not simply in terms of *quantitative* change, of an increase in the amount of economic activity. As the prominent English economic historian Eric Hobsbawm points out, the important point to grasp is that the Industrial Revolution was '…not merely an acceleration of economic growth, but an acceleration of growth because of, and through, economic and social transformation', culminating in '…self-sustained economic growth by means of perpetual technological revolution and social transformation' (Hobsbawm, 1969, p. 20).

This concept of **social transformation**, or changes in the social structures that regulated human life, is the cornerstone of the process of development and social change. This process dramatically altered the everyday life of the population of England, and also altered the nature of the relationship between newly industrialised countries such as England and the rest of the world, with profound consequences for patterns of health and disease.

One example of the changes in social structures occurring during the process of industrialisation in England involved the use of land and of agricultural labour. At the beginning of the eighteenth century, at least half of the agricultural land in Britain was farmed on an open-field system. This system gave equal shares of good and bad land to each farmer in a community, with no physical barrier between the farmed strips, and with each farmer's cattle grazing together on common pasture. 'The system', writes the economic historian Michael Flinn, 'originating almost a thousand years before, was devised to ensure livelihoods for all members of the communities. In protecting the weak, it inevitably hampered the strong and enterprising.' (Flinn, 1965, p. 170). Weeds spread easily, as did cattle disease, and there were few incentives to improve or innovate.

During the second half of the eighteenth century, however, the need to feed England's rapidly rising population placed farmers under intense pressure to expand production, and this open-field system was pushed aside by Acts of Parliament and commercial pressure. The land was enclosed into compact areas of fenced land, and customs of access and use were renounced. In the 34 years up to 1760, a mere 70 000 acres were enclosed, but between 1760 and 1792 the total jumped by half a million, and by 1812 had increased by a further million acres. In consequence, a large number of people no longer had any direct access to the produce of the land, their means of subsistence was cut away, and many became destitute paupers.

It would be impossible to put any figure on the mortality or morbidity that may have resulted from this dislocation, but it is quite plausible to argue that, from being poor but relatively comfortable, large numbers of people became poor and frequently desperate about getting enough to eat. In 25 of the 37 years from 1811 to 1848, for example, the agricultural areas of England witnessed widespread rioting and disorder, and their plight is summed up in the words of a rioter from the Fens in 1816: 'Here I am between Earth and Sky, so help me God. I would sooner lose my life than go home as I am. Bread I want and bread I will have.' (quoted in Hobsbawm, 1969, p. 74).

Accompanying these changes in land ownership and land use, an entirely different kind of labour force was created. In modern industrialised countries such as

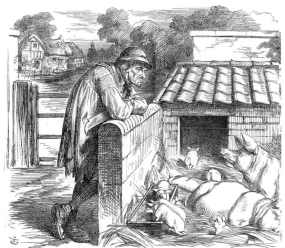

THE PIG AND THE PEASANT.
PEASANT. "AH! I'D LIKE TO BE CARED VOR HALF AS WELL AS THEE BE!"

According to this Punch *cartoon, agricultural destitution was still an issue in the 1860s.* (Punch, 19 September 1863)

Britain, the great majority of people make a living for themselves and their dependants by obtaining work from an employer in return for a wage or salary. Such paid employment normally takes place separated from home- and family in offices or factories where quite large numbers of people work. In pre-industrial England the contrast is striking. Although wage-labour was not uncommon—even in the sixteenth century perhaps two-thirds of all households earned some part of their living from wages—nevertheless, far fewer households were dependent on wages for all of their living all of the time. Instead, they worked the land tied to the home and exchanged the produce for other necessities. And in the home they carried out 'industrial' activities such as spinning or weaving.

Because agricultural work is seasonal, large numbers of people would have spent part of the year looking for other forms of employment, and some would fail to find any and become beggars. But, as the British historian Peter Laslett has observed:

> the trouble then…was not so much unemployment, as under-employment, as it is now called…the comparison is with the countries of Asia in our own century. Too many members of a family were half-busied about an inadequate plot of infertile land; not enough work could be found for the women and children to do around the cottage fire, in some districts none at all, for there was no rural industry in them. (Laslett, 1971, p. 33)

□ What similarities strike you between this description of pre-industrial England and the case study of village life in Bangladesh in Chapter 4?

■ Temporary migration to casual labouring jobs, pavement-dwelling in cities and short-term unskilled employment are features of life for the rural population in Bangladesh and for pre-industrial England.

During the Industrial Revolution in England, therefore, another change in social structures was the transformation of the work-force into much larger groupings of employees dependent on wages. Without this transformation, it would not have been possible to organise production in factories and the industrial towns they gave rise to, or to increase the specialisation of tasks and the division of labour, or to practice the rapid hiring and firing of labour that accompanied technical innovation. A mass of labouring people was created, depending for their livelihood on selling their labour. Only this wage relationship stood between the labourer and destitution, and if jobs were scarce destitution was rife. Even with a job, there was no guarantee that the wage the employer chose to pay would adequately sustain the labourer.

These changes in the position of land and labour would not have been possible without a series of even more profound and subtle social transformations. An economy based on commodity exchange and markets can only operate with the use of money, and the role of money had been increasing in English society since at least the Tudor period. Shakespeare frequently mentions the growth in the importance of money, and in *Timon of Athens* he was scathing about the 'common whore of mankind, that putt'st odds among the rout of nations…. Thus much of this will make black, white; foul, fair; wrong, right; base, noble; old, young; coward, valiant…. This yellow slave will knit and break religions'. (IV. iii. 28–44)

A final example of the changed social structures that occurred during the Industrial Revolution is provided by the historian Edward Thompson in a study of changing perceptions of time. Thompson begins by noting the way in which clock time was irrelevant and disregarded in any pre-industrial fishing, crafting or farming community, '…whose framework of marketing and administration is minimal, and in which the day's tasks (which might vary from fishing to farming, building, mending of nets, thatching, making a cradle or a coffin) seem to disclose themselves, by the logic of need, before the crofter's eyes.' He perfectly illustrates his point with an observation made by the Irish writer J. M. Synge on a visit to the Aran Islands, off the coast of County Clare:

The general knowledge of time on the island depends, curiously enough, upon the direction of the wind. Nearly all the cottages are built…with two doors opposite each other, the more sheltered of which lies open all day to give light to the interior. If the wind is northerly the south door is opened, and the shadow of the door-post moving across the kitchen floor indicates the hour; as soon, however, as the wind changes to the south the other door is opened, and the people, who never think of putting up a primitive dial, are at a loss…. When the wind is from the north the old woman manages my meals with fair regularity; but on the other days she often makes my tea at three o'clock instead of six. (Quoted in Thompson, 1967, p. 59)

Clearly, such nature-dependent rhythms of life and work were incompatible with the operation of a large factory using powered machinery and employing several hundred workers, or with the running of a railway network or school. And so the Industrial Revolution witnessed a complete restructuring of the whole rhythm of life, with clocks and bells, timetables and schedules, set times for eating, sleeping, working and resting, and a sharp distinction between work and the rest of life.

In short, the whole process of industrial development meant much more than a growth in the national product: the kinds of processes outlined above make it clear that development cannot be seen as simply a quantitative increase in economic activity brought about by technological changes. Development did eventually bring massive improvements in health to England, which will be looked at in much more detail in Chapter 6 of this book. But these were only one facet of a complete social, political, cultural and economic upheaval, which caused massive social dislocation, which did not happen overnight, and which was accompanied for a long period by great hardship and misery among the rural and especially the urban populations before general improvements in the standard of living and levels of health began to appear.

At the time, many people were horrified at the consequences of the Industrial Revolution in England. Some, like the Romantic poets, recoiled from it and wished to reject it completely. Others, like Charles Dickens and his illustrator, Paul Gustave Doré, devoted their lives to exposing its cruelties. And some, like the German social revolutionary Frederick Engels, condemned the conditions that the Industrial Revolution had created as part

RULES AND REGULATIONS
TO BE OBSERVED BY THE
WORKMEN
EMPLOYED BY
SAMUEL BASTOW,
CLIFF HOUSE IRON WORKS.

I.
The Engagement of each Workman shall be subject to a Fortnight's Notice, such Notice to be given at the Office on the pay day only, except in Cases of Dismissal for misconduct.

II.
Each Workman to enter and leave Work by the Office Door, where he must put his Ticket in the Box in the Morning, and at each Meal-time, or he will not have any time allowed for such neglect, the Box being open Five Minutes for that purpose, previous to the time of commencing Work; and in the Morning Five Minutes after the time for commencing Work.

III.
Any Workman absenting himself from his Employment for a longer period than 2 Working Days, without leave, shall be held to have left his service, and dealt with accordingly.

IV.
Work to commence at 6 o'clock in the Morning, and to end at 6 o'clock at Night, except on Saturdays, when the Days Work shall end at 4 o'clock, and on the Pay Saturday at 2 o'clock, no Dinner hour being allowed.

V.
Meal Hours to be from 8 to ½ past 8 o'clock, for Breakfast; and 12 to 1 o'clock, for Dinner. No Dinner Hour being allowed on Pay Saturdays.

VI.
Time to be kept by the *Hour*.—10 Working Hours to be a day's work.

VII.
The Door shall be closed every Morning when the Bell Rings, at 6 o'clock; but, should any Workman over-sleep himself, he may be admitted at 10 minutes past 6 o'clock, forfeiting ½ an hour.

The new work disciplines of the Industrial Revolution: factory regulations in Hartlepool, 1857. (Source: R. Wood, from Shellard, P., 1970, Factory Life in 1774–1885, Evans Bros.)

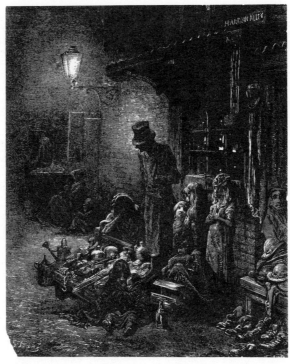

A London night scene by Gustav Doré, 1871. Doré's images have been a major influence on the twentieth century's view of the cruelties of the Industrial Revolution. (Source: The Mansell Collection)

of a critique of the whole social order. An extract from the book he published in 1845, *The Condition of the Working Class in England*, is included (as 'Health: 1844') in the Reader[4]. This extract examines the results of the Industrial Revolution in terms of the health of city dwellers, and you should now read it.

☐ In the statistics he quotes, Engels concentrates on two particular aspects of the pattern of health and disease: social class differences and differences between town and country. What findings does he make?

■ Engels notes that scarlet fever, rachitis (rickets) and scrofula were confined largely to the working classes, and did not seriously afflict the middle and upper classes. He also draws on evidence that the mortality rate in lower-class streets was up to twice as high as in upper-class streets. He then observes that the death rate in the industrial cities—at around one in thirty—was substantially higher than in rural districts, where it was around one in forty.

[4]*Health and Disease: A Reader*, (Open University Press, 1984; revised edition 1994).

☐ Within an historical perspective, what other dimension of health and disease patterns not considered in the extract would be of particular interest?

■ Perhaps the most important is some comparison of health and disease patterns around 1844 with patterns before the Industrial Revolution.

Intense controversy surrounds the question of the initial health consequences of the Industrial Revolution. This controversy is part of a wider dispute about trends in the standard of living of the population for, although it is plain that from the 1840s onwards average standards of living were definitely rising, the pattern before then is not at all clear. The fact that there is no obvious answer to this question suggests that there can have been very little if any general improvement for at least half a century.

But, whatever the short-term consequences of the Industrial Revolution in England, a giant break with the past had clearly occurred, involving among many other things health and disease patterns, populations and food. The next step, therefore, is to look in more detail at the impact of the Industrial Revolution on the health and the population of England.

OBJECTIVES FOR CHAPTER 5

When you have studied this chapter, you should be able to:

5.1   Summarise the available information on disease patterns in early human societies up to and including the first Agricultural Revolution.

5.2   Sketch the broad history of human population growth to the mid-nineteenth century.

5.3   Outline the Malthusian population model, and the alternative views of Godwinian optimists and evolutionary biologists. Then assess evidence from the pre-industrial world about the validity of these views of population change.

5.4   Outline the principal features of the Industrial Revolution in England, giving due emphasis to changes both in economic activity and social structures.

5.5   Describe the initial impact of the Industrial Revolution on the living conditions in English cities and among the rural peasantry.

QUESTIONS FOR CHAPTER 5

Question 1 (*Objective 5.1*)

We have almost no hard data on how disease patterns altered during the first Agricultural Revolution. Why is it possible to state fairly confidently that infectious diseases were a much bigger threat after this revolution than before?

Question 2 (*Objective 5.2*)

'Stability punctuated by sudden changes.' How accurate is this as a description of human population history in the eighteenth century?

Question 3 (*Objective 5.3*)

In the Malthusian population model, population and real wages are linked in two ways. Describe them briefly.

Question 4 (*Objective 5.4*)

In the eighteenth and nineteenth centuries, many public buildings in England began to display clocks, and there was a big expansion in the manufacture of cheap pocket watches. What does this tell you about changes in English society at the time?

Question 5 (*Objective 5.5*)

According to Engels, life in England's nineteenth-century cities was one of 'toil and wretchedness, rich in suffering and poor in enjoyment'. And yet many people were migrating to the cities from rural areas. How would you account for this?

6

The decline of infectious diseases: the case of England

During this chapter you will be asked to read two extracts contained in Health and Disease: A Reader[1]. *The first is 'The medical contribution' by Thomas McKeown, taken from his book* The Modern Rise of Populations. *The second is 'The importance of social intervention in Britain's mortality decline, c. 1850–1914: a reinterpretation of the role of public health' by Simon Szreter.*

The rise of industrial society sketched in the previous chapter has profoundly affected the world in which we live. This chapter looks in more detail at the effects of the Industrial Revolution on health. Focusing on just one country, England, the chapter surveys what is known of changes over time in disease patterns and demographic structure. England makes a good subject for this survey, because it had a pioneering role in the Industrial Revolution and has good records of disease and demography covering a relatively long period of time. (Scotland and Wales, which also made a pioneering contribution to industrial society, have population histories which are equally interesting and display many similar features, but which are less comprehensively documented and researched.) However, just as the introduction to the description of village life in Bangladesh (in Chapter 4) warned of the dangers of generalising from one case study, so the same applies in this chapter. Although England is, in many respects, a typical industrialised country, it is also in other ways unique, not least because it was the first industrial nation.

The chapter is divided into three sections. The first begins with the earliest available quantitative data on

[1]*Health and Disease: A Reader* (Open University Press, 1984; revised edition 1994).

population size—the Doomsday Book of 1086—and stops around 1680. All such historical 'book-marks' are a little artificial, but the reason for picking 1680 is that it is believed that at around this time the population size started to increase rapidly, considerably faster than during the preceding centuries. The end of the seventeenth century also marks the end of the second pandemic of plague (1666). The second section of the chapter continues from 1680 to 1850, around which date accurate and reliable information on cause of death became widely available. The final section deals with the period from 1850 to the present.

Infection, famine and mortality crises, 1086–1680

The period from the first agricultural communities to the end of the seventeenth century is significant for the consistency rather than the changes in the pattern of diseases that affected humans. Despite the passage of about 8 000 years, the main threats to health remained infectious diseases and food shortages. These two, together with violence, both accidental and deliberate (such as warfare), accounted for almost all deaths. Their relative contribution and demographic impact are our main concern when considering this period. Much of our knowledge is speculative, based on a variety of different sources: from archaeology, diaries, chronicles and other texts, parish registers of births and deaths since the sixteenth century, and Bills of Mortality from the following century. Most of the information on disease tends to be limited to records of mortality: the ages at which people died; the numbers dying at a particular time; and the causes of their deaths. This is a problem you have already encountered in earlier chapters, that our picture of the spectrum of disease is biased towards the more lethal diseases. In addition, because of the limitations of epidemiological information on mental illness, throughout this chapter the emphasis will be on physical (often termed 'somatic') illness.

Population 1086–1680

England is especially interesting to students of historical demography because records of its population are so detailed: parish registers of births, marriages and deaths were introduced in 1538, and form a set of records that begins earlier and is wider in coverage than in any other country. Estimates of population before this date are much less reliable, although sources such as the Dooms-day Book of 1086 and the poll-tax returns of 1377 are very useful. From figures recorded in the Doomsday Book, the population of England has been estimated as numbering about 1.75 million in 1086, and that is taken as the starting point for Figure 6.1, which shows estimates of changes in the size of the population of England from 1100 to 1820.

□ Consider Figure 6.1 and describe the features of population change during the years (a) 1100–1348, (b) 1348–1480, (c) 1480–1620, and (d) 1620–1700.

■ You should have noted that: (a) from 1100 to 1348 the population appears to have trebled in size; (b) from 1348 to 1480 there was an overall decline in size, including a possible 50 per cent reduction between about 1348 and 1375; (c) from 1480 to 1620 there was a rapid expansion of population; and (d) that 1620–1700 was a period in which popu-lation expansion came almost to a halt.

Though the population figures shown in Figure 6.1 prob-ably represent the current view of most historians, it should be noted that some estimates of the population during the fourteenth century before the Black Death caused the collapse shown in (b) above range as high as 5 to 7 million.

Figure 6.2 shows some other aspects of English population during the period from 1541 right up to the present: the crude birth and death rates and the average annual rate of growth averaged over each decade. From 1541 to 1871 these data are based on estimates from a detailed analysis of many thousands of parish registers, a vast project from which the historians E. A. Wrigley and R. S. Schofield have reconstructed the history of England's population since 1541.

The figure shows that over the period 1541 to about 1631 the birth rate generally exceeded the death rate by a substantial margin, so the rate of population growth was fairly rapid: around 1 per cent per annum on average. But from 1641 to around 1741 birth and death rate are almost in line, so that population growth almost comes to a halt and for a period is reversed.

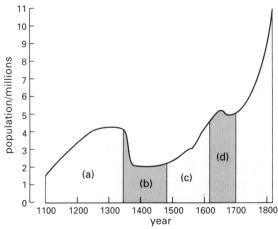

Figure 6.1 *Population of England 1100–1820. (Data for 1100–1540 from Chambers, I. D., 1972, Population, Economy and Society in Pre-Industrial England, Oxford University Press, Oxford, Figure 1; for 1540–1820 from Wrigley, E. A. and Schofield, R. S., 1989, The Population History of England 1541–1871: a Reconstruction, Cambridge University Press, Cambridge, Table A3.1)*

□ What other feature of the birth and death rates in Figure 6.2 strikes you?

■ They seem to be constantly fluctuating from one decade to another.

These fluctuations become even more marked when annual rates are considered, and the reasons for these fluctuations, especially in the death rate, have attracted a great deal of interest. Let us now look in more detail at these mortality crises.

Mortality crises: frequency and cause

Mortality crises are events where there is a sudden increase in the mortality rate for a fairly short duration. The definition adopted by Wrigley and Schofield is any year in which the crude death rate was at least 10 per cent above the average for the 25 years around that date.

Using this definition, Wrigley and Schofield ident-ified 31 years between 1541 and 1701 in which a mor-tality crisis occurred in England, or roughly once every 5 years. After 1701 the frequency of such crises fell to once every 13 years on average, although they could be equally severe when they did occur.

□ What limitations of the definition of mortality crises used above can you think of?

■ Because it is annual, this definition may miss sudden surges in mortality that last only a month or two. And because it is national it may miss local mortality crises.

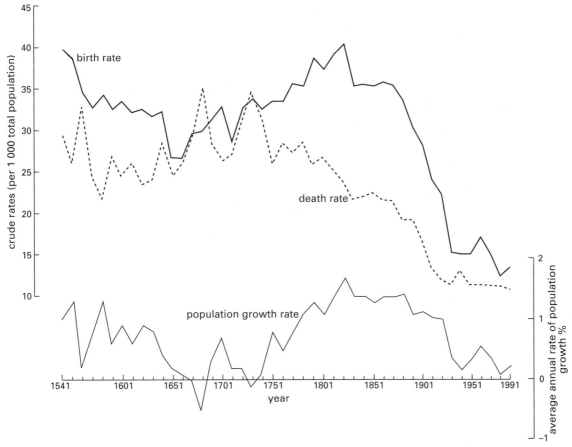

Figure 6.2 *Crude birth rate, crude death rate and average annual rate of population growth, England 1541–1991. (Data up to 1871 from Wrigley, E. A. and Schofield, R. S., 1989,* The Population History of England 1541–1871: a Reconstruction, *Cambridge University Press, Cambridge, Table A3.1; from 1871 Registrar-General, various years,* Annual Abstract of Statistics, *HMSO, London)*

Using monthly mortality rates from hundreds of parishes, Wrigley and Schofield have been able to throw some light on these *local* mortality crises. They found that in every year around 2 or 3 per cent of all parishes experienced a mortality crisis, but that in years of *national* crisis this rose to 15 or 20 per cent. However, even in the very worst national crises no more than 40 per cent of parishes were involved. On average a parish might be affected by a mortality crisis six times every century. It would last on average for just over two months, and during it there would be five times the usual number of deaths. Some parishes appeared to be more prone to these crises than others, but less than 1 per cent managed to avoid them completely. Crises were more likely in parishes with a large population, and less likely in parishes that were remote from market towns.

An obvious question posed by these crises is: what caused them? One useful piece of evidence would be to discover whether specific diseases were responsible, and if so, which particular diseases. However, death certificates were not introduced until the nineteenth century, and parish registers seldom entered a cause of death. Therefore, discovering the diseases responsible requires a study of the demographic features of each crisis: the seasonal pattern of deaths, the ages and social background of the victims, the duration of the crisis or the size of the geographical area affected. For example, diarrhoeal diseases such as dysentery are most likely to occur in late summer and early autumn. A crisis that spreads rapidly and widely suggests an airborne infection such as influenza. Deaths of more adults than children would suggest typhus, whereas deaths occurring only among children suggest a smallpox epidemic in an area where smallpox was endemic (i.e. adults would have built up some resistance to the disease).

However, knowledge of the main causes of death from disease during a mortality crisis goes only part way to answering the question of what caused the mortality crisis in the first place: in particular, in trying to establish whether it was related to a shortage of food or a fall in real wages, or simply resulted from an infectious disease that reached epidemic proportions and then died down. The occurrence of mortality crises at times of adequate food supplies would lend support to the notion of **autonomous infectious epidemics** (sometimes called **exogenous epidemics**). By this is meant an infectious disease that strikes down large numbers of people *independently* of other factors internal to that society that render the population more vulnerable or trigger the epidemic. By contrast, **endogenous epidemics** are related to social factors such as famine, warfare or **crises of subsistence** (a collapse of the ability to procure food and shelter).

☐ What evidence on the social backgrounds of the victims of a mortality crisis would suggest autonomous infections as the cause of a mortality crisis, rather than (say) a shortage of food?

■ Deaths occurring in all social sections of the population and not just the poorest and weakest would point to an autonomous infectious epidemic, such as the plague.

In a few cases it is not possible to distinguish autonomous infection from food shortage as being primarily responsible: sometimes they simply coincided—a likely event given the frequency with which they both occurred; or a crisis of subsistence may have stoked an existing outbreak of an infectious disease, particularly if famine and starvation caused an increased number of people to move from rural to urban areas, thus favouring the spread of an infection. Similarly, if the population was weakened by an epidemic infection, this could lead to, or at least exacerbate, a failure to produce sufficient food. However, in most cases it appears that mortality crises were not related to harvest failures or more generally to falling real wages, but were indeed due to autonomous infectious epidemics. It has also been estimated that the mortality rate in a crisis resulting from a lack of food tended to be about three to four times the 'normal' rate, whereas that resulting from an infectious disease outbreak was up to a twelve-fold increase.

The 'Golden Age of Bacteria'

Infectious diseases are caused by micro-organisms such as bacteria and viruses. Although information is limited, we do know something about those diseases responsible for the epidemics during the five or six hundred years up to 1680; about earlier times, however, we can only speculate. One of the most dramatic causes of mortality was plague. Although many recorded cases attributed to plague were almost certainly not due to infection with the plague bacterium (*Yersinia pestis*), this organism *was* responsible for many of the most devastating mortality crises between 1348 and 1666 in Britain.

The first hundred years of that period (1348–1448) is sometimes referred to as the '**Golden Age of Bacteria**' in recognition of the repeated infectious epidemics that held back any growth in population. It should, however, be noted that not all such infections were caused by bacteria—some (such as smallpox) were the result of viruses. Between 1348 and 1375 the population may have been reduced by half, as successive local epidemics occurred. Apart from plague, the other main causes are thought to have been smallpox, typhus and dysentery. There is considerable difficulty in recognising the true nature of past epidemics. Moreover, despite high death rates associated with epidemic infections such as plague, they may have had less effect on the general level of mortality than the constantly high death rate from endemic infections, such as tuberculosis. Unfortunately, the steady, unchanging impact of endemic infections makes accurate quantitative assessment of their contribution to mortality rates in the past impossible.

The pattern of infectious diseases was not static in pre-industrial Europe: plague appeared suddenly in 1348 and disappeared just as suddenly in 1666. Another example is leprosy, a disease which affects particularly the skin and nerves, and which, without treatment, can destroy nerves, thus leading to gross deformities. Leprosy appears to have been prevalent throughout Europe and the Mediterranean for many centuries, with around 19 000 leprosaria (institutions for sufferers of leprosy) in existence in 1300. However, the arrival of plague in Europe was associated with a massive decline in the number of lepers, an association that so far lacks any widely accepted explanation.

One important feature of historical research is that, although the events themselves may be long over, information and theories about them are constantly changing. For example, interpretations of historical outbreaks of disease have been updated in recent years by a greater understanding of the ability of micro-organisms to change their characteristics and hence the pattern of

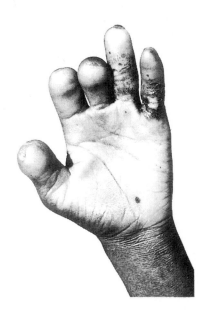

A hand badly deformed by leprosy. Its decline in Europe remains something of a mystery but it is still a health problem in many Third World countries. (Source: C. J. Webb, London School of Hygiene and Tropical Medicine)

disease that they cause. A good example of the ability of micro-organisms to adapt to changing circumstances is the causation of three diseases—*yaws, pinta* and *syphilis*—by the same bacterium in different circumstances. All three diseases are found in parts of West and Central Africa, Latin America and Asia, and are distinguished by the type and location of ulcerating skin lesions, the extent of damage to internal organs and the route of transmission. Yaws, pinta and so-called endemic syphilis are transferred by any contact with open sores, whereas venereal syphilis is transferred by sexual contact. In warm climates and conditions of overcrowding and poverty, direct skin contact is so common that the bacteria most commonly multiply in the non-sexually transmitted diseases. But it is thought that the bacterium had to adapt to sexual transmission in the temperate climates of northern Europe and North America, because casual contact with the skin of an infected person is limited by clothing.

Another problem for the medical historian is that historical accounts of some illnesses have proved insufficient to identify them in terms of modern categories of disease. The best example of this is the 'English Sweat' or 'sweating sickness' which first struck in London in 1486, and then spread across England, without ever reaching Wales or Scotland. In 1529 it crossed to the Netherlands,

Germany and Switzerland, and by 1551 had disappeared from England completely, its true nature lost in the mysteries of time. From contemporary descriptions it was probably a disease caused by a virus (some historians have suggested it may have been an early form of influenza) that affected the heart and lungs, causing rheumatic pains, fits of shivering and profuse sweating. Victims were often dead within hours of its onset, though in demographic terms it rarely caused more than a doubling of the mortality rate, compared with ten- to twelve-fold increases during plague epidemics. The appearance given by contemporary records that the disease particularly struck the eminent and famous (unlike almost all other infections) probably reflects the chroniclers' interest and concern rather than its true social distribution.

Local patterns of disease

Only a few parish registers survive that are complete enough to indicate the pattern of mortality in a whole community, and we have no way of knowing if these are representative even of the part of the country they came from, much less of the country as a whole. One such example is for the parish of St Botolph without Aldgate in London for the years 1583–99. As the size of the population of the parish for this period is not known (the first census was not taken in England until 1801) it is neither possible to determine the *incidence* of deaths for specific ages and sexes, nor the mortality *rates* for specific diseases.

□ How could the number of deaths from a particular disease in 1583–99 be meaningfully compared with the number occurring in the present day?

■ One way in which this has been done is to compare the *percentages* of all deaths that were caused by the particular disease.

This is known as the *proportional mortality*, and was discussed in Chapter 3. Note that this measure does not express the risk of dying from the disease, only the proportion of all deaths caused by that particular disease. For example, the number of deaths occurring at different ages in the Parish of St Botolph in 1583–99 can be compared with similar data for England and Wales, and Zimbabwe, at present, and this is done in Figure 6.3 (overleaf).

□ What are the main differences between the mortality experiences in St Botolph at the end of the sixteenth century and England and Wales in 1990?

■ There was a much higher infant and childhood mortality, and a higher mortality in young adulthood

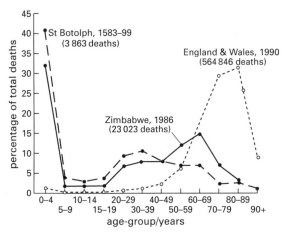

Figure 6.3 *Proportional mortality by age-group; St Botolph without Aldgate 1583–99, England and Wales, 1990 and Zimbabwe, 1986. (Data for St Botolph derived from Forbes, T. R., 1979, By what disease or casualty: the changing face of death in London, in Webster, C. (ed.) Health, Medicine and Mortality in the Sixteenth Century, Cambridge University Press, Cambridge, p. 124; England and Wales, 1990, derived from OPCS, 1991, Mortality Statistics: Cause 1990, OPCS Series DH2, No. 17, HMSO, London, Table 2; Zimbabwe, 1986, derived from United Nations, 1991, United Nations Demographic Yearbook 1989, UN, New York, Table 19)*

Table 6.1 Proportional mortality (per cent) from ten most common 'causes' of death, St Botolph's, 1583–99

plague	23.6
consumption convulsions }	22.2
(not stated)	14.1
pining, decline	13.2
ague, fever	6.1
flux, colic	2.5
smallpox	2.4
childbed	1.5
teeth	1.1

Data from Forbes, T. R. (1979) By what disease or casualty: the changing face of death in London, in Webster, C. (ed.) *Health, Medicine and Mortality in the Sixteenth Century*, Cambridge University Press, Cambridge, Table 2, p. 127.

during the earlier period. Over 40 per cent of all deaths occurred before the age of 5. In contrast, most deaths in England and Wales in 1990 occurred in people aged over 70 years—an age that few people reached in the sixteenth century.

☐ How does the pattern of mortality in St Botolph at the end of the sixteenth century compare with that in Zimbabwe in 1986?

■ In both cases there is a high proportion of deaths in infancy and childhood: 41 per cent in the sixteenth century, and 32 per cent in modern Zimbabwe. However, a proportionally much greater number of people in Zimbabwe than in the St Botolph records survive middle age and die after the age of 60.

Proportional mortality for the ten most common 'causes' of death in the parish of St Botolph is shown in Table 6.1.

These data once again raise an issue already encountered in this chapter: the problem of interpretation. Plague, for example (which the table indicates to be responsible for a higher proportion of deaths than any

other cause), was often used to denote any epidemic disease rather than specifically that caused by plague bacteria (*Yersinia pestis*). Similarly, consumption and convulsions could be confused because records often only state the abbreviation 'con', and finally the meaning of a term such as 'pining' is open to misinterpretation, though it is thought to refer to tuberculosis.

The notion of 'cause' has also altered since the sixteenth century. 'Infancy' was seen as sufficient explanation for dying (though the current use of 'cot death' could be viewed as a modern equivalent, in the sense that the underlying biological cause is unknown).

Although plague only occurred intermittently it was nevertheless responsible for almost a quarter of all deaths. The impact of plague epidemics at the end of the sixteenth century can be seen in the fluctuation in the annual number of burials at that time (Figure 6.4). No other disease caused such fearful loss of life in relatively short periods of time. In contrast, tuberculosis, a chronic infection (recorded as 'consumption' and 'pining'), showed no epidemic pattern.

Returning to Table 6.1, the dominance of infectious causes is striking, particularly when it is considered that the apparently non-infectious causes probably conceal an infectious basis. These include 'childbed' (maternal mortality) which led to the death of 23 women per 1 000 deliveries, and 'teeth' which denoted deaths in infancy. Of every 100 babies born in St Botolph's parish, about 30 died before their first birthday, a further 22 died in the next 4 years, and only about 30 survived to the age of 15.

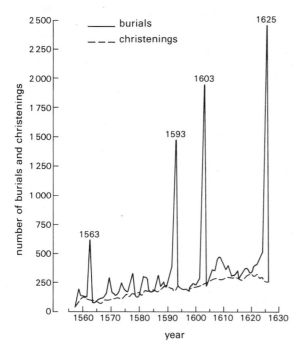

Figure 6.4 *St Botolph without Aldgate, burials and christenings 1558–1626. (Data from Forbes, T. R., 1979, By what disease or casualty: the changing face of death in London, in Webster, C. (ed.)* Health, Medicine and Mortality in the Sixteenth Century, *Cambridge University Press, Cambridge, p. 126)*

The difficulties of interpreting historical information on diseases are especially well illustrated by one of the few historical records from before 1680 that tell us about non-fatal diseases and conditions (i.e. morbidity): the diary kept by a country physician named Richard Napier, who lived and worked in the area approximating to modern Milton Keynes. His diary is not only a rich source of data on the prevalence of conditions but also on how people described their complaints. Uniquely in such diaries, Napier recorded his patients' own descriptions of their illnesses.

Two examples of consultations (from the many thousands he wrote) reveal both the ease and the difficulty of interpreting such data in modern terms. The first example is the case of Alice Billington of Fenny Stratford (see Figure 6.5 overleaf), 60 years old, who was seen by Napier on 10 June 1605 at 6.50 p.m.

> Hath complained of sickness at her hart this week this morning fell into a swoone and now lyes speechless.

This woman had probably suffered a stroke, and was prescribed 'cinamon water an ounce'. Contrast this with the case of Joane Nickson (also Figure 6.5) aged 38, of Wavendon. Seen earlier the same day, she complained of:

> A payne in her hart
> hath had worms of late
> yesterday voided some downwards
> had an Impostume brake upwards 9 yeeres since
> feares the like agayne
> had them last week
> her breath very strong.

The worms were probably roundworms (still common throughout the Third World today), but the nature of the 'Impostume' she fears (some sort of abscess) is not clear to us. We should of course remember that random scrutiny of the present-day records kept by a general practitioner could be equally puzzling!

☐ Before leaving Napier's diary, can you suggest what the strange diagrams in his records might represent? (Remember this was written in 1605 when medicine still contained many traditional beliefs.)

■ They are astrological charts. Napier used astrology to augment his clinical methods in deciding on a diagnosis and suitable treatment.

Unfortunately, few such records of morbidity before 1680 survive (or maybe ever existed).

You have seen that, despite the existence of historical data on mortality and population size that are better than for almost any other country, our understanding of the health and disease experience of pre-industrial society in England is still hampered by a lack of knowledge. However, our knowledge has deepened considerably in recent years. This suggests that lack of interest, as much as lack of data, has been a reason for our previous ignorance and doubts about the interaction of population, disease, and food. Peter Laslett, a contemporary historian who has done a great deal to assert the importance of such interactions, has summed up the position as follows:

> Why is it that we know so much about the building of the British Empire, the growth of Parliament, and its practices, the public and private lives of English kings, statesmen, generals, writers, thinkers and yet do not know whether all our ancestors had enough to eat?. . .

Why has almost nothing been done to discover how long those earlier Englishmen lived and how confident most of them would be of having any posterity at all? Not only do we not know the answers to these questions, until now we never seem to have bothered to ask them. (Laslett, 1971, p. 134)

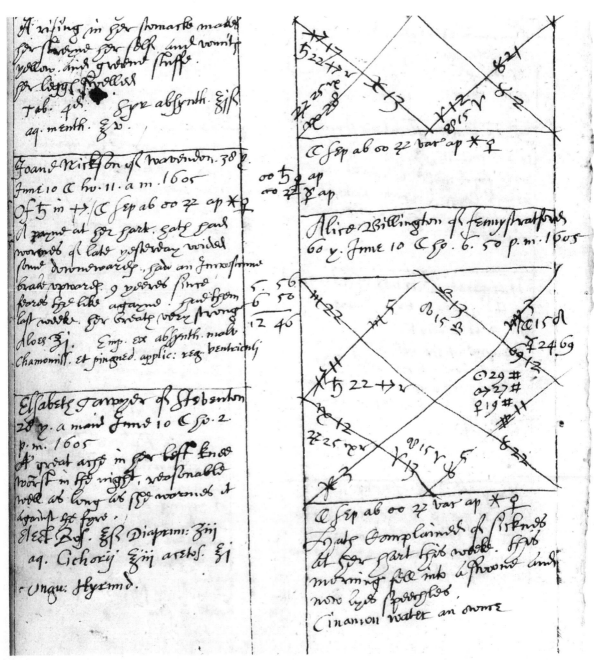

Figure 6.5 *Extracts from the diaries of Richard Napier, seventeenth-century physician (Bodleian Library, MS Ashmole 216, Folio 116')*

Disease and population, 1680–1850

The transition from the disease and mortality patterns of pre-industrial society in which infectious diseases and food shortages were the main causative factors, to the present pattern dominated by chronic non-infectious diseases (such as heart disease and cancers) took place over a period of about 250 years. This was accompanied by an unprecedented increase in the size of the population. As you have seen, the population of England in 1680 was around 5 million (Figure 6.1), and birth and death rates were roughly in balance. Over the following 170 years however, the population is estimated to have trebled to reach almost 17 million by 1851, and in the later part of this period the growth rate is thought to have been the highest in Europe. Whether this surge of growth was the result of a fall in mortality, a rise in fertility, or both, has been the subject of much debate.

Trends in fertility and mortality 1680–1850

Let us now return to Figure 6.2 and pick up the story of fertility and mortality trends in England between 1680 and 1850.

☐ Describe the main features of Figure 6.2 between about 1680 and 1850.

■ The crude birth rate increased throughout the eighteenth century, and reached a peak in the first half of the nineteenth century. The crude death rate moved erratically during most of the eighteenth century, showing no clear sign of a trend, but in the early nineteenth century appeared to begin a long but erratic decline.

Over the same period, the expectation of life at birth also fluctuated erratically, as Figure 6.6 shows, but started to rise at some point towards the end of the eighteenth century to reach almost 40 years by 1851.

☐ List as many factors as you can think of that could have contributed to the rise in the crude birth rate.

■ Some of the factors are:

(i) An increase in the proportion of women of childbearing age in the population.

(ii) Earlier age for marriage, leading to more pregnancies during a woman's reproductive life.

(iii) A greater proportion of women marrying and having children, that is, increased nuptiality.

(iv) Shorter intervals between successive pregnancies.

(v) Improvements in the health of women, leading to greater fecundity (reproductive capacity), earlier onset of menstruation (menarche), later menopause, and fewer stillbirths.

Investigation of parish registers and marriage documents have demonstrated that the rise in the birth rate during the eighteenth century was due primarily to changes in marriage patterns, in particular earlier and more universal marriage. Average age at first marriage in those parishes studied dropped from 26 to 23 years and the proportion of unmarried women fell from 15 to 7 per cent.

It appears, therefore, that the expansion in population between 1680 and 1850 resulted from both a rise in fertility and a decline in mortality. The birth and death

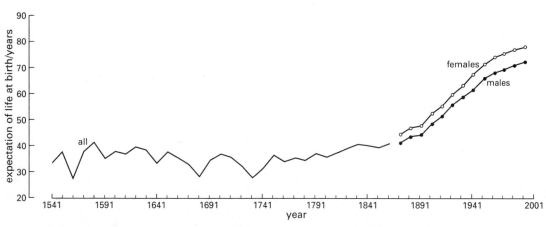

Figure 6.6 *Expectation of life at birth, England, 1541–1991. (Data up to 1871 from Wrigley, E. A. and Schofield, R. S., 1989,* The Population History of England 1541–1871: a Reconstruction, *Cambridge University Press, Cambridge, Table A3.1; from 1871, Registrar-General, various years,* Annual Abstract of Statistics *, HMSO, London)*

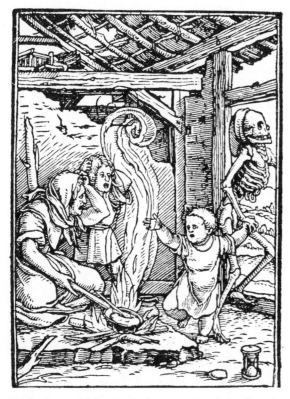

Death takes a child victim in this engraving, dating from the early eighteenth century. There is little evidence of a sustained decline in English death rates until the mid-eighteenth century. (Source: Royal Collection)

rates quoted above are of course crude rates that do not take into account the population's age structure, but once this has been done it can be calculated that the rise in the birth rate contributed two and a half times as much to the increase in population as did the decline in the death rate.

Explaining fertility and mortality changes, 1680–1850

Although it is now clear that rising fertility was a much more important reason than declining mortality for the increasing population during the period 1680–1850, the latter reason has been debated much more extensively than the former. One reason for this emphasis is that until recently many historians believed that falling mortality was the main reason for population growth. Another reason may be that it is relatively more straightforward to explain rising fertility: the most recent evidence indicates that the changes in nuptiality that underlay rising fertility were fairly strongly and consistently related to changes in real incomes, broadly in accord with the Malthusian model: as real incomes rose, so nuptiality rose, and vice

versa. But possible explanations for any decline in mortality are more complex, in part because of a lack of solid information on causes of death, and in part because the decline was not regular, but took place towards the end of a long sequence of erratic movements. It is precisely such irregularities and unpredictable series of events that models—such as the Malthusian one—tend to be bad at accommodating.

As the main causes of death in the early eighteenth century were infectious diseases, it is fairly certain that the main reason for the decline in mortality towards the end of the period 1680–1850 was a fall in the number of deaths from infectious diseases, though fewer deaths resulting from chronic food shortages may also have contributed. Potential explanations for a decline in deaths from infectious diseases can be grouped into three broad types:

(i) Biological—such as a decrease in the virulence of the micro-organisms, or an increase in immunity or resistance.

(ii) Environmental and social—such as less exposure to infections, for example through improvements in living conditions such as housing and water supplies, in turn related to a rising standard of living.

(iii) Medical—such as an improvement in the effectiveness of medical intervention in the treatment of infectious diseases.

We shall look at each in turn. First, as you have seen, biological explanations of historical changes in disease patterns are difficult to establish. The best evidence is often simply the failure to substantiate any other explanation. However, it is sometimes possible to provide circumstantial evidence, such as a decrease in the reported case-fatality rates, which may suggest that, for instance, the virulence of a micro-organism had changed. This is thought to have been the case with the decline of scarlet fever, and may also have been true of plague and some other infectious diseases.

Second, changes in the social environment that are claimed to have been responsible for the decline in mortality in this period were improvements in nutrition and in general social conditions. A leading advocate of the importance of nutrition has been Thomas McKeown, a doctor and prominent sceptic about the impact of health care. However, his arguments have been made with particular force in relation to the nineteenth century, and we will return to them below. McKeown has argued that other social improvements had little or no impact until after 1820, but some historians have suggested otherwise. They have pointed to such factors as the drainage of land which led to less malaria (though this was never more than a localised problem in Britain), the replacement of wooden with brick or stone buildings after the urban fires of the seventeenth century, leading to improved domestic hygiene and control of vermin; and the introduction of mechanised cotton cloth manufacture, which may have contributed to reducing the incidence of typhus, a disease spread by body lice, as a result of the greater availability of cotton clothes which could be boiled during washing.

Whatever the balance of evidence on these factors, it has become increasingly clear in recent years that there is no good evidence of a strong link between long-term economic trends and mortality levels in England during this period. Real wages, which were introduced in Chapter 5 as one measure of the standard of living, rose during some periods when mortality was also increasing, and were falling during some periods when mortality was declining. One possible explanation for these findings is that, although rising wages may improve the standard of living and reduce mortality if the social and economic environment remains otherwise unchanged, it is likely that rising wages over a period of time will be associated with other changes, such as a growth in urbanisation or in industry, which may initially tend to increase rather than lower mortality.

The third possible explanation of the decline of mortality towards the end of the period 1680–1850 is an improvement in medical intervention. Most commentators have considered the contribution of medicine during the eighteenth century to have been slight or even in some instances harmful. However, the historian Peter Razzell has argued that the introduction from Turkey of smallpox inoculation in 1717, and its widespread use from 1760, helped to reduce mortality from this condition long before the introduction of Edward Jenner's cowpox vaccine from 1796 onwards. Some researchers have also suggested that hospitals—especially the voluntary general hospitals which spread during the eighteenth century—were not as harmful as is generally supposed, and may in fact have contributed to the falling death rate. However, hospital populations were probably too small to be of demographic significance in the eighteenth century.

On balance, Wrigley and Schofield (whose work is increasingly used as the basis for discussion of this period) provide the following assessment of influences on mortality trends during this period in England:

It is doubtful…whether the course of real wages was ever the dominant influence on mortality trends. A slowly changing balance between infective parasites and their human host was probably a weightier factor, a balance which

tilted to and fro largely outside the consciousness of men and, with few exceptions, quite outside their power to influence. (Wrigley and Schofield, 1989, p. 416)

Finally, it is important to bear in mind that over the period 1680–1850, and especially up to the end of the eighteenth century, there is less of a decline in mortality to be explained than has often been thought.

Mortality and fertility since 1850

Returning to Figure 6.2, let us complete this account of mortality and fertility changes in England by examining the period from 1850 to the present.

☐ Describe the main features revealed in Figure 6.2 for the period 1850–1990.

■ Death and birth rates began to fall even more steeply around 1861 and continued to do so until well into the twentieth century. The rate of population growth fell from its peak of approximately 1.5 per cent per annum around the mid-nineteenth century to its present value close to zero.

Referring back to Figure 6.6, you will also see that the expectation of life at birth rose at an accelerating rate: from an average of approximately 40 years in 1850, to 50 years by 1911, 60 by 1931 and over 70 by 1971.

The difference in life expectancies between males and females is apparent in Figure 6.6 from 1871 onwards. Although the expectation of life has increased for both sexes, the increase for males has been slightly less than that for females. The consequence of this has been a widening of the difference between the sexes. Some further evidence on this subject will be discussed in Chapters 8 and 9.

Changes in the cause of death since 1850

In contrast to the situation pre-1850, fairly reliable information on cause of death is available from around 1850 onwards as a result of the introduction of death certification in 1838. In addition, the establishment of a decennial (10-yearly) census in 1801 provided the means of determining mortality rates not only for the whole population, but for specific age groups, for each sex, and, from 1921, for social classes. However, this only represents a relative improvement in our knowledge of the causes of death, and many problems can still arise unless care is taken in interpreting the evidence:

Problems arise both from vagueness and inaccuracy of diagnosis and from changes in nomenclature and classification. For example, there must be doubts about the diagnosis of tuberculosis at a time when it was not possible to X-ray the chest or identify the tubercle bacillus. In the Registrar-General's classification scarlet fever was not separated from diphtheria until 1855, nor typhus from typhoid before 1869. Even the less exacting task, so important for the present discussion of distinguishing infectious from non-infectious causes of death, presents difficulties. For example, deaths attributed to diseases of the heart and nervous system included a considerable but unknown number due to infections such as syphilis. (McKeown, 1976, p. 50)

Some of these problems can be avoided by adopting a simple classification based on groups of conditions rather than specific causes. Table 6.2 groups causes of death under four broad headings: infectious disease caused by airborne, water- or food-borne and other micro-organisms, and all other (that is, non-infectious) diseases. In the first column, it shows the percentage contribution of each disease to the decline in the death rate between 1848–54 (that is, the average sampled over these 6 years) and 1971, standardised for changes in the age and sex structure of the population between these dates. In the second and third columns, it then sub-divides this period of roughly 120 years into the period 1848–54 to 1901, and the period 1901 to 1971. This allows a comparison of the extent to which a cause of death was declining in the period *before* 1901 and that *after* that date. For example, the table shows that the decline in deaths from cholera and diarrhoea accounted for 11 per cent of the total fall in the death rate between 1848–54 and 1971, and that 3.5 per cent of this reduction occurred *before* 1901 and the remaining 7.5 per cent *afterwards*.

□ Overall, what was the relative contribution of infectious diseases and non-infectious diseases to the fall in death rates between 1848–54 and 1971?

■ Between 1848–54 and 1971 three-quarters of the improvement in death rates was due to the decline in infectious diseases, while non-infectious conditions accounted for the remaining quarter.

□ For each of these two broad categories of disease, how much of the contribution to falling death rates came (a) before, and (b) after 1901?

■ For both categories of disease, most of the contribution came *after* 1901. This is especially the case with the non-infectious diseases.

Table 6.2 Reasons for the reduction in Standardised Death Rates in England and Wales between 1848–54 and 1971

Cause of death	Percent contribution to total fall in Standardised Death Rate between:		
	1848–54 and 1971	of which	
		1848–54 to 1901	1901 to 1971
airborne micro-organisms			
respiratory tuberculosis	**17.5**	9.0	8.5
scarlet fever; diphtheria	**6.0**	4.0	2.0
smallpox	**1.5**	1.5	0
bronchitis, pneumonia, influenza	**7.0**	3.0	10.0
other	**6.5**	1.0	5.5
water/food-borne micro-organisms			
cholera; diarrhoea	**11.0**	3.5	7.5
typhoid; typhus*	**6.0**	5.0	1.0
other (e.g. dysentery)	**4.5**	1.0	3.5
other micro-organisms	**12.5**	4.5	8.0
sub-total all micro-organisms	**74.5**	27.5	47.0
other conditions:			
(not micro-organisms)	**25.5**	2.5	23.0
total (all causes)	**100**	30	70

*Typhus should be in the 'other micro-organisms' category, but was not distinguished from typhoid before 1869. (Data from Szreter, S. (1988) The importance of social intervention in Britain's mortality decline, c. 1850–1914: a re-interpretation of the role of public health, *Journal of the Social History of Medicine*, p. 8)

Within each of these two groups of causes there was considerable variation in the pattern of the decline of different diseases. Of the airborne infections, respiratory tuberculosis was the single most important disease to decline, accounting for as much as 17.5 per cent of the fall in overall mortality (from all causes) between 1848–54 and 1971. Whereas deaths from tuberculosis fell throughout this period, there was actually a small increase in deaths from bronchitis, pneumonia and influenza between 1848–54 and 1901, with a decline only occurring during the twentieth century. Before 1901 water-borne infections (such as typhoid) declined more than those which were food-borne (such as dysentery).

Though the mortality rate for all infectious diseases and all non-infectious diseases fell between 1848–54 and 1971, this was not true of some

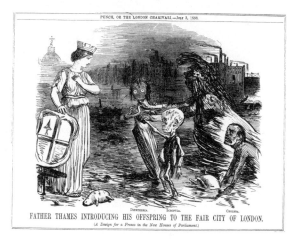

PUNCH, OR THE LONDON CHARIVARI.—July 3, 1858.

FATHER THAMES INTRODUCING HIS OFFSPRING TO THE FAIR CITY OF LONDON.
(A Design for a Fresco in the New Houses of Parliament.)

A cartoon drawn by Tenniel in 1858 shows a keen awareness of the hazardous state of the River Thames. The 'offspring' are named Diptheria, Scrofula and Cholera (Punch, 3 July 1858)

non-infectious causes of death. In particular, the death rates for cardiovascular disease and cancers increased substantially.

The overall effect of all these changes in the causes of death can be seen in Figure 6.7. Infections (infectious diseases with tuberculosis shown separately) have undergone a spectacular decline and are now responsible for

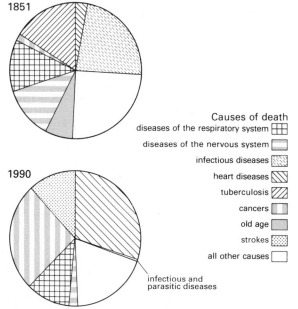

1851

1990

Causes of death

diseases of the respiratory system
diseases of the nervous system
infectious diseases
heart diseases
tuberculosis
cancers
old age
strokes
all other causes

infectious and parasitic diseases

Figure 6.7 *Causes of death in England and Wales, 1851 and 1990. (Data for 1851 from Registrar-General, 1855, England and Wales Report; for 1990 from Registrar-General, 1992, Annual Abstract of Statistics 1992, HMSO, London, Table 2.20, p. 37)*

less than 2 per cent of all deaths. The decline of diseases of the nervous system was because of changes in diagnosis and classification: in 1851 many people were certified as dying from convulsions, others from insanity and delirium tremens, none of which would be commonly recognised as causes of death today.

These principal causes of mortality have been replaced in recent years by three categories in particular: heart disease, strokes and cancers. Though most of their increase is relative, due to the decline of other causes and the survival of more people to ages in which these diseases occur, some of the increase is thought to have resulted from an absolute rise in incidence. The current pattern of causes of death in the United Kingdom will be considered in greater detail in Chapter 9.

A final comment on the historical changes in patterns of disease in England must be made. Most of the discussion has been concerned with mortality and changing causes of death. This is unfortunate as it provides only one indication of the health of a population. In particular, it ignores two aspects of ill-health—morbidity and disability—which may also be important indicators of the health of a population. The reason for their omission is simple and no doubt obvious—a lack of historical data. However, they are considered in the discussion of contemporary epidemiology in Chapter 9.

In summary, it seems that the decline in mortality since 1850 has followed a very broad sequence as regards the type of condition causing death: first water-borne and then food-borne infections declined, followed by air-borne infections, and finally some non-infectious conditions. Of course, these changes in mortality rates have not been mutually exclusive and, as you have seen, within some categories the incidence of specific diseases has actually increased at times. The timing of these changes should help us to understand how they came about but, as you will see, fierce controversy continues to surround this area.

Explanations of the modern decline in mortality

As you saw earlier in this chapter, explanations of falling mortality in the period from 1680 up to 1850 did give credence to the possibility of a biological explanation—changing virulence of infectious organisms, for example. However, the influence of biological factors on the *overall* pattern of change has largely been dismissed on the grounds that the virulence of many different micro-organisms would have had to decline more or less simultaneously—an event that is regarded as most unlikely to have happened, even though changing virulence of some micro-organisms is quite likely. The debate on the **explanations of the modern decline in**

75

mortality and, in particular, reasons for the dramatic decline in mortality rates attributable to infectious diseases since 1850, have had a different emphasis, concentrating on three points:

(i)   the impact of medical intervention;

(ii) the establishment of public health administration and legislation;

(iii) improvements in nutrition and standards of living.

For many years, the major contribution to the decline in mortality was considered to have been from medical advances. However, from the 1960s this view was challenged vigorously, largely as a result of the work of Thomas McKeown. An account of his views on this subject appears in *Health and Disease, A Reader*[2] and you should now read his article, 'The medical contribution'.

☐ On what grounds does McKeown argue that medical measures made only an insignificant contribution to the overall decline of mortality from infectious diseases since 1850?

■ He does this principally by demonstrating that mortality had declined or was declining before the introduction of relevant medical measures (e.g. in the cases of measles and respiratory tuberculosis).

☐ Despite this, medical measures appear (a) to have made a dramatic contribution to the decline of one infection, and (b) to have accelerated the decline in mortality from two others since the 1940s. Which diseases are these?

■ These are (a) smallpox, in which the decline was mainly due to vaccination, and (b) respiratory tuberculosis, with the introduction of chemotherapy, and diphtheria, with the widespread use of immunisation.

☐ As an assessment of the contribution that doctors have made to the overall decline in mortality, what are the main limitations of this article?

■ Quite explicitly, McKeown is only concerned with the decline in infectious diseases, ignoring the possible effect doctors may have had on the other types of condition that account for 26 per cent of the overall decline. However, a more important limitation is that he concentrates on the biomedical role of medicine and ignores the preventive work carried out by doctors, both in the area of individual advice to people and in the establishment of public health measures.

McKeown not only rejected the importance of medical intervention, but attributed the decline in mortality to improvements in nutrition and standard of living. This so-called **McKeown hypothesis** rapidly acquired the status of the new orthodoxy, but it has itself come under increasingly critical scrutiny. The historian J. M. Winter, for example, has argued that

> …when a doctor advises a change in diet or the removal of unsanitary debris, he may very well improve the survival chances of his patients. Simply because doctors do not require a medical education to make such statements is no reason to conclude that such indirect medical intervention was unimportant in the process of mortality decline. (Winter, 1982, p. 111)

A more sustained critique has been mounted by the historian Simon Szreter, and extracts from his work are also reprinted in *Health and Disease: A Reader*. You should read his article ('The importance of social intervention in Britain's mortality decline, c. 1850–1914') now.

The objective of Szreter's work is not to question McKeown's *negative* conclusion, that modern scientific medicine cannot be awarded much credit for the historical decline of mortality, but to counter McKeown's *positive* conclusion that nutritional improvements and a rising standard of living were the main causes of declining mortality. Szreter's argument proceeds on a number of fronts. First, he argues that McKeown reached his conclusions about the importance of nutrition and the standard of living on methodologically suspect grounds, by eliminating other possible causes so that, by default, only nutrition and rising standards of living could have been responsible for the decline in mortality, through improving the natural defences of individuals to infectious diseases, especially airborne diseases. He also accuses McKeown of subsuming far too much under the term 'standard of living', and as a result implying incorrectly that a whole range of social, cultural and political factors are the automatic corollary of changes in a country's per capita real income. Second, he argues that McKeown misinterpreted the evidence on the contribution of different diseases to declining mortality, and on the chronology of the decline.

☐ Which particular airborne disease does McKeown's argument heavily rely on, according to Szreter?

[2]*Health and Disease: a Reader*, (Open University Press, 1984; revised edition 1994).

■ Respiratory tuberculosis, which in the mid-nineteenth century was the single most important cause of death.[3]

□ In what ways is McKeown's reliance on the decline of this disease to substantiate his thesis flawed, according to Szreter?

■ First, respiratory tuberculosis was only one of a group of important airborne diseases. Two of these declined for reasons not related to nutrition: smallpox as a consequence of the spread of inoculation, vaccination and isolation procedures; and scarlet fever probably as a result of immunological changes in the population or in the micro-organism's virulence. A third group of airborne diseases—bronchitis, pneumonia and influenza—actually *increased* substantially during the second half of the nineteenth century. Thus respiratory tuberculosis cannot be taken as typical of the airborne diseases. Second, Szreter claims that McKeown places too much faith on unconvincing evidence of the *early* decline of tuberculosis. Third, he argues that the prevalence of tuberculosis might best be viewed as a *consequence* of other debilitating diseases, and therefore declined as a result of the decline of other diseases. (An interesting modern parallel of this final point is the resurgence of tuberculosis as a consequence of the AIDS epidemic.)

Having moved the focus of attention from the airborne to the water- and food-borne diseases, Szreter argues that these probably *rose* earlier in the nineteenth century as the population of urban areas expanded rapidly, and experienced conditions such as those described by Engels and discussed in Chapter 5. But these water- and food-borne diseases were finally pushed back towards the end of the century as the result of a whole series of *public health measures* undertaken primarily by local authorities, and including sanitation and clean water supplies, and the increasing regulation of food and drink. The air-borne diseases took longer to decline, perhaps because of the lack of effective public health intervention directed against them until the twentieth century.[4] Szreter thus concludes that there is no automatic reason to think that a growing economy will be translated into health gains: if it results in rapid urbanisation, poor working conditions and growing pollution it might be harmful to health. The key factor, therefore, is how the consequences of economic growth are used: Here Szreter emphasises strongly the role of public health measures in improving the urban environment, but he also stresses the issue of distribution: unless such measures, and other benefits of economic growth, are distributed widely across the population, the health gains will be reduced.

If Szreter's analysis and conclusions are broadly correct, they may be of some wider significance: they suggest that McKeown's thesis, which has been so influential, may mislead countries which are still attempting to lower their population mortality. Social and medical intervention, and especially public health measures, may be a more reliable route to lowering mortality than the straightforward pursuit of national income growth, while the *distribution* of such interventions becomes an important issue of public policy. Moreover, an improved technology and science of social and medical intervention since the nineteenth century is likely to make the historical lesson drawn by Szreter even more pertinent today. These are issues we will return to in the following two chapters.

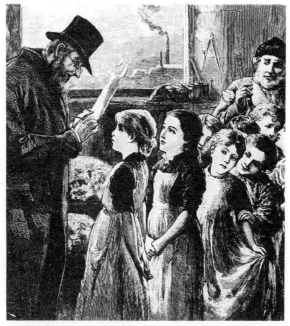

A factory inspector checks the age of children at work. The factory inspectorate was one example of the public health measures introduced throughout the eighteenth century. After 1833 it was illegal to employ children below the age of nine in factories.

[3] The history of tuberculosis and factors contributing to its decline are fully discussed in *Medical Knowledge: Doubt and Certainty* (Open University Press, revised edition 1994).

[4] The history of the public health movement in the United Kingdom is described in *Caring for Health: History and Diversity* (Open University Press, revised edition 1993).

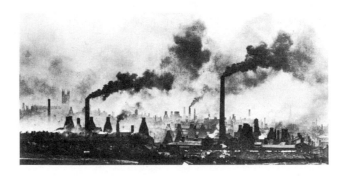

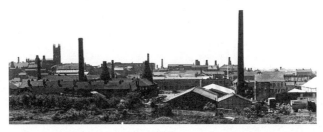

Factory chimneys in Longton, Staffordshire, in (a) 1910, and (b) 1970. Clean air legislation was not effective until the second half of the twentieth century. (Source: Oxford University Press)

Health transition and demographic transition

Finally, does the English case examined here provide a broader insight into links between population change, health, and social and economic development? First, you have seen how the transition from an agricultural society to an industrial society was accompanied by a complete change in disease and mortality patterns, in which infectious diseases and diseases caused by food shortages gave way to the chronic non-infectious diseases such as heart disease and cancers which now predominate. Increasingly this process of change has come to be described as the **health transition.**

Demographers and epidemiologists argue that the health transition has two main components:

> ...the first is the epidemiologic transition strictly speaking, which is defined as the long-term process of change in the health conditions of a society, including changes in the patterns of disease, disability, and death. The second component, which may be called the health care transition, refers to the change in the patterns of organised social response to health conditions. (Frenk *et al.*, 1991, p. 23)

As the case of England demonstrates, this health transition is associated with many different factors: demographic, socio-economic, biological, technological, political and cultural changes were all involved in one way or another. Because of this complexity, it would be misleading to generalise across countries about the health transition. It should also be noted that even within a population, the health transition may be at different stages, with infectious disease still dominant in some groups while chronic and degenerative diseases predominate in others. Finally, as with all such models, it is all too easy to assume that the health transition inevitably proceeds in just one direction. In fact, it is possible that infectious diseases may undergo resurgences which increase their importance in the pattern of disease and death.

☐ Can you recall from Chapters 2 and 3 any examples of changes in disease patterns that run counter to the general direction of the health transition?

■ The global emergence of the viral disease AIDS during the 1980s is a particularly striking example. Even in countries such as the USA which made the health transition many years ago, this infectious disease has become a leading cause of death. Malaria is an example of an infectious disease that has not declined steadily, but rather has undergone a widespread resurgence. Another infectious disease that may be on the increase is tuberculosis, the resurgence of which is partly related to the AIDS epidemic.

Despite these qualifications, the concept of the health transition is a useful reference point from which to view the experience of individual countries.

The English case, then, provides evidence relevant to the health transition. But it also throws some light on another link between population change, health, and social and economic development. As the Industrial Revolution progressed in England and spread to other countries, so evidence accumulated that the massive social and economic changes involved were accompanied by changes in birth and death rates that first accelerated and later retarded population growth. In the 1930s and 1940s, attempts were made to construct a more formal theory linking population change to industrialisation—this came to be known as the **theory of demographic transition**. And although this theory was originally intended to fit the demographic experience of industrialised countries such as England, it has been used to try to explain demographic trends in the Third World.

Figure 6.8 depicts the demographic transition for a hypothetical population before and after industrialisation. In this model, the demographic transition has four stages. Stage 1 is characterised by a high death rate and a high birth rate, so any population growth is very slow. This is the pre-industrial stage in the model. In Stage 2, the death rate starts to fall sharply, but the birth rate remains high.

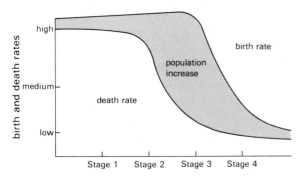

Figure 6.8 *A model of the demographic transition. (The Open University, 1982, D301 Historical Data and the Social Sciences, Units 5–8 Historical Demography: Problems and Projects, The Open University, Milton Keynes, Figure 3, p.19)*

□ What hypothesis could you suggest to explain this stage?

■ One hypothesis that could be supported from the evidence in the previous chapter is that increases in agricultural productivity have removed the Malthusian 'checks' of famine and disease, allowing the population to expand.

By the third stage of the transition, the birth rate also falls sharply, while the fall in the death rate begins to level off. The fourth stage is reached when both the birth rate and the death rate have levelled off at a low level, and the total population size is again fairly stable, but much larger.

This hypothetical model of demographic change can be compared with Figure 6.2, which shows changes in the birth rate and death rate in England between 1541 and 1990. It is clear that the model is a considerable simplification of what actually happened. In particular, the sixteenth and seventeenth centuries, when the birth rate was falling and the death rate if anything rising, do not appear to fit the model very well. However, from the early eighteenth century onwards it is possible to discern periods that correspond approximately to the four stages of the demographic transition model. From 1700 to 1740 the birth and death rates are both high and are quite similar (Stage 1). Then the death rate begins to fall while the birth rate remains high and in fact rises to a peak around 1821 (Stage 2). The death rate continues to fall, and around 1861 the birth rate also begins to decline (Stage 3). Finally, from around 1941, both birth and death rates come together again and start stabilising at a much lower level (Stage 4).

This four-stage model of demographic transition has been criticised, as some aspects do not fit the facts of population change in many of the now industrialised countries: for example, in France it appears that the birth rate began falling before there was any significant industrialisation. In this respect the demographic transition model is little different from models in many other science and social science areas, which are often criticised for failing to deal with exceptional cases, erratic and irregular sequences of events, or simply with individual cases: simplification of the real world is simultaneously their strength and their weakness. Critics have also argued that there is no real theoretical basis for the theory of demographic transition, even if it does have some descriptive value. Despite these criticisms, however, and returning to the starting point of this chapter, it can be seen as a valuable descriptive account of the link between social and economic development and population change. The model is a useful starting point from which to consider demographic trends, and experience to date does support it as a generalisation. The following two chapters will take up its relevance for the Third World countries of today.

OBJECTIVES FOR CHAPTER 6

When you have studied this chapter, you should be able to:

6.1   Explain what is meant by a mortality crisis and describe the features of (a) a mortality crisis caused largely by a shortage of food, and (b) one resulting from an autonomous infectious epidemic.

6.2   Discuss the difficulties of estimating mortality and interpreting the cause of death and illness in historical sources such as parish registers and personal accounts.

6.3   Describe the main change in English population size since 1680, and the accompanying changes in life expectancy, mortality and fertility.

6.4   Describe the main changes in the causes of death since 1850, and summarise and comment on different explanations for the decline in mortality in England during the nineteenth and early twentieth centuries.

6.5   Describe the model of demographic transition, and be able to analyse data on birth and death rates from specific countries using its main stages.

QUESTIONS FOR CHAPTER 6

Question 1 (*Objective 6.1*)

Looking at Figure 6.4, what do you think were the likely causes of the mortality crises in the parish of St Botolph in 1593, 1603 and 1625? What features of these crises determined your answer?

Question 2 (*Objective 6.2*)

Can you suggest three reasons why it is impossible to compare meaningfully the prevalence of a condition such as hysteria in 1550 with its prevalence today?

Question 3 (*Objective 6.3*)

Assess the relative contributions of changes in mortality and in fertility between 1680 and 1850 to population expansion.

Question 4 (*Objective 6.4*)

Why does the critique of McKeown mounted by Szreter rely to a degree on drawing a distinction between air-borne and water-borne diseases as contributors to mortality decline during the nineteenth century?

Question 5 (*Objective 6.5*)

To what extent can the model of demographic transition be fitted to the trends in birth rates and death rates in England between 1541 and the start of the eighteenth century?

7 Health in a world of wealth and poverty

During this chapter you will be asked to read an extract contained in **Health and Disease: A Reader**[1] — *'Entitlement and Deprivation' by Jean Drèze and Amartya K. Sen, taken from their book* **Hunger and Public Action.**

Only a few countries in the world were involved in the first wave of the Industrial Revolution, and the majority of the world's population still lives in countries that are not fully industrialised. As the example of England has shown, health and disease are intimately related to processes of social change and development, and it is clear that the solution to the health problems of Third World countries must involve some kind of social and economic development. How this might come about, however, is one of the biggest problems of our time, and raises a series of questions about the origins and present features of the Third World's problems, and the relationship between social and economic development and health. Let us begin by considering the origins of the **Third World**.

The Industrial Revolution and the Third World

Before the Industrial Revolution, the differences in economic wealth between the major regions of the world were almost certainly much smaller than they are today. If we go back several hundred years, fragments of evidence come to us from the observations of travellers on the condition of the population and the wealth or poverty of the lands they visited. Most famous of all, perhaps, was Marco Polo, who in the late thirteenth century spent 24 years travelling widely throughout the Middle East and Asia taking detailed notes on what he saw.

[1]*Health and Disease: A Reader* (Open University Press, 1984; revised edition 1994).

☐ Marco Polo was a merchant and a business traveller. Why might this background be of interest when reading his account?

■ Because he was a successful merchant and trader (a merchant of Venice, no less), he had a seasoned eye for the details of commercial life and the clues and signals of economic activity.

In his travels, Marco Polo was 'quick to notice the available sources of food and water along the route, the means of transport, and no less quick to observe the marketable products of every district, whether natural or manufactured, and the channels through which flowed the interlacing streams of export and import'. (R. E. Latham, in Introduction to 1968 edition, p.xix)

Following Marco Polo through his travels, the picture which emerges is not at all one that might be obtained today in the Third World, which now includes many countries he passed through: Armenia: 'a land of many villages and towns, amply stocked with the means of life'; Northern Persia: a ride 'through a fine plain and a fine valley and along fine hillsides, where there is a rich herbage, fine pasturage, fruit in plenty, and no lack of anything'; Cathay (North-East China): 'when harvests are

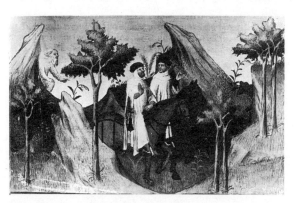

Marco Polo travelling through lands of plenty. (Source: The Mansell Collection)

bountiful corn is accumulated in huge granaries, along with wheat, barley, millet, and rice to be distributed when crops fail'; Bengal: 'the people live on meat, milk and rice. They have cotton in plenty. They are great traders, exporting spikenard, galingale, ginger, sugar and many other precious spices'; and Northern India: 'They live by trade and industry. They have rice and wheat in profusion. The staple foods are rice, meat and milk. Merchants come here in great numbers by sea and by land with a variety of merchandise and export the products of the kingdom'.

Venice may have been a 'jewel on the shores of the Adriatic', about to take its place in the forefront of the Renaissance, but Marco Polo at least gives no indication that it was unimaginably more advanced than many other places he passed through.

Even between 1750 and 1800, as the Industrial Revolution was getting well under way in Britain, the economic historian Paul Bairoch has calculated that the average levels of production and wealth in what are now Third World countries were not so very different from those in the countries that are now industrialised: in China they may have been higher.

However, as the Industrial Revolution gathered pace in a small number of countries, it gave them a tremendous advantage over the rest of the world in economic, technological and military power, and a gap rapidly opened and widened. Propelled by an immense increase in trade and exchange between different parts of the world, there began a great wave of colonisation, empire-building, and annexation of territories. As every British schoolchild used to be taught, for a time the sun never set on the many countries of the world that were part of the British Empire, and there were very few areas of the world in which control or influence was not exercised or fiercely contested by the newly industrialised countries, including France, Germany, Italy, Belgium and Holland.

Overseas expansion was not of course a phenomenon new to the period of industrialisation. We have only to think of the Romans, whose influence and power in Europe and much of Asia is witnessed even today, not only by the many relics of buildings, but by the location of towns, the routes taken by roads, the language, laws, currencies and measurements that still mould our lives. We must also note that other examples of European conquest, which have already been mentioned (for example the conquest of the Americas by the Spaniards) occurred from the sixteenth century onwards, well before the Industrial Revolution reached full speed.

However, the expansion that occurred in the wake of the Industrial Revolution was unprecedented in scope and scale. Between 1846 and 1930 over 50 million Europeans migrated to other parts of the world in a great wave of humanity, settling in the Americas and Australasia, and temporarily taking control of most of Africa and much of Asia. Pushed by the rapidly growing population of Europe and pulled by the prospect of open lands and escape from hunger and poverty, they helped to diffuse the Industrial Revolution and to transform the world. While the population of Europe was growing at more than double the rate of the rest of the world, the rate of growth in these newly settled lands was almost unchecked, with relatively low death rates coupled to some of the highest fertility rates ever recorded.

One consequence of this expansion was that the 'white' or 'Caucasian' population of the world surged from around one-fifth of the global total in 1800 to over one-third by 1930. And, although this share of population was not long held, the surge in their population did give the Europeans a more permanent advantage: the settlement of territories comprising almost one-quarter of the world's land surface. What's more, these newly settled territories, including the United States of America, Canada, Argentina, Uruguay, New Zealand and Australia, turned out to be vastly productive agricultural lands, able to feed not only their own burgeoning populations, but also to produce huge surpluses for anyone able to purchase them.

Of course the lands settled by European emigrants were not empty of other inhabitants, who were dispossessed and often suffered demographic collapse as a result of the devastating impact on native populations of infectious diseases imported with the European settlers.[2] In New Zealand, for example, the native population of Maori, estimated to number around 150 000–180 000 at the beginning of the nineteenth century, had collapsed to barely 40 000 by the end of that century as a result of infectious diseases such as measles and venereal disease introduced by the Europeans, and also as a result of social and economic collapse manifesting itself in alcoholism, infanticide, malnutrition and sheer despair.

As Europe's rush of colonial acquisition proceeded, key aspects of the political, social and economic systems prevailing in these territories were greatly altered in a way that was essentially geared to the needs of the colonialists rather than the local populations. In the Americas and

[2]The reciprocal influences on health care in the colonies and in the European countries which controlled these territories is discussed in *Caring for Health: History and Diversity* (Open University Press, revised edition, 1993).

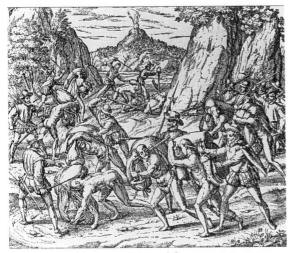

Contemporary engraving depicting ill-treatment of native Americans by the Spanish colonialists in the sixteenth century.

Caribbean, the first major change introduced was the establishment of plantations to provide cotton, and later coffee and tobacco, for Europe. In the first instance, this required the importation of labour on a massive scale, in large part to compensate for the collapse of the native population through the epidemics. These were the origins of the slave trade, which not only dislocated the social and economic system of much of Africa, but again set off new waves of infectious disease.

The other important aspect of this process was that the entire pattern of agriculture and farming was changed beyond recognition, with the most fertile land being devoted to the production of crops that were grown for export rather than to meet the needs of local populations. As the economic, technological and political predominance of the industrialised countries grew, many parts of the world were transformed into satellite economies producing the raw materials and foodstuffs required by the industrial countries: tea from India and Ceylon (Sri Lanka), coffee from Brazil and Kenya, rice from Burma and Thailand, rubber from Malaya, guano fertiliser from Peru, and so on. For these countries, whether formally administered as colonies or informally administered by European commercial enterprises, the needs of distant industrial economies were placed foremost, and the needs of the local populations and of indigenous development were very much secondary considerations. This dependence on the export of raw materials has continued to the present day: in 1990 only 21 per cent of the total

exports of the high-income countries were comprised of raw materials and foods, compared with 48 per cent in the low-income countries, and no less than 89 per cent in the Sub-Saharan countries.

The industrialised countries have thus exerted a powerful influence over agriculture around the world. But, in addition to this role as producers of foodstuffs and raw materials, the colonised or partly colonised countries of the world were affected in other ways as a world economy developed around the industrialised countries. In particular, they became markets for the industrial goods being manufactured in Britain and elsewhere. The frequent result of this need for new markets, and of the technological superiority of the industrial countries, was that traditional manufacturing industries in the colonised countries were destroyed. India's textile industry, for example, was devastated as cotton fabric imports from Britain soared from one million yards in 1814 to 51 million yards by 1830.

In an attempt to calculate the effects of this process on the Third World as a whole, the economic historian Paul Bairoch has assessed changes in total world manufacturing production from 1750 onwards, and some results are shown in Table 7.1 (overleaf). The figures are expressed in terms of an index in which the volume of production in the United Kingdom in 1900 is taken as equal to an index number of 100. Thus, in 1880, manufacturing production in the USA had an index number of 47, which means that it was approximately equal to 47 per cent of United Kingdom production in 1900.

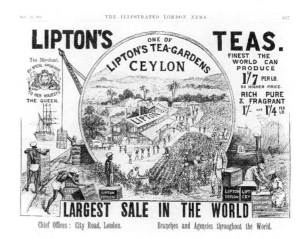

An advertisement for Lipton's Teas depicts Ceylon (Sri Lanka) as the 'tea garden' for the British consumer. (Illustrated London News, 21 November 1896)

Table 7.1 The development of world manufacturing production, 1750–1980 (United Kingdom in 1900 = 100)

| Year | Industrialised countries | | | Third World |
	UK	USA	All	
1750	2	–	34	93
1800	6	1	47	99
1830	16	5	73	112
1850	45	16	143	83
1880	73	47	253	67
1900	100	128	481	60
1913	127	298	863	70
1928	135	533	1 258	98
1938	181	528	1 562	122
1953	262	1 373	2 870	200
1963	334	1 804	4 699	439
1973	471	3 089	8 432	927
1980	454	3 475	9 718	1 323

Data from Bairoch, P. (1982) International industrialization levels from 1750 to 1980, *Journal of European Economic History*, **11** (2), pp. 269–333, Table 2.

☐ Look at the column for the Third World. What happens from 1750 onwards?

■ From 1750 to 1830 the Third World index rose from 93 to 112 (in other words, by 1830 it exceeded by 12 per cent the production of the United Kingdom in 1900). From 1830 onwards, however, as the process of colonisation we have described gathered pace, manufacturing production in these countries started to fall, and by 1900 was barely half the level it had been at the beginning of the nineteenth century. Not until 1938 did Third World manufacturing production regain its earlier level. After 1938, manufacturing production in the Third World grew more rapidly.

It seems clear, therefore, that the social and economic development of the Third World has been influenced powerfully by the Industrial Revolution, and in particular by the countries that are now industrialised. In order to explore the implications of this for health and disease patterns, let us now take stock of the differences in social and economic development in the world today.

Measuring social and economic development

One way of looking at the world, already encountered in this book, is to draw up a list of countries and then order them into a league table according to some indicator such as life expectancy or infant mortality. International agencies such as the World Health Organisation present data in this way, and so also do organisations such as the World Bank, which publishes data on social and economic development. Such league tables are therefore a convenient starting point, although they have limitations which we shall be discussing later.

One of the most commonly used indicators of social and economic development is **Gross National Product (GNP)** per capita (per head). The GNP is a measure of the total output of a national economy expressed in money terms. It includes wealth produced abroad but brought into a country, and excludes wealth produced in a country but taken abroad. For example, millions of people— 'migrant workers'—go abroad to earn money and send remittances back to relatives in the country they left. Their remittances are included in the GNP of the country the remittances are sent to, and excluded from the GNP of the country the remittances were earned in. Profits which companies earn in one country and move to another are included in the GNP of the country that receives them. The GNP is thus an attempt to place a figure on the total wealth that accrues to the residents of a particular country, and GNP per capita is simply the total GNP divided by the number of residents in the country.

The Gross National Product and other national accounts have been described as one of the most significant social inventions of the twentieth century, and their influence is pervasive. They are used to divide and describe the countries of the world; politicians use the GNP as a measure of national potency, of their successes and their opponents' failures; small changes in GNP can trigger policy changes and influence public mood by determining whether a country is in or out of recession, growing steadily or 'overheating'.

Despite the tremendous influence of national accounts, they have defects and weaknesses. For example, one of the limitations of using GNP to measure wealth is that it only includes goods or services exchanged by a financial transaction in a market, and excludes goods and services which contribute to wealth but are not bought or sold.

☐ What common examples of goods and services can you think of that contribute to wealth but would be excluded from GNP?

■ In all countries of the world a great deal of cleaning, washing, cooking and other domestic work is done in households, mainly by women. Because no formal payment is made for this work it is not included in the GNP.

Housework is probably the largest single item excluded from GNP, and it has been estimated that including this sort of work might increase measured GNP by anything up to 30 per cent. This kind of measurement problem can be found in all countries, but is particularly acute in Third World countries: subsistence farming, for instance, is by definition an activity in which food is consumed by the people who produce it. As they do not sell it in a market, it is not included in the GNP.

Another criticism sometimes levelled at the GNP as a measure of economic progress is that it does not reflect the depletion or despoliation of natural resources. For example, if a country's main source of wealth was its forests, and it felled them and sold them while making no attempt to replace them or use them in a sustainable way, its GNP would for a while increase. However, it would in fact be destroying the basis of its future prosperity, rather like a factory owner tearing up the floor-boards to feed the boilers. Thus the GNP would give a very misleading impression of economic progress. A variety of ways of dealing with this problem have been proposed, but so far none has been adopted.

For these reasons, GNP measurements should not be accepted uncritically as a measure of wealth: like measures of health such as mortality they have the advantage of being relatively easy to arrive at, but they present only one part of the story.

Figures for GNP per capita and various other social and economic measurements are published by the World Bank for almost every country in the world—180 countries. (The countries for which no information on GNP was available in 1992 are all socialist or formerly socialist countries: Albania, Cuba, the former German Democratic Republic, the People's Democratic Republic of Korea and the Commonwealth of Independent States—formerly the USSR). The reported countries are grouped by the World Bank into five categories, as shown in Table 7.2.

The 'low-income' countries are those with an annual GNP per head of up to $580 in 1989; they include China and India, which are shown separate from the others. The 'middle-income' countries had an annual GNP per head greater than $580 but less than $6 000, and are shown split into a 'lower' and an 'upper' category. The lower-middle-income group of countries includes, for example, Egypt, Turkey and Poland. Examples of countries in the upper-middle-income group include Brazil, Korea and Greece. The high-income countries all had an annual GNP per head of $6 000 or above; they include the United Kingdom, USA, Japan and Canada.

□ What proportion of the world's population live in countries with low-income or lower-middle-income economies (broadly, the Third World)?

■ Three-quarters of the world's population lives in these countries (mainly in the low-income countries).

Table 7.2 World shares of population and GNP, 1990

Country group	GNP per head/US dollars	(Of which foreign aid/US dollars)	Percentage of world* population	Percentage of world* GNP
Low-income economies	**(less than $580)**			
1 China and India	350	(2)	39.9	3.7
2 other low-income	300	(17)	20.5	1.6
Middle-income economies	**($580–6 000)**			
3 lower-middle-income	11 360	(17)	13.9	5.0
4 upper-middle-income	3 150	(2)	8.7	7.2
High-income economies	**(more than $6 000)**			
5 all high-income	18 330		17.0	82.4

*'World' excludes the following countries, for which no recent information is available on GNP: Albania, Cuba, former German Democratic Republic, People's Democratic Republic of Korea, and former USSR. (Data derived from World Bank, 1991, *World Development Report 1991*, Oxford University Press, Oxford and New York, Tables 1 and 19)

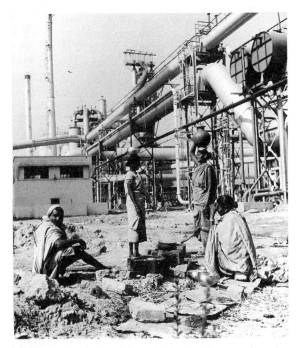

Preparing a mid-day meal outside the Durgarpur Steel Works, India. The uneven process of development which creates such contrasts is typical of many Third World countries. (Photo: Terry Fincher, Camera Press)

Perhaps the most striking thing about Table 7.2, however, is the final column showing the share of total world GNP taken by each group of countries.

☐ What proportion of world GNP is taken by the countries with upper-middle-income and high-income economies (broadly the industrialised countries), and how does this compare with the share taken by the low-income countries?

■ The 25 per cent of the world's population living in the upper-middle-income and high-income economies take almost 90 per cent of the world's GNP, whereas the 60 per cent of the world's population in low-income countries take only a tiny 5 per cent of the world's GNP.

Many measures other than GNP per head are often used to illustrate differences in social and economic development, and Table 7.3 shows a number of these **development indicators**, using the same income groupings used in Table 7.2.

☐ What patterns emerge from studying Table 7.3?

■ The table reveals that although adult literacy and secondary education are the norm in the high-income countries, they are common to only half or less of the population in low-income countries. The average daily supply of calories per person in the high-income countries is 40 per cent higher than in the low-income countries. And over three-quarters of the population in the high-income countries live in towns and cities, two or three times the proportion in the low-income countries.

☐ What evidence does the table contain of a gender gap?

■ In terms of literacy and access to secondary education, women do much worse than men in the low-income countries, but the gap narrows or disappears as we move up the national income scale.

Table 7.3 Selected development indicators, 1991

Country group	Percentage of adults who are literate (1985)		Average daily calorie (kcal) supply per person (1988)	Percentage of relevant age group in secondary education (1988)		Percentage of population living in large towns and cities (1989)
	All	Women		All	Women	
low-income economies						
China and India	58	46	2 407	43	34	42
other low-income	49	38	2 182	25	20	25
middle-income economies						
lower-middle-income	74	68	2 738	54	54	53
upper-middle-income	76	72	2 990	58	58	66
high-income economies	>95	>95	3 398	93	94	77

Data from World Bank (1991), *World Development Report 1991*, Oxford University Press, Oxford and New York, Tables 1, 28, 29, 31 and 32. > = greater than.

Table 7.4 Human development: North–South gaps

Indicator	North (industrialised countries)	South (non-industrialised countries) All	Least developed
total population in millions (and as a percentage of world population), 1990	1 210 (23%)	4 070 (77%)	440 (8%)
life expectancy at birth (years)	75	63	51
infant mortality rate (per 1 000 live births)	15	76	120
population with access to safe water (%)	>95	62	34
population with access to sanitation (%)	>95	46	23
scientists and technicians per 1 000 people	139	9	not known
radio sets per 1 000 people	1 021	173	88
daily newspapers per 1 000 people	342	34	12
percentage of labour force in agriculture	12	61	73
expenditure per person (taking North as index = 100) on			
food	100	34	19
health services	100	8	3
education	100	27	18
ratio of military to education + health spending	38 : 1	109 : 1	96 : 1

Data from United Nations Development Programme (1991) *Human Development Report 1991*, Oxford University Press, Oxford and New York, Tables 2, 3, 5, 7, 8, 14, 16, 19. > = greater than.

Looking across all the development indicators listed in the Table, the general pattern is that each indicator is better when national income is higher. This suggests that the World Bank's approach of classifying countries strictly on the basis of GNP per head does give a fair guide to many features of development. Nevertheless, a number of attempts have been made to devise alternative classifications. One of the simplest is 'North' (industrialised) and 'South' (non-industrialised), a split that was popularised in the 1980 'Brandt Report' on international development. Table 7.4 shows a variety of development indicators for 'North' and 'South'. The 'South' category has been split to show a group of **least developed countries**: these have been identified by the United Nations as suffering from one or more of the following: a GNP per head of less than $300 in 1990, a land-locked position, remote insularity, desertification and exposure to natural disasters. They include 39 countries, almost three-quarters of which are in Africa south of the Sahara.

The table first of all confirms the now-familiar pattern: that three-quarters of the world's population live in non-industrialised countries and have a substantially poorer health experience. No fewer than 440 million people live in the least developed countries.

☐ How many people in the South do not have access to safe water or sanitation?

■ Around 1 550 million people (38 per cent of the total population) are without access to safe water, and 2 200 million do not have access to sanitation, whereas there is almost universal access to these essential services in industrialised countries.

The other numbers and proportions in the table reveal just some aspects of the many differences that exist between industrialised and Third World countries. The bottom row of the table shows one final burden of the Third World, that military spending actually exceeds spending on education and health combined. Apart from the sheer financial cost and lost opportunities this represents, it also reflects a great human cost of war: on one estimate, there have been 106 civil or international wars since 1950, and all but 11 000 of the 19.5 million deaths that followed were in the Third World (Sivard, 1989).

Before leaving this survey of measures of social and economic development, let us look at an attempt to construct a more general 'Human Development Index'. The United Nations in 1990 published the first in a series of reports which argued that development was essentially the process of increasing people's options:

...the most critical choices that people should have include the options to lead a long and healthy life, to be knowledgeable and to find access to the assets, employment and income needed for a decent standard of living. (United Nations Development Programme, 1991 p. 88)

Taking this view, development cannot be measured by income alone, and so the UN proposed a new **Human Development Index** based on three separate components: life expectancy, educational attainment, and a measure of income which gives a progressively lower weight to income above the poverty level (the thinking behind this last component being that above a certain level the contribution of an extra unit of income to human development begins to decline).

☐ Consider the main components of the Human Development Index. Can you think of any important items that are omitted?

■ One important omission is that the index does not embrace any measure of human freedom: freedom of speech or assembly, enfranchisement, freedom from arbitrary rule or illegal arrest or torture, and so on.

Despite this and other limitations, the Human Development Index has proved a useful innovation. In all, the UN has applied the index to 160 countries, and when they are ranked from best (= 1) to worst (= 160) using the index it is perhaps not surprising to find that the overall ranking is broadly similar to that which would be obtained if the same countries were to be ranked simply on the basis of GNP per head. However, some interesting differences do emerge: some countries had a human development ranking well *below* their GNP ranking, while others did much *better* on the Human Development Index than might have been predicted on the basis of their GNP per head. Figure 7.1 attempts to illustrate these discrepancies for a small sample of countries.

If GNP rank and human development rank are the same, the country will be on the diagonal line. Below the line, countries are doing worse in terms of human development than their GNP per person would indicate, suggesting that they have the resources to improve their performance in life expectancy and educational provision. Above the line, human development is higher than would be predicted on the basis of GNP, suggesting that health and education have been higher priorities, or that resources have been used more effectively.

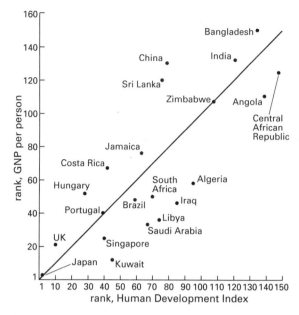

Figure 7.1 *Scattergram showing relationship between GNP rank and Human Development Index rank, 1992. Rank ordering: best = 1; worst = 160. (Data derived from United Nations Development Programme, 1992,* Human Development Report 1992, *Oxford University Press, Oxford and New York, Table 1)*

☐ Looking at the figure, how would you describe the broad association between GNP and human development?

■ The association is strongly positive for most countries in the sample. Countries with a high ranking on GNP per person also tend to have a high ranking on the Human Development Index, and those with a low ranking on one index also tend to rank low on the other.

☐ Which countries appear to diverge most markedly from this pattern?

■ Sri Lanka and China, for example, are ranked in terms of GNP per head at a point close to the Central African Republic, but their rank on the Human Development Index is much better. Hungary has a rank of GNP per head almost the same as South Africa's, but does significantly better on the Human Development Index (in fact life expectancy is 9 years longer and the infant mortality rate is only a quarter of South Africa's—17 compared with 68 per 1 000 live births in 1989). And Saudi Arabia and Kuwait have very high GNP per head ranks, but do no better in human development terms than a much poorer country such as Jamaica.

Those countries which do diverge from the more general pattern of health and development give some interesting clues as to the limitations of the 'league-table' approach. In the first place, it can be grossly misleading to talk about national averages. South Africa, for example, had a per capita GNP of US $2 470 in 1989, putting it in among the 'upper-middle-income' group of countries. But within South Africa the consequences of apartheid are that 5 million whites have health and income levels comparable with those of Western Europe, whereas the 30 million black and 'coloured' (mainly Asians) peoples have health and income levels more similar to the pattern in low-income countries: in 1985 the IMR per 1 000 live births in South Africa was 12.3 among whites, 51.9 among 'coloureds' (mainly Asian), and approximately 109 among blacks. Similarly, in Brazil, over the period from 1960 to 1983, the share of national income taken by the poorest 50 per cent of the population fell from 17 per cent to around 13 per cent, while the share of the wealthiest 1 per cent rose from 12 per cent to 18 per cent. Thus, although the average per capita GNP of Brazil grew relatively rapidly, the distribution of income within the country became even more unequal. In turn, the average values of Brazil's health indicators conceal very wide variations between a wealthy elite and a great mass of rural poor and urban shanty dwellers.

By contrast, one of the reasons for Sri Lanka's relatively good health indicators is that, although per capita GNP is not high, attempts have been made to pursue a more equitable distribution. In particular, the Sri Lankan government has long operated a food-distribution programme, issuing ration books or coupons for essential commodities, running a state system of food subsidies to the low-income sections of the population, and providing special protein-enriched food supplements to school children. In Chapter 8 we will look in a little more detail at the policies for improving health which low-income countries such as Sri Lanka have pursued.

Distribution, therefore, is as important as any average figure or total amount of wealth, and although this is particularly so of poor countries, it is also true of industrial countries, as you will see when you study the United Kingdom in Chapters 9 and 10 of this book.

Another facet of the relationship between health and development can be seen in the experiences of the countries of central and eastern Europe, including the former USSR—the **Second World**. Until the late 1980s, when communist rule in these countries collapsed, they had been run for many decades as 'command' economies. In effect, planners in government offices attempted to direct the economy by issuing directives and decrees which laid down wages, prices and levels of production. This system seemed for a time to produce rapid rates of economic growth and industrialisation, but at a cost of tremendous inefficiency and profligate energy use, resulting in extensive environmental pollution and degradation, and in widespread social malaise which eventually contributed to the collapse of the old regimes. These problems in turn seem to have had a significant impact on the health of populations in these countries (although detailed documentary evidence on this only began to be made available after the collapse of communist rule, and was still emerging when this book was being written in 1992). For example, the eastern part of Germany failed to keep up with the health improvements in West Germany after 1945. And Figure 7.2 shows some data from the USSR on trends in average life expectancy.

The figure shows that average life expectancy in the USSR seems to have improved rapidly until the mid-1950s. This then slowed down, and during the later 1970s and early 1980s appears to have gone into reverse, with life expectancy actually falling. By 1986 the deterioration has ended, but average life expectancy by this date is no better than it was 15 years previously.

This pattern of falling average life expectancy during the 1970s has been documented in every one of the 17 Republics of the USSR. The reasons are still being researched, but were almost certainly a combination of factors including environmental pollution and occupational hazards, lagging standards of medical care, an

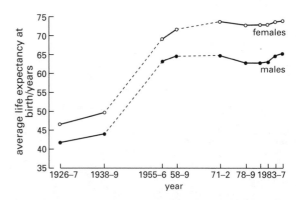

Figure 7.2 *Average life expectancy (in years) of men and women in the USSR, 1926–27 to 1986–87. Each point on the graph represents the average over a two-year period, the last four being 1983–4, 1984–5, 1985–6 and 1986–7. (Data from Rockney, B. P., 1991, Soviet Statistics since 1950, Dartmouth, Aldershot, Table 38, p. 81)*

epidemic of alcoholism, and possibly the long-term consequences of injuries, wounds and deprivations sustained during World War II. But the essential point, following on from the previous discussion, is that economic growth and industrialisation do not automatically translate into health gains, and indeed have within them the potential to damage health unless they are properly managed.

So far, you have seen that the link between national wealth and measures of human development such as education and health is much less straightforward than is sometimes claimed. This is crucially important when considering policies to improve health, as you will see in the following chapter. However, another major issue is that GNP league tables suggest a ladder of progress, with different countries on different rungs but all heading in the same direction (upwards), and separated only by the time they set off. How true is this?

Closing the gap?

Clearly there are very wide differences in both wealth and health between industrialised and Third World countries. It could be argued, however, that this is the inevitable short-term consequence of some countries industrialising before others, that where there are pioneers there must also be late-comers, but in time the late-comers will catch up. We can begin to explore the validity of this catching-up concept by looking at the relative rates of growth of GNP in different countries.

The first column of Table 7.5 shows the average annual rate of growth of total GNP for each of the three main groups of countries over the period from 1965 to 1989.

Table 7.5 World rates of economic growth, 1965–89

	Average annual growth rate (%) in	
	GNP, 1965–89	GNP per person, 1965–89
low-income economies	5.1	2.9
(of which) China	7.9	5.7
all others	4.2	1.6
middle-income economies	4.5	2.5
high-income economies	3.6	2.4

Data derived from World Bank (1991), *World Development Report 1991*, Oxford University Press, Oxford and New York, Tables 1.5, A.2 and 2.

□ What light does the first column of Table 7.5 cast on the idea that the non-industrial countries of the world are catching up with the industrial countries?

■ The average annual growth rate of GNP was higher in the low-income and middle-income groups of countries than in the high-income group, suggesting that there was some narrowing of the gap.

□ Now look at the second column of Table 7.5, which shows the average annual rate of growth of GNP *per person* over the same period. What is the reason for the difference between the first and second columns?

■ The GNP per person is calculated by dividing the total GNP by the population. The differences are explained by population growth.

If the population of a country is increasing, the GNP per person will not grow as quickly as total GNP. The bigger the difference between the two columns the higher the increase in population must be. For the high-income group of countries the difference between GNP growth and GNP per person growth is around 1 per cent, but for the other groups of countries it is much wider: between 2.2 and 2.6 per cent. The effect is that, although the total GNP in the lower-income countries grew substantially more rapidly than in the high-income group, the gap between the lower-income countries and the high-income group in GNP per person hardly closed.

It is important to remember that by bundling many countries into just three groups many differences will be lost among average figures. Looking more closely at Table 7.5, for example, you can see that the growth in GNP per person in the low-income countries has been strongly influenced by the above average performance of China, and that, excluding China (which contains about one-third of the population of the whole low-income group), the rate of growth of GNP per person was in fact much lower than in the middle- or high-income groups. For these countries, therefore, containing around 2 billion of the world's poorest people, the gap dividing them from the rest of the world appears to have been growing.

One last step in this exploration is taken in Figure 7.3.

It shows that, overall, the low- and middle-income countries of the world experienced a higher rate of growth in GNP per person than the high-income countries during much of the 1960s and 1970s. But during the 1980s, when the pace of growth quickened in many countries, some groups of low- and middle-income countries began falling behind not only relatively but in

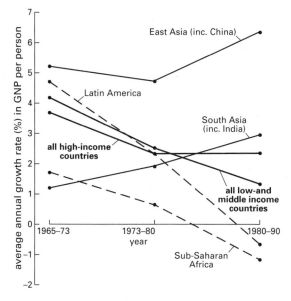

Figure 7.3 *World rates of economic growth, by region, 1965–90. (Data derived from World Bank, 1991,* World Development Report 1991, *Oxford University Press, Oxford and New York, Table A)*

absolute terms. The populations of Latin America and the Caribbean (and also those in eastern Europe and the Middle East and North Africa) experienced falling incomes. And for the countries of Sub-Saharan Africa the 1980s were especially grim. There, around 500 million of the poorest people in the world have been getting poorer, with everything that implies for their health, welfare and prospects for survival.

There is no single reason for the experience of these latter countries; in some, wars or revolutions have caused economic and social dislocation, others have been affected by droughts or other ecological changes to which they have been unable to respond unaided. But an underlying problem has been that their growth in total GNP, which in most cases averaged over 2 per cent each year during the 1980s, was outstripped by a rate of growth of population which exceeded 3 per cent. Once again, therefore, we can see that population change is inseparable from social and economic development, which in turn is linked to health and disease patterns, but that—in the Third World as in the case of England—these links are not straightforward. Many of the same issues arise when we consider one aspect of economic activity that is fundamentally important to health: food production.

Food production

Measuring a country's **food production** raises many of the same difficulties encountered in measuring GNP. The normal procedure is to estimate the amount of food which comes onto the market in a country, by first calculating for each type of food crop the total area planted multiplied by the yield per unit of area. Then all types of food crops and all the producers in a country are added together to obtain a total. Imported food is added, and exports and any food grains fed to animals are subtracted. A correction is then made for losses in storage and during milling and processing and the remainder is converted into equivalent amounts of nutrients (protein, fat, etc.) and energy, using average figures for the chemical composition of each foodstuff. Finally, the result is divided by the current estimate of the total population of the country to give an estimate of food supplies per person.

Some of the pitfalls in this method are obvious. In Third World countries, where a large part of production is in the hands of small family farms, many of these stages are a source of systematic under-reporting: farmers the world over are conservative and pessimistic about their prospects and wary of giving information which might be used to assess land and production taxes. Their estimates of food retained for their own families tend to be minimal. Many countries have long and poorly regulated borders and, if price differences across these borders provide incentives to import or export illegally, there may be large volumes of unreported food movement. And when times are bad, because of drought or recession, large numbers of small farmers may simply withdraw from the market, return to a subsistence pattern of life and wait for better times.

In industrialised countries, the basic statistics of land use, yields, imports and exports are probably much more accurate and the numbers of producers very much smaller. The problems are more in the distribution system. Somewhere in between primary production and the purchase of food by households, around 20–30 per cent of food measured by its energy value goes astray. The more highly industrialised the food processing and retailing system, the greater the losses. Probably a good deal of this is not actual waste, but represents a diversion of some by-products of the food industry into other non-food processes. These systematic errors in the recording of food production create a tendency to underestimate available food in predominantly agricultural populations and to their overestimation in industrial countries.

Table 7.6 Total food production of the world, developed (including the 'Second World') and developing countries, 1989

| Food type | Total annual production (million tonnes) | | | | | |
	World	%	Developed	%	Developing	%
cereal (wheat, rice, coarse grain)	**1 940.8**	100	928.7	48	1 012.1	52
meat	**170.1**	100	103.3	61	66.8	39
milk	**543.6**	100	288.0	53	155.7	47
sugar	**108.1**	100	44.5	41	63.6	59
population/millions	**(5 280)**	100	(1 210)	23	(4 070)	77

Data from Food and Agriculture Organisation (1991), *The State of Food and Agriculture 1990*, FAO, Rome, Table 1.3.

Bearing these problems in mind, what is the current pattern of food production in the world? Table 7.6 shows the way in which world production of a variety of foods is split between developed and developing countries.

☐ What strikes you about the distribution in 1989 of food production compared with population, as shown in Table 7.6?

■ The developed world, with less than one-quarter of the world's population, produces almost half of the world's most important foodstuffs (cereals) and well over half of the world's milk and meat.

This dominance of the developed world as a whole in global food production is paralleled in the world trade in foodstuffs. The developed countries have a dominance of the international food trade greater than the Middle East has ever attained in the oil trade: for example, during the 1980s they accounted for almost three-quarters of wheat exports.

Although the developed world dominates global food production and trade, there was a large increase in food production in the Third World as a whole during the 1970s and 1980s: between 1965 and 1988 the production of cereals and of meat, milk and fish more than doubled, while root crop production increased by more than 50 per cent. However, these average figures disguise many variations in different regions and countries of the world and, as with GNP growth, they have to be adjusted to take into account population growth. Figure 7.4 shows an index of food production per person for major regions of the Third World, taking the level of production in 1970 as an index number of 100, and covering the period to 1990.

☐ Summarise the main features of Figure 7.4.

■ In four of the five regions shown, there has been an increase in food production per person since 1970, although in some regions, such as Latin

America and the Near East, there has been little increase during the 1980s. However, in Africa there has been a long-term decline in food production per person, going back to the 1970s.

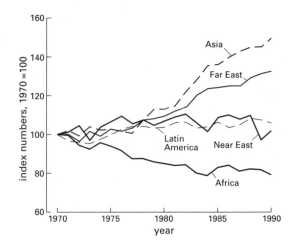

Figure 7.4 *Index of food production per person in Third World regions, 1965–90 (1970 = 100). (Data from World Resources Institute, 1992,* World Resources 1992–93, *Oxford University Press, Oxford and New York, Figure 7.6, p. 96)*

The difficulties of measuring accurately a country's food production were noted earlier, and these should be borne in mind when considering the data in Figure 7.4. In particular, there is an argument that food production in Sub-Saharan Africa has deteriorated *less* than the official figures indicate, and that a substantial amount of food production, exchange and consumption goes unrecorded. If the official figures were telling the whole story, continues this argument, then one would not expect to observe life expectancy continuing to rise and infant mortality rates continuing to fall in the region. And yet this has happened, as Chapter 2 indicated.

Despite these qualifications, it does seem that Sub-Saharan Africa faces uniquely difficult problems: as you saw earlier in this chapter, GNP per person also declined during the 1980s, and many other indicators of health and development are the worst of all the world's major regions. And as with the GNP decline, there are many possible reasons why it might be difficult for food production to keep pace with population growth.

One factor is the physical environment, which is very poor for farming: a large portion of the continent is desert or too sandy to farm, much of the land is almost unusable because it is infested with tsetse flies, which transmit to humans and cattle the parasites (*Trypanosoma* species) that cause sleeping sickness (*trypanosomiasis*)— a slowly progressive infestation of the nervous system resulting eventually in abnormal behavioural patterns, coma and death. Rainfall is low and droughts are normal.

Historically, farmers in Africa have adapted their farming methods to these conditions, for example by leaving land fallow sufficiently long for it to recover from cropping. However, these sustainable farming methods have been jeopardised by growing population pressures, so that, for example, land is given insufficient time to recover from cropping, or vegetation is removed for fuelwood, which is the major source of energy in this region.

Another factor has been damaging policies, such as price controls on foods, which give farmers little incentive to increase production, or too much investment in urban areas at the expense of rural roads and towns.

Finally, a substantial number of countries in this region have been afflicted since the 1970s by political instability and at worst by civil or international wars: the list includes Angola, Chad, Ethiopia, Mozambique, Nigeria, Somalia, Sudan and Uganda. These wars have disrupted food production, created large numbers of refugees, hindered aid efforts, and diverted scarce resources into military expenditure.

However, the countries of Sub-Saharan Africa affected by this gap between population growth and food production would not necessarily be headed for crisis if they were able to purchase food from other countries. After all, many countries of the world—the United Kingdom is a good example—no longer grow enough food to feed themselves, but do not have any problem feeding their populations because they are able to export other commodities in exchange for food imports. It could be argued, therefore, that the fundamental problem in the Sub-Saharan region is not so much that food production in this part of the world has failed to keep pace with population growth, as that the region is not earning enough from its exports to afford to import enough food to meet its requirements.

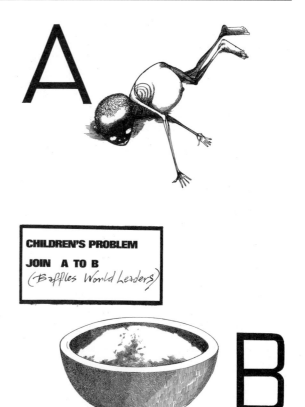

Gerald Scarfe, 1970.

This raises a general issue: if we are interested in the ability of a nation to feed itself, it is misleading to focus on national food production without taking into account the ability of that nation to obtain its food requirements from elsewhere. And what is true at the national or regional level is also true of individuals: obtaining food does depend in part on what is produced, but it also depends on such crucial issues as distribution, access and 'entitlement'. As you will see below, this important point is dramatically illustrated by famines.

Entitlement, food and famine

One image of Third World countries that is all too familiar is probably that of a black child with arms and legs of skin and bones and a swollen belly, caught in the middle of drought, famine or simply pervasive and chronic malnutrition and poverty. Insufficient food is a major contributory cause of much death and disease, and seems to be another defining characteristic of the Third World.

Famines raise in a tragic and acute way the need to take into account the social and economic circumstances in which they occur. They have been the subject of a great deal of research, and one theory which helps to explain their occurrence and the persistence of other forms of food insecurity has been developed by the economist Amartya Sen. An extract from a book by Sen and Jean Drèze entitled *Hunger and Public Action* is included in *Health and Disease: A Reader.*[3]

☐ Before reading this extract, write down as briefly as possible your own view of why famines occur. Then read the extract before continuing with this chapter and compare your view with Sen and Drèze's comments on how famines occur. How does it differ?

■ Of course we can't claim to know what your earlier views were. But most probably you would have held to the common assumption that famines occur because of a shortage of food. However, Sen and Drèze argue that it is quite misleading to focus only on food supply; what is much more important, they argue, is the ability of people to procure food, or entitlement.

The system of **entitlement relations**, which govern whether or not people can get hold of food, is of central importance to Sen and Drèze.

☐ Why do Sen and Drèze claim that it is misleading to focus only on the *supply* of food?

■ Famines can occur even if there is no overall shortage of food, as a consequence of some groups having no 'entitlement' to what is available.

To illustrate their argument, Sen and Drèze examine a famine that occurred in Bangladesh towards the end of 1974. You have already seen that it is often extremely difficult to obtain reliable health statistics in Third World countries, and not surprisingly there is no agreement over how many people may have lost their lives as a consequence of this famine: the absolute minimum is approximately 26 000 deaths, but the estimates range up to 1.5 million deaths.

Between June and August in 1974 severe flooding occurred in northern Bangladesh as the Brahmaputra river burst its banks, and this event seemed to point to the common-sense conclusion that the food supply had been

[3]*Health and Disease: A Reader* (Open University Press, 1984; revised edition 1994).

badly hit and people went hungry in consequence. Once again, however, a careful look at the data reveals a much more complex picture.

☐ Table 7.7 shows the average availability per capita of all food-grains in Bangladesh for the years 1971–5, measured in ounces per day. What do you notice about 1974, the year the famine occurred?

■ The availability of food-grain in this year was actually higher than in the surrounding years.

Table 7.7 Availability of food-grains in Bangladesh, 1967–76, compared with availability in 1967 (given an index value = 100)

Year	Grain availability per day/ounces per person	Index (1967 = 100)
1967	15.0	100
1968	15.7	105
1969	16.6	111
1970	17.1	114
1971	14.9	99
1972	15.3	102
1973	15.3	102
1974 (famine)	15.9	106
1975	14.9	99
1976	14.8	99

Data from Drèze, J. and Sen, A. (1989) *Hunger and Public Action*, Clarendon Press, Oxford, Table 2.1, p. 27.

Not only was 1974 the least likely year for a famine to have occurred if we look at total food supply, but the districts of Bangladesh most seriously affected by famine tended to be those which, if anything, had *increased* their food supply in 1974 by more than the average for the country as a whole.

In fact the Bangladesh famine of 1974 is a good illustration of the way in which an initial event can trigger a series of changes which may compound and magnify the consequences, further destabilising the situation instead of returning it to equilibrium. In the language of systems technology, we might think of **positive and negative feedback loops**: a thermostat which responds to an increase in an oven's temperature by reducing power to the oven and so maintaining equilibrium is an example of negative feedback, whereas a thermostat which responds to a rise in the oven's temperature by further increasing the supply of power to the oven and thus

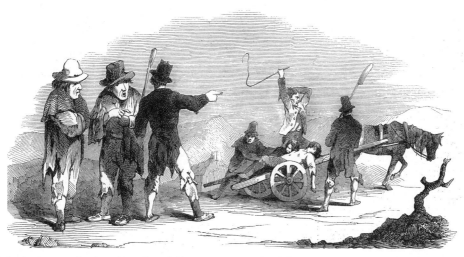

The famine in Ireland—a funeral at Skibbereen. (From a sketch by Mr H. Smith, Cork; Illustrated London News, *30 January 1847)*

accentuates the disequilibrium is an example of positive feedback. Complex models of biological systems such as the human body have now been devised, with many coexisting positive and negative feedback loops.[4] But some simpler models fail to acknowledge that positive feedback may occur. For example, the Malthusian population model outlined in Chapter 6 suggests a world of negative feedback loops which automatically restore equilibrium.

In the Bangladesh famine of 1974, those most seriously affected by the famine were the wage-labourers, and their employment opportunities and therefore income were severely reduced by the flooding. At the same time, the price of food rose very sharply in response to an expectation of a damaged harvest in 1975, and also perhaps because of panic buying or hoarding. These price rises compounded the reduction in the entitlement to food of this part of the population, leading to destitution, famine and, for many, death.

One of the best-known famines occurred in the nineteenth century—the potato famine in Ireland of 1845–9. During this period, it seems likely that the population of Ireland fell by almost one-third, from roughly 9 million to 6.5 million. Of this 'lost' 2.5 million, nearly one million people emigrated, and the rest died of hunger, disease

and fever. A conventional view of this event would be that the potato crop, a staple in the diet of most of the Irish population at the time, had been ruined several years in a row by a blight or disease, leading to a straightforward food shortage.

The closer we look at this event, however, the more the facts seem to fit the 'entitlement' approach. In the first place, large quantities of cattle, corn and other foodstuffs were being produced normally throughout the famine years and exported to England in quantities that would have been sufficient to avert the famine had the Irish population had the means to obtain them. Second, although the English Parliament cheapened the price of grain in 1846 by repealing the Corn Laws in a proclaimed attempt to make grain more accessible to the Irish, the reality of the situation was that the Irish tenant farmers grew grain to pay rent to the landowners, and the falling price of grain increased their rent and thus their poverty, and made them liable to eviction through an inability to meet the landowners' demands. Again, the social and economic organisation of Ireland, and its colonial relations with England, were of more importance than the absolute quantity of food being produced in Ireland at the time. Hence the Irish saying 'God sent the blight; but the English landlords sent the Famine!'.

[4]These models are discussed in *Studying Health and Disease* (Open University Press, revised edition, 1994) and *The Biology of Health and Disease* (Open University Press, 1985; revised as *Human Biology and Health: An Evolutionary Approach*, 1994)

Famine, of course, is only the most spectacular instance of a breakdown in the system of entitlements to food, and these systems can vary widely from one country to another with correspondingly different consequences. In India, for example, periodic famine no longer occurs, but substantial sections of the population suffer from chronically inadequate access to food. In China, by contrast, the normal lot of the population is much better, and entitlement to food is comprehensive. But it now seems clear that occasional large-scale famines have occurred. In 1959–61, for example, it has been estimated that up to 15 million people may have died in China because of famine conditions to which the government was unable to respond rapidly. (The impact of this event on the subsequent demographic structure of the Chinese population was noted in Chapter 3.)

Sen has suggested that this difference may be caused by the political processes which affect and influence the system of entitlements. In India, relatively independent media and competing political parties act to ensure that sudden famine is at least newsworthy and considered a political liability to be avoided, but chronic long-term hunger is neither newsworthy nor politically intolerable to the main parties. In China, the state is committed to and can ensure regular access and a more equal entitlement to food. But because its political system is centralised, Sen argues, it can pursue policies which may have completely unintended and (for a time) unknown consequences. Indeed not until 1983, over 20 years after this famine, was its occurrence officially acknowledged by the Chinese Government, following publication of a detailed account by a Chinese economist in the *New York Review of Books*.

One other aspect of entitlement that requires greater emphasis relates to gender. Chapter 3 discussed the phenomenon of 'missing' women, and noted that it occurs mainly in areas of the world (especially in the Indian sub-continent and China) where, in comparison with men, women have restricted access to paid employment, fewer land rights, and less freedom of movement. They thus have fewer opportunities to secure entitlement to goods and services, and, although there is no conclusive evidence that in countries such as Bangladesh the division of food within families is to the disadvantage of women and girls, there is a good deal of evidence that they receive less parental attention and that their entitlement to health care is impaired.

In conclusion, therefore, the concept of entitlement seems to be a valuable way of helping to understand the relationship between health and disease patterns and social and economic development. Equipped with this concept, it no longer seems so paradoxical, for example, that during the 1980s no fewer than 42 of the 77 countries

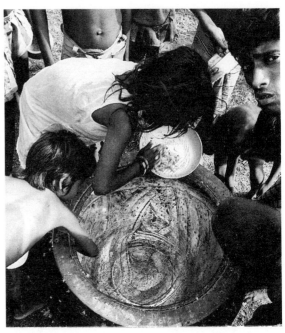

Scraping the bowl. A government feeding programme averts famine in Jinjira, near Dhaka, Bangladesh, following floods in August 1980. (Photo: Tom Learmonth)

in the world which had inadequate food supplies for their own populations were also net food-exporters.

The entitlement approach also opens a new perspective on the contribution of Malthus to the debate on the relationship between population and food. By rejecting Malthusian pessimism on the grounds that food production at the global level is keeping ahead of population growth, we may run the risk of falling into an equally unwarranted trap of Malthusian optimism: that as long as food production is keeping ahead of population growth there is nothing to worry about. The point is that food production is just one of a range of factors determining entitlements, and to focus on some ratio of food to population as Malthus and many others have done is to see only one element of a much more complex picture.

Similarly, as you saw earlier in this chapter, it cannot be assumed that the level or rate of growth of GNP per person can be equated with levels of health or human development: again, there is some connection, but it is much less direct than is sometimes thought.

Finally, it should be clear from the evidence in this chapter that population growth remains a crucial factor in understanding trends in GNP and in food production in different regions of the world. The next chapter therefore begins by examining these population trends.

OBJECTIVES FOR CHAPTER 7

When you have studied this chapter you should be able to:

7.1 Discuss some of the main consequences of the Industrial Revolution for the countries that now form the Third World, particularly in agriculture and industry.

7.2 Explain what GNP and the Human Development Index (HDI) measure and what their main limitations are.

7.3 Evaluate the evidence on whether the gap in income per head between rich and poor in the world is narrowing or widening.

7.4 Outline recent trends in food production in different areas of the world, and some of the problems in interpreting these data.

7.5 Describe and illustrate the entitlement approach to famine.

QUESTIONS FOR CHAPTER 7

Question 1 *(Objective 7.1)*

The United Kingdom during the Industrial Revolution was often described as 'the workshop of the world'. From Table 7.1, how true was this?

Question 2 *(Objectives 7.2)*

The United Nations Development Programme has argued that the Human Development Index broadens the development dialogue from a discussion of mere *means* (GNP growth) to a discussion of the ultimate ends. To what extent do you think the HDI does succeed in doing this?

Question 3 *(Objective 7.3)*

'The Third World may be a lot poorer, but by sheer weight of numbers it must account for a big share of total world economic activity. After all, India is one of the top ten world industrial producers.' How valid is this line of reasoning?

Question 4 *(Objective 7.4)*

In what ways do the measurement of food production per person and the measurement of GNP per person face common difficulties?

Question 5 *(Objective 7.5)*

The entitlement approach argues that food availability is an inadequate and misleading way of viewing famine. Does this mean that food availability and entitlement are not linked?

8 Population and development prospects

In Chapter 7 you saw that there is no simple link between national wealth and levels of health or human development. Some countries have lower mortality and longer life expectancy than might be predicted on the basis of their GNP per person, others do less well. This chapter begins by placing such findings in a broader context: it looks in more detail at population change in the Third World, then considers the evidence of a link between economic development and the demographic transition described in Chapter 6. It then looks at some of the ways in which countries have attempted to promote the demographic transition, not simply by relying on economic development, but by pursuing policies explicitly aimed at lowering their birth rates and their mortality rates. The chapter concludes with a brief survey of some of the major obstacles to development facing Third World countries.

Population change in the Third World

Global trends

As Chapter 7 illustrated, rates of **population growth** are a crucial factor in understanding trends in GNP and in food production in different regions of the world. They also represent one of the main differences between the industrialised countries and the Third World. Figure 8.1 shows some features of the rate of population growth in the more developed and less developed countries, based on United Nations estimates.

Comparing the 1950s with the 1990s, perhaps the most striking thing about changes in the growth rate of the world's population as a whole is that it has hardly changed, being only fractionally lower in 1985–90 than forty-five years earlier.

☐ Compare the growth rates of the more and less developed countries. How have they changed over time?

■ The growth rate in the less developed countries is substantially higher than in the more developed countries. For example, in the years 1985–90, it averaged 2.1 per cent per year in the less developed countries, and 0.5 per cent in the developed countries. The difference appears to be widening, mainly because population growth rates in the developed world have fallen, while in the less developed countries they have remained fairly constant.

However, although the average annual rate of growth has not changed very much, the actual number of additional people per year in the world has been rising steadily: 1.7 per cent of 5.3 billion in 1990 is a lot more than 1.7 per cent of 2.5 billion in 1950. In fact, whereas in 1950 the annual increase in the world's population was around 45 million, by 1990 this had risen to an extra 93 million people every year. This is equivalent to a new Mexico every 12 months, or another United Kingdom every 7 months.

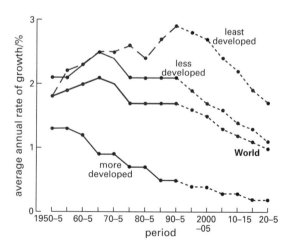

Figure 8.1 *World population growth rates, 1950–2025. (Data from United Nations, 1989,* World Population Prospects 1988, *Population Studies No. 106, UN, New York, Table 2.2, and United Nations, 1990,* World Population Monitoring 1989: Special Report: the Population Situation of the Least Developed Countries, *UN, New York, Table 1)*

Population projections

On the basis of current trends, it is estimated that between 1990 and 2025 the world's population is likely to increase by 60 per cent, from 5.2 billion to 8.5 billion, even though the rate of growth is projected to slow everywhere (Figure 8.1). And, as you saw in Table 2.1, most of this increase—in fact more than 95 per cent of the growth—will take place in the less developed countries.

In 1992 the United Nations Population Division produced some much longer term world **population projections**, stretching into the middle of the twenty-second century. Figure 8.2 shows three of these projections. (The main difference between them concerns the assumptions made about the pace of change in birth rates, especially after the year 2025, and we will discuss birth rates in more detail shortly.)

Using the medium projection, the global population would eventually stabilise at 11.6 billion people in the second half of the twenty-second century, a little more than double the population in 1990. Most of this increase (almost 90 per cent) would be between the years 1990 and 2050, with an increasingly rapid slow-down after that date. In the high projection, the population would have reached 28 billion in the year 2150 and would still be rising rapidly. Finally, using the low projection, world population would reach 7.8 billion by the year 2050 and would then decline, so that by the year 2150 it would stand at 4.8 billion, or some way below the figure in 1990.

To give some idea of the way in which population growth might affect individual countries, we can look at some estimates by the World Bank of the hypothetical size of countries on reaching a stationary state *if current trends continue*: many countries will not reach a state in which their population is stable until the twenty-second century, by which time, for example, the population of Bangladesh would have risen from around 111 million in 1992 to over 295 million at steady state, of Uganda from 17 million to 119 million, and of Ethiopia from 49 million to 435 million. These are not *predictions*; they are simply projections of current trends, but they do illustrate very forcefully the impact of a population growth rate when compounded over time.

Of course, such long-term projections are highly speculative, and the passage of a fairly short time can lead demographers to change their assumptions and forecasts quite substantially. The eventual world population in the 1992 medium forecast is about 10 per cent higher than the previous UN long-term projection made only ten years previously in 1982, mainly because the declining trend of birth rates during the 1960s and 1970s slowed down during the 1980s. Nevertheless, as you will recall from the discussion of population pyramids in Chapter 2,

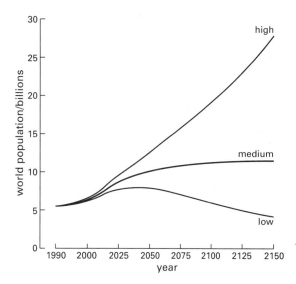

Figure 8.2 *The projected population of the world, 1990–2150. (Data from United Nations Population Division, 1992,* Long-range World Population Projections: Two Centuries of Population Growth 1990–2150, *UN, New York)*

a population structure does have a tremendous amount of in-built momentum, so that even quite rapid changes in birth rates or death rates take time to feed through into changes in growth rates and age structure. Consequently, although forecasts beyond the middle of next century are very uncertain, it *is* certain, barring calamities, that the world's human population by 2025 will be several billion more than in 1990.

One possible such calamity is the AIDS epidemic, which gained ground throughout the 1980s. As you saw in Chapter 3, some of the countries most affected by AIDS are in Sub-Saharan Africa; in 1992 estimates of the total number of people with HIV in Africa ranged as high as 10 million. Various attempts have been made to project the impact of the AIDS epidemic on the population of countries in Sub-Saharan Africa, and one such exercise is shown in Table 8.1 overleaf.

□ According to Table 8.1, what impact would AIDS have on the likely population growth between 1987 and 1997?

■ It would reduce population growth by around a third in urban areas, but by less than 3 per cent in the rural areas. Overall, population growth would be only 7 per cent less than it would have been in the absence of the epidemic, despite the fact that almost half a million people would die from the disease in this hypothetical country of 20 million people.

Table 8.1 Potential impact of AIDS on population growth in a hypothetical central African country, 1987–97

	Urban/millions	Rural/millions	Total
population in 1987	2.943	16.712	**19.655**
likely population growth, 1987–97 assuming no AIDS impact	0.895	5.700	**6.595**
likely population in 1997 assuming no AIDS impact	3.838	22.412	**26.250**
probable AIDS deaths, 1987–97	0.320	0.159	**0.479**
likely population growth, 1987–97, allowing for impact of AIDS	0.575	5.541	**6.116**
likely population in 1997 allowing for impact of AIDS	3.518	22.253	**25.771**
per cent reduction in likely population growth as a result of AIDS	35.8%	2.8%	**7.3%**

Data from United Nations (1990) *World Population Monitoring 1989: Special Report: the Population Situation in the Least Developed Countries*, UN Population Studies No. 113, UN, New York, Table 48.

However, there is very little consensus among experts on such projections, and some projections do indicate an impact so drastic as to reverse population growth in some countries. And whatever the demographic impact, the AIDS epidemic is likely to impose a very heavy financial burden on some of the poorest countries in the world.

Mortality and fertility trends

What factors have most influenced the population changes that have occurred in recent decades in the Third World? Arithmetically, population growth occurs when the crude birth rate exceeds the crude death rate. As Figure 8.3 shows, the birth rate has been falling around

the world for many years and is projected to continue falling, but the crude death rate has also been falling at around the same rate, so the population has continued growing.

In the more developed countries, however, most of the major reductions in mortality have already occurred, so the falling birth rate has greatly slowed the rate of population growth. In the less developed countries a similar flattening off in mortality decline is projected to occur from the 1990s onwards, in time slowing the rate of population increase.

Turning to birth rates, we encounter a familiar measurement problem, namely that the crude birth rate

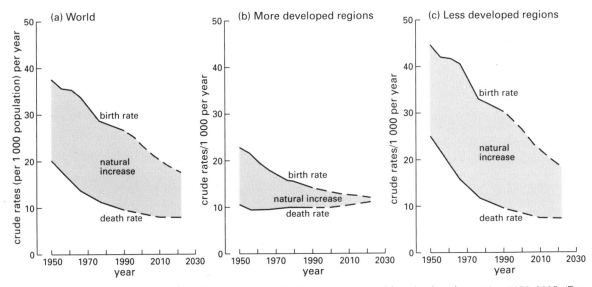

Figure 8.3 *Crude birth and death rates for the world, more developed countries and less developed countries, 1950–2025. (Data from United Nations, 1989,* World Population Prospects 1988, *Population Studies No. 106, UN, New York)*

is influenced by the age-structure of the population, as is the crude death rate. To overcome this problem, a good measure of the underlying trend in the birth rate is the **total period fertility rate (TPFR)**—the average number of children a woman would give birth to if she experienced the prevailing age-specific birth rates as she passed through the child-bearing ages. When a population has a low overall mortality rate, it will replace itself if each woman has 2.1 babies on average. If the overall mortality is high, as it is for example in most of the least developed countries, the replacement rate would be around 2.7 babies per woman. Figure 8.4 shows this fertility rate and how it is changing.

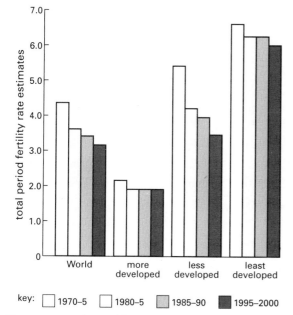

Figure 8.4 *Total period fertility rate estimates, 1970–5 to 1995–2000. (Data from United Nations, 1989,* World Population Prospects 1988, *Population Studies No. 106, UN, New York)*

☐ How would you summarise the data in Figure 8.4?

■ The total period fertility rate is much higher in the less developed than in the more developed countries (which have fallen below their replacement level of 2.1, although this takes time to feed through to actual population decline), and highest of all in the least developed group, where the rate is well above the replacement rate of 2.7 and in consequence produces strong population growth. The TPFR has been falling in all groups of countries, including the less

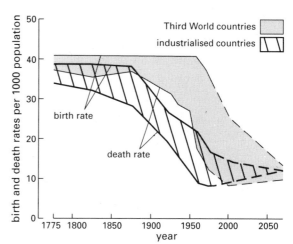

Figure 8.5 *Demographic transition? Birth and death rates in Third World and industrial countries, from 1775 to 1980 and projected to 2100. (Data from World Bank, 1982,* World Development Report 1982, *Oxford University Press, Oxford and New York, Figure 3.4)*

developed group as a whole, and this is projected to continue. But the decline is much less pronounced in the least developed group.

The countries in the 'least developed' group, as you have already seen, are mainly in Sub-Saharan Africa. There has been almost no change in TPFRs in Africa since the 1950s, but the UN projections assume that even there a fairly sharp decline will take place in the near future. By the year 2025 the UN projects that only Africa and Latin America will still be above the replacement level of fertility. If this does not happen, then it is more likely that the course of world population will be well above the medium projection of Figure 8.2.

Demographic transition?

How do changes in birth rates and death rates in the Third World compare with the pattern of change laid out in the model of demographic transition? The World Bank has assembled the available data on birth and death rates to produce a graph for the industrialised and Third World countries from 1775 onwards. This is shown in Figure 8.5, although it should be emphasised that the estimates for earlier periods, especially those for the Third World, are fairly speculative.

Using the model of demographic transition shown in Chapter 6 (Figure 6.8), it is possible to try to fit the four different stages of transition onto Figure 8.5. For the industrialised countries, it looks as if Stage 1 is at the left-hand edge of the figure, that is, up to the late eighteenth century. By 1800 the death rate is clearly falling while the birth rate remains high: this approximates to Stage 2. By around 1880 the birth rate has also started falling, while the decline in the death rate continues to accelerate: this is the broad pattern of Stage 3. By 1960 the death rate and the birth rate are beginning to stabilise at a much lower level—Stage 4 of the transition. Among the Third World countries, it seems that high birth rates and death rates (Stage 1) existed until around 1880. Then the death rate began to fall, but the birth rate remained high (Stage 2) until about 1960, when it too started to fall in a number of countries (Stage 3).

Although there are some apparent similarities between the past experience of the industrialised countries and present trends in the Third World, a number of differences should also be noted. First, the rate of growth of the Third World's population in the post-war period is unprecedented. Even at its peak, the average annual rate of growth of England's population did not go above 1.7 per cent, and for most of the Industrial Revolution was well below this, as Figure 6.2 showed. In some Third World countries the annual rate of population growth has gone as high as 4 per cent. Birth rates were never as high in England as they still are in much of the Third World. Mortality decline in England and other industrialised countries took place over a long period of time, whereas in the Third World it has happened quite rapidly. And the industrialising countries of the nineteenth century were able to export a large portion of their population growth in the form of international migration.

These differences help to explain why rapid population growth has sometimes been seen as an obstacle to development in the Third World, in a way which generally was not the case in the history of the industrialised countries.

Problems of population growth

Despite almost two centuries of research and debate, opinion on the relation between population and economic development is still divided much as it was in the age of Malthus and Godwin. Pessimists, such as the biologist Paul Ehrlich, argue that if population continues to grow it will inevitably collide with finite resources at some not-too-distant point, and the result will be a return on a grand scale of the old Malthusian checks of epidemic and famine (Ehrlich *et al.*, 1970). Optimists, of whom the most extreme is possibly the American economist Julian Simon, argue that resource limits are not fixed, but depend on technology, which is constantly advancing. From this perspective, human beings are the 'ultimate resource', and population growth could actually augment economic growth in the Third World (Simon, 1981).

So far, any evidence on the impact of population growth on economic development has been much less strong than are the opinions of these different protagonists. However, most recent surveys have concluded that, on balance, '...economic growth in many developing countries would have been more rapid in an environment of slower population growth' (Kelly, 1988, p. 1715). Examples of the negative consequences of rapid population growth are not hard to find: overgrazing and other land pressures have led in many areas to land degradation, erosion, deforestation (also caused by the search for fuel) and sometimes the creation of desert. Unemployment and underemployment lead to migration to the cities and the break-up of families. Apart from the human costs, high birth rates in countries where child mortality remains high have economic consequences. For example, a substantial portion of agricultural output may be consumed by people who die before reaching an age when they can contribute their labour.

Development prospects and problems

In addition to these population pressures, the development prospects of many Third World countries are uncertain. You saw in Chapter 7 that rates of economic growth vary widely across the Third World, with some of the lowest rates of growth—and indeed some absolute declines in GNP per person—among the world's poorest countries. Looking to the future, it seems likely that this pattern will persist. In 1992 the World Bank predicted that, as a whole, the countries of the Third World might anticipate more growth in the 1990s than they achieved in the 1980s, but that the growth of GNP in

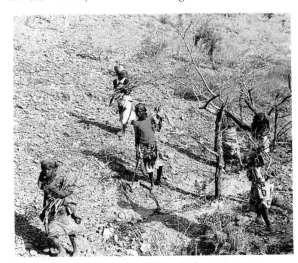

People collecting firewood in Africa. Deforestation is increasingly recognised as a major problem in many areas of the world. (Photo: OXFAM/Mark Edwards)

Sub-Saharan Africa would barely keep up with population growth during the 1990s, even on fairly optimistic assumptions (World Bank, 1992).

However, as with population projections, such forecasts of economic growth are based on a range of assumptions which may or may not prove valid. One such assumption is that the world's poorest countries will be able to export many more goods and services. At present, Third World exports often face trade barriers, which the industrialised countries use to protect their own industries and farmers. These trade restrictions have been growing rapidly in recent decades, and now affect more than a fifth of all imports from the Third World to industrialised countries. Another barrier to Third World exports is the vast amount industrialised countries spend on farm-subsidies, amounting to over $300 billion in 1990, or almost ten times their aid to the Third World. On one estimate, the restrictions on exports of goods and services alone were costing Third World countries almost $60 billion each year in 1990.

Another unsolved problem many Third World countries face is indebtedness to the industrialised countries. For most of the post-war period there was a net flow of resources from private banks and government agencies in the industrialised countries to the Third World. This grew rapidly during the 1970s, but much of the money was poorly invested or was simply used to buy consumer goods, while world interest rates rose, so that it became very difficult for many countries to repay these loans. They began sliding further and further into debt, until by 1990 total Third World debt was well over 1 trillion (thousand billion) dollars. In consequence, the traditional flow of resources from North to South has been reversed since 1982, and the less developed countries by 1990 were making a net transfer of almost $60 billion per year to the richest countries of the world. No fewer than 19 countries in the Third World had total external debts bigger than their entire Gross National Product, and the debt of Sub-Saharan Africa—$150 billion in 1990—was the same as the regions's total GNP.

Numerous proposals have been made to deal with this debt problem, but none offer the prospect of a rapid solution. Meanwhile, many Third World countries burdened by debt have been obliged to reduce expenditure on health, welfare and social support programmes, with health consequences that may only become fully apparent in the future.

One final problem faced by Third World countries (and another difference compared with the historical experience of the industrialised countries) is that these countries have to find their place in a world whose natural resources have already been depleted and whose environment has already been degraded by the first waves of industrialisation. In 1989, for example, energy consumption per person in the high-income countries of the world was almost 40 times greater than in the least developed countries (World Bank, 1991, Table 5), so that the 16 per cent of the world's population in these countries contributed around one half of the 'greenhouse' gases implicated in global warming.

Looked at another way, these figures indicate that the gulf in wealth between rich and poor countries is so great that the 5 per cent or so of total population growth attributable to the industrialised countries will consume approximately the same volume of the world's natural resources as the 95 per cent of the increase located in Third World countries. In this sense, many of the global problems of pollution are still primarily the responsibility of the industrialised countries.

If consumption of raw materials per person were to rise in the Third World to the levels currently prevailing in the industrialised world, then many of these raw materials would be exhausted in just a few years. And, while the industrialised world's profligacy creates one set of environmental problems, another arises from the Third World's poverty and inability to control its environment. Population pressure and poverty coupled with climatic change, for example, have led to desertification in many areas, notably the Sahel in Africa, resulting in an estimated 14 million environmental refugees.

This tension between the desire of three-quarters of the world's population to participate fully in industrialisation and the many pressing environmental problems already confronting the world has been well stated by the economic historian Carlo Cipolla:

> In order to improve their miserable standards of living, the underdeveloped and developing countries must undergo the Industrial Revolution. If they fail, they are condemned to abject misery. If they succeed, they will add greatly to the problems of pollution and depletion plaguing our planet today. (Cipolla, 1974, p. 120)

These are some of the most complex and possibly intractable problems that humanity has had to face so far: all that can be said with any certainty is that present trends cannot continue indefinitely. But, if they are to be stopped by the adoption of some more stable and sustainable relationship between humans and their natural environment, many observers believe that it will be necessary actively to promote policies to accelerate the decline in fertility rates in Third World countries. And, given the uncertain development prospects facing some major regions of the world, and the many obstacles to development that have to be overcome, it will also be necessary to look for ways of trying to improve health and further reduce mortality. In short, economic development cannot be relied upon alone to propel the demographic transition. Let us look first at policies to reduce fertility rates.

Promoting the decline of fertility rates

Influences on fertility

As you saw in Chapters 5 and 6, there are a number of influences on fertility, including marriage patterns, breast-feeding customs (breast-feeding suppresses ovulation and makes a woman significantly less likely to become pregnant), and the availability and reliability of contraception. The factors that might be related to fertility decline have been extensively studied in recent decades, and three broad areas have been identified: general socio-economic development, the cultural setting including prevailing religious beliefs, and government population policy.

Although these studies confirm that the overall level of development has the strongest influence in reducing fertility rates, they also show that some aspects of development are more important than others. In particular, higher levels of education (especially for women) and better child survival seem to be especially powerful influences. When these are coupled to energetic family planning programmes, most of the variation in fertility rates from country to country can be explained. Other measures of development, such as economic indicators of production or income, appear to add very little.

The powerful contribution of improved child survival to reducing fertility rates has been quantified by some studies, which have indicated that this factor has an impact on fertility decline up to three times stronger than that of family planning programmes.

□ Why might child survival rates be such an important influence on fertility rates?

■ When child survival rates are low, parents are likely to adopt an 'insurance' strategy, having more children than they actually want in case some die. As child survival improves, parents are more likely to have additional children only if existing ones die. In addition, lower infant mortality is likely to mean lengthened periods of breast-feeding, and this in turn increases the intervals between pregnancies.

As for government policy, the United Nations (1989) has reported that, in 1988, 68 countries in the world did not have any policies designed to alter their fertility rate, 61 had policies to lower their rate and 20 had policies to maintain their current fertility level. In addition, 21 countries were **pronatalist**, or wished to see a higher fertility rate and had policies to promote this objective (normally involving financial incentives and/or legal restrictions on abortion and contraception). Among this latter group were several European countries, including France, Hungary and Romania, and countries elsewhere including Argentina, Bolivia, Burma, Israel and Kampuchea.

Although **family planning programmes** are by no means the only or even the foremost influence on fertility rates, they are nevertheless an essential component of effective population policies. Table 8.2 summarises data on the current prevalence of contraceptive use in the world.

The table indicates that there is a substantial gap in contraceptive prevalence between the industrialised countries, where 70 per cent of married women of child-bearing age or their partners practice contraception, and the developing countries, where the comparable proportion is barely one-half. The contrast with the least developed countries is especially marked: there, fewer than one in five women of child-bearing age or their partners currently use contraception.

Table 8.2 World use of contraceptives, 1985–7

Country group	Contraceptive prevalence rate*, 1985–7	TPFR, 1990	Annual population growth rate, 1960–90
all developing countries	52	3.9	2.3
least developed	19	6.1	2.5
Sub-Saharan Africa	15	6.5	2.8
industrialised countries	70	1.9	0.8
world	**56**	**3.5**	**1.8**

* The percentage of married women of child-bearing age who are using, or whose husbands are using, any form of contraception: that is, modern or traditional methods. (Data from United Nations Development Programme, 1991, *Human Development Report 1991*, Oxford University Press, Oxford and New York, Tables 12 and 21)

Contraceptive prevalence rates for a number of individual countries are shown in Figure 8.6, which also indicates each country's Gross National Product per person.

☐ What is the relationship between contraceptive prevalence and GNP per person?

■ There seems to be a broadly positive relationship, but it is quite weak.

On the evidence of these data, it seems that there is a clear relationship between contraceptive prevalence and broad level of development, but that there is a great deal of variation between countries that are at similar levels of economic development. This suggests that there is substantial scope for expanding contraceptive prevalence and thus reducing fertility rates and population growth.

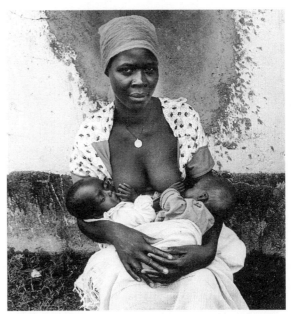

A Kenyan woman breast-feeding twins. Breast-feeding has major advantages for child health and for birth-spacing. (Photo: Panos Pictures/Paul Harrison)

Population planning

Among the countries that have achieved greatly improved access to education and increased child survival, and that have ensured a wide availability of family planning programmes, are China, Costa Rica, Jamaica, Korea, Thailand, Sri Lanka and Mexico (see Figure 8.6). These have all attained rapid declines in fertility rates. Conversely, countries with poor child survival, low levels of education and poor family planning services, such as Afghanistan and many countries in the Middle East and North and Sub-Saharan Africa, have shown few signs of fertility decline.

Such data suggest that a range of measures to accelerate falling fertility rates can be a highly effective means to slow the growth in world population, and that effective methods of birth control are an essential component of any such strategy. Of course, there are many cultures in which a large family size may bring greater social or political prestige in a community, and increase the likelihood of favourable settlement of disputes over land or water rights, legal disputes, or straightforward feuds. Economically, children may be highly valued from a very early age as agricultural and domestic workers. It must also be borne in mind that in many Third World countries social security provision against unemployment, old age, or sickness is either negligible or non-existent. Children may therefore be valued for the financial support they could eventually provide. In other words, large

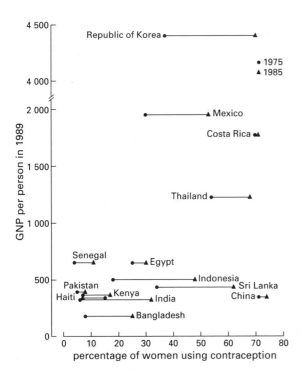

Figure 8.6 *Percentage of women of child-bearing age using contraception in 1975 and 1985 (or nearest dates) in various countries, compared with the GNP per person in those countries. (Data from United Nations, 1990, World Population Monitoring 1989: Special Report: the Population Situation of the Least Developed Countries, Population Studies No. 113, UN, New York, Table 33)*

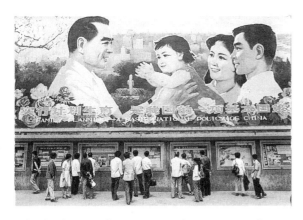

A family planning advertisement in China. Despite its low GNP per person, China has one of the highest contraceptive prevalence rates in the Third World. (Photo: Sally and Richard Greenhill)

family size is a positive choice in many areas of the world, and not an accident or mistake. This view is supported by attitude surveys in Indonesia, the Philippines, Nigeria, Ghana, Kenya and elsewhere. In Zimbabwe, for example, women on average say they want five children and in fact do give birth to an average 5.3 babies.

Family planning programmes should not raise any issues of compulsion or removal of individual rights and liberties. The compulsory sterilisation campaign mounted in parts of India during the Emergency of 1975–7 did have a dramatic effect on fertility, but the policy could not survive the return to democracy and the reductions on fertility were not sustained. In many parts of the Third World people face obstacles that restrict or prohibit the use of modern and effective contraceptive practices. Potential users may be deterred by the cost. And there may be legal or religious obstacles to the use of contraception. This is especially so in areas of the world where a substantial amount of political power is exercised by the religious hierarchies of Islam or Roman Catholicism: Central and Southern America, parts of North Africa and the Middle East, Pakistan, Bangladesh and the Philippines.

In other countries the problems are more to do with information, availability and access. In Zimbabwe, according to the Demographic and Health Survey of 1988, 34 per cent of married women did not want any more children or wanted to delay their next birth by two or more years, but were not using contraception. This may well be typical of many low-income countries: in fact, the Zimbabwean family planning programme is

relatively well developed, to the extent that the country has the highest contraceptive prevalence in Sub-Saharan Africa. Globally, if everyone who wished to control their family size by the most effective means possible were enabled to do so, so that such unmet need was eradicated, there is little doubt that the world-wide decline in fertility rates would be significantly accelerated.

This in turn would feed through to population growth: as was noted earlier, the long-range population projections in Figure 8.2 were crucially dependent on various assumptions about the future trend of fertility rates. These projections do in fact assume that contraceptive prevalence will continue to increase, from the 52 per cent in the developing countries as a whole in 1987 to 56 per cent by the year 2000 and 70 per cent by 2025. In Africa in particular, these figures require a significant increase in the rate of growth of contraceptive prevalence achieved so far. Despite this, there is evidence that funding for family planning programmes has fallen in real terms during the 1980s, and by the late 1980s international assistance was actually below the level achieved during the 1970s.

Routes to low mortality?

As you have seen at various points in this book, mortality decline—like fertility decline—is related in a broad way to economic development, but there are many countries performing better or worse than might be predicted on the basis of their national income per person. Let us now look at these countries, and try to discover why their mortality is exceptional.

Inferior and superior health achievers

The way we have identified the countries that are furthest above or below average has been to rank each country in terms of GNP per person in 1989 and in terms of life expectancy at birth in 1990. The bigger the difference between the two rankings, the more exceptional the country's mortality in relation to its income level. The ten countries with the highest life expectancy in relation to income level form one group (referred to hereafter as *superior health achievers*), and the ten with the lowest life expectancy relative to income form another (*inferior health achievers*). To ensure that the comparison between the two groups is not distorted by the presence of very small countries, only countries with a population of 10 million or over are included. Table 8.3 shows the results of this exercise.

Table 8.3 Countries with high and low mortality relative to level of income, 1990

	Low mortality relative to income level	High mortality relative to income level
countries (with populations of 10 million or over)	China, Sri Lanka, Viet Nam, Myanmar (Burma), Cuba, Tanzania, Nepal, Madagascar, Chile, India	Saudi Arabia, South Africa, Angola, Iraq, Cameroon, Iran, Brazil, Algeria, Côte D'Ivoire, Sudan
average GNP per person, 1989/US dollars	561	2011
average life expectancy at birth, 1990/years	61.4	59.1
average infant mortality rate, 1990/per 1 000 live births	72	83
average female literacy rate, 1989/per 100 women	66	43

Data derived from United Nations Development Programme (1992), *Human Development Report 1992*, Oxford University Press, Oxford and New York, Tables 1 and 11; World Resources Institute (1992), *World Resources 1992–93*, Oxford University Press, Oxford and New York, Tables 16.1, 16.2 and 16.5.

☐ Summarise the health indicators relative to income in the two groups of countries shown in Table 8.3.

■ The superior health achievers have an average GNP per person of just $561, not much more than one quarter of the average GNP per person among the inferior health achievers. The table is intended to show the *relative* performance of the two groups, but even in absolute terms, and despite their poverty, the superior health achievers have longer life expectancy, and lower infant mortality rates than the inferior health achievers.

If the table had not excluded countries with populations smaller than 10 million, then Costa Rica, Jamaica and the Dominican Republic would have been near the top of the list of superior health achievers, while Oman, Qatar, Libya, Gabon, Senegal and the United Arab Emirates would have been to the fore in the list of inferior health achievers.

How have this group of superior health achievers been able to transcend their very low income levels and achieve their success, and can they teach the rest of the Third World some lessons? This question has been asked repeatedly, and some of the countries in this group have been studied extensively. In particular, a report commissioned by the Rockefeller Foundation (Halstead *et al.*, 1985) reported in detail on the way in which mortality was reduced in four populations—China, Sri Lanka, Costa Rica and Kerala (a state of India)—and has been very influential in promoting a message of 'good health at low cost'.

'Good health at low cost'

The way in which countries such as China, Sri Lanka, Costa Rica and Kerala State have reduced their mortality rates despite their low income levels seems to have four main elements.

1   political and social will;

2   education for all with emphasis on primary and secondary schooling;

3   equitable distribution throughout the urban and rural populations of public-health measures and primary health care;

4   assurance of adequate calorific intake for all (Halstead *et al.*, 1985, p. 246)

Not all of these elements have been present in equal measure in the countries which have reduced their mortality despite low income levels. But combinations of them can be found in all the superior health achievers listed in Table 8.3.

First, a number of the countries have had long histories of political radicalism and grass-roots activism, or have experienced revolutionary governments dedicated to various forms of egalitarianism and welfare in the post-war period.

Second, women generally hold more equal social positions in the countries which have been superior health achievers, reflected in higher rates of female access to employment, health care and education: the female literacy rate in 1990 averaged 66 per cent in these countries, compared to only 43 per cent among the inferior health achievers listed in Table 8.3. Kerala State has achieved a much higher female literacy rate than is the norm in the rest of India; this may be one reason why there are no 'missing' females in Kerala State, unlike the situation in the remainder of India.

Third, the essential feature of public-health measures and health-care provision among the superior health achievers has not on the whole been a higher level of spending (although this has also been true of some of the group), but services that are more equally distributed between the rural and urban areas than is often the case in Third World countries, that give more equal access to females, and that therefore are more efficient at producing health improvement for a given level of resources.

And, finally, most of the superior health achievers have publicly supported nutrition programmes. These embrace a variety of mechanisms: for example, free school meal systems; food supplements distributed to expectant and nursing mothers and other social groups; public distribution systems and voucher schemes; food subsidies; and schemes of social insurance and assistance and of public employment to maintain income and hence entitlement.

In reference to these common elements in the experience of the superior health achievers, the demographer John Caldwell has stressed the striking parallels between Sri Lanka, Kerala and Costa Rica:

> These parallels include a substantial degree of female autonomy, a dedication to education, an open political system, a largely civilian society without a rigid class structure, a history of egalitarianism and radicalism and of national consensus arising from political contest with marked elements of populism. (Caldwell, 1986, p. 182)

However, these similarities are so striking and so rooted in historical experience that, as Caldwell goes on to observe, '...they give pause to any belief that low mortality will be achieved easily in most other countries' (Caldwell, 1986, p. 182). In other words, the characteristics of the countries that have succeeded in lowering mortality despite their low incomes may be so strikingly different to those pertaining in the group of inferior health achievers that the idea of drawing lessons and transferring them from one group to the other is far too simplistic. And this view tends to gain support when the characteristics of the inferior health achievers are also examined. Of the ten such countries listed in Table 8.3, seven are either predominantly Muslim countries (Saudi Arabia, Iraq, Iran, Algeria, Sudan) or have substantial Muslim minorities (Cameroon, Côte D'Ivoire); so are most of the

smaller countries in this group but not listed in the table. In contrast, none of the superior health achievers have anything other than small Muslim minorities.

Why might these differences of religion between the two groups of countries be related to their mortalities? Just as you have seen that a country's mortality is not determined by its level of income, so it would be wrong to think that it is determined by its religion. Some predominantly Muslim countries are doing better in terms of mortality than their levels of income might suggest. However, one of the most important features of Islamic societies concerns the position of women. Relatively good female access to education and health care is a feature of the countries that have managed to reduce their mortality despite their low incomes. These same factors seemed also to be a crucial factor in reducing fertility rates, as you saw above. And, as Chapter 3 showed, female education was strongly related to childhood mortality, while the position of women and their ability to obtain employment and hence entitlement was an important factor in explaining differences in female–male population ratios in different areas of the world (there are no 'missing' females in Kerala State, unlike the situation in the remainder of India). In Islamic countries, women tend to have quite restricted autonomy in a number of spheres, and in particular the secular education of females historically has not been encouraged. This is certainly not the only explanation for the over-representation of Islamic countries among the inferior health achievers, but it is of undoubted importance.

Aid

One obvious way to promote the human development policies outlined above, with their emphasis on basic education, primary health care, family planning and nutrition programmes, is by means of **Official Development Assistance (ODA)**, that is, donations of money from the industrialised countries to the Third World. ODA amounted to $54 billion in 1990, or 0.35 per cent of the combined GNP of the industrialised countries. This is just half the level set by the UN and agreed by most donor countries as an aid target. Meanwhile, the total amount of aid to the Third World is about the same as the net debt payments from the Third World to the industrialised countries, and also similar to their probable lost export earnings due to trade barriers.

The distribution of official aid is not related in any obvious way to the poverty of the recipient countries. In fact the United Nations Development Programme has estimated that the richest 40 per cent of the Third World's population receives more than twice as much aid per person as the poorest 40 per cent (UNDP, 1992, pp. 45–6). And only a very small share of official aid is directed into the basic human priority areas identified in this book as being most relevant to health. Basic education, primary health care, safe drinking water, family planning and nutrition programmes together are allocated less than 8 per cent of all aid, the great bulk of which is directed to industrial projects, agriculture and infrastructure. Once again, this illustrates that some concepts of development, for example those which guide official development assistance, fail to recognise human development.

Summary

In summary, the social, cultural and historical differences between the superior and inferior health achievers are often profound, and challenge the idea that there are easy routes to low mortality by simply transferring a few policies from one setting to another. But the steps taken by countries such as China, Sri Lanka or Kerala State to lower mortality have been documented in detail, and do demonstrate that low mortality potentially is within the reach of most countries, few of which are poorer than these high achievers. Perhaps above all, the lesson is that low mortality is unlikely to be attained simply as a side-effect of rising income levels. Because a country is poor it does not follow that the only way health can be improved is to become richer. As the economists Amartya Sen and Jean Drèze noted, in a summing-up of the performance of the superior health achievers:

> At the risk of oversimplifying the problem, it can be argued that a high level of GNP per head provides an *opportunity* for improving nutrition and other basic capabilities, but that opportunity may or may not be seized. In the process of transforming this opportunity into a tangible achievement, public support in various forms…often plays a crucial role. (Drèze and Sen, 1989, p. 181)

In a number of Third World countries facing falling income per person, the degree to which improvements in mortality can be separated from levels of income may be put to a severe test during the 1990s.

In the final chapter of this book we shall look in more detail at nutrition, which has been a recurring theme in our explorations of contemporary Third World health and of health changes in the past of the industrialised countries. Before that, the next two chapters complete our account of world health and disease patterns with a detailed look at contemporary health and disease in an industrialised country: the United Kingdom.

OBJECTIVES FOR CHAPTER 8

When you have studied this chapter you should be able to:

8.1 Outline the main features of the projected future world population, and the evidence in present trends for a demographic transition in the Third World.

8.2 Discuss the determinants of fertility decline, and describe the prevalence of family planning and other population policies.

8.3 Give examples of countries that seem to have exceptional (high or low) mortality in relation to their income levels, and discuss some of the characteristics of these countries.

QUESTIONS FOR CHAPTER 8

Question 1 (*Objective 8.1*)

'There are so many uncertainties concerning human population growth that making projections of the future world population is a futile exercise'. Discuss.

Question 2 (*Objective 8.2*)

According to most research evidence, what are the main factors that influence fertility decline, and how would you rank them in terms of importance?

Question 3 (*Objective 8.3*)

'Some poor countries may have achieved exceptionally low mortality in relation to their income levels, but this is irrelevant when the objective of most Third World countries is not low *relative* mortality, but low mortality in *absolute* terms'. How true is this statement?

9

Contemporary patterns of disease in the United Kingdom

During this chapter you may find it useful to refer to **Studying Health and Disease**[1]. *A television programme ('A Tale of Four Cities') is associated with this chapter. It looks at the impact of the living and working environment on health in the United Kingdom and examines the interaction of social factors such as poverty with 'lifestyle' factors. Details can be found in the Broadcast and Audiocassette Notes.*

This chapter contains a considerable amount of data, presented in several different ways: tables, graphs, pie diagrams, histograms and maps. They have been included partly for illustrative purposes and partly as a useful source of reference, and it is important to realise that you are not expected to memorise the details. This is the longest chapter in the book, so allow adequate time for it.

So far in this book we have examined differences in the patterns of health and disease between industrialised and Third World countries, and looked at how these are related to the social and economic environment. We have also traced the historical changes in the health of the people of England, from a pattern which in some ways resembled that of a present-day Third World country, to that of a modern industrialised state. This chapter now considers in more detail the patterns of health and disease experienced by different social groups in the United Kingdom today.

The chapter begins by describing the overall patterns of mortality, morbidity and disability. It then discusses both the nature of the epidemiological approach to

[1] *Studying Health and Disease* (Open University Press, 1985, revised edition, 1994).

understanding how such patterns arise, and some limitations of this approach that should be borne in mind when examining the data it generates. In the remaining six sections we consider the main biological and social determinants of health and disease under six broad headings: gender; age; marital status; ethnicity; geography; and occupation and social class.

You may already be aware of some examples of the epidemiological approach to investigating disease. For instance, during the 1980s two reports on inequalities in health in the United Kingdom received a great deal of attention. The first, published in 1980, was the report of a Department of Health and Social Security (DHSS) working group entitled *Inequalities in Health* (often referred to as the 'Black Report' after the group's chair and at that time President of the Royal College of Physicians, Douglas Black). In 1988 the report was updated by Margaret Whitehead in a book entitled *The Health Divide*. These two reports, and other work on the distribution of health and disease in the population, have tended to concentrate on a single biological or social dimension that seems to be associated with disease patterns. In the case of the 'Black Report' and *The Health Divide*, the main dimension was social class, with less attention to such factors as gender, ethnicity and marital status. The approach adopted in this chapter is unusual in that several important dimensions of inequality are considered alongside one another.

The main causes of mortality, morbidity and disability

In Chapters 2 and 3 you saw how epidemiology and demography interact in Third World countries. In the United Kingdom and other industrialised countries, changes in the pattern of many diseases have gone hand in hand with alterations in the age structure of the population. And, as Figure 9.1 shows, these changes in the age

110

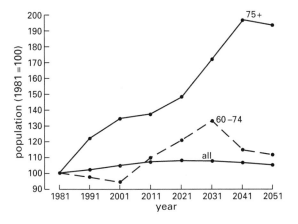

Figure 9.1 *1989-based projected population changes by age-groups (60–74, 75 and over, and all), England and Wales (1981 = 100). (Data from OPCS, 1991,* National Population Projections, 1989-based, *OPCS Series PP2, No. 17, HMSO, London)*

structure of the population are expected to continue into the foreseeable future. The figure shows population changes by age-group, in the form of an index beginning at 1981 = 100 for each group. Thus the total population rises from an index of 100 in 1981 to 108 in the year 2021: that is, an increase of 8 per cent.

☐ Describe the projected changes in size of the three population categories shown by the year (i) 2001, and (ii) 2051.

■ From Figure 9.1:

(i) By 2001 the size of the total population is projected to increase only slightly; the numbers of those aged 60–74 will have decreased by about 5 per cent compared with 1981, whereas the 75 and over group will increase by 35 per cent.

(ii) By 2051 the total population will have increased by 6 per cent compared with 1981, but there will be 12 per cent more people aged 60–74, and the numbers of those aged 75 and over will have almost doubled.

These trends reflect the probability of surviving to any given age, but they also reflect the actual numbers of people born in the past. For example, the fall in the number of people in the age-group 60–74 during the 1980s and 1990s results from a fall in the birth rate during and after World War I.

Mortality

In Chapter 6 you saw how life expectancy in the United Kingdom has increased rapidly from the late nineteenth century onwards. By 1991 males born in the United Kingdom could expect to live for about 73 years, and females for 79 years. One consequence of this improvement in survival has been that **degenerative diseases** (due to the wearing out of tissues) have become a leading cause of death, as Figure 9.2 indicates.

This figure shows the proportional mortality, i.e. the percentages of all deaths in England and Wales attributable to leading causes of death. (In 1990 the total number of deaths in England and Wales from all causes was 564 846.) Two groups of chronic disease associated with degeneration of the arteries together accounted for about 42 per cent of all deaths in 1990: those caused by deterioration of the arteries supplying the heart muscle (coronary arteries), and cerebrovascular disease, in which a similar process of deterioration causes part of the brain to be damaged or destroyed by losing its blood supply, known as a stroke. The proportion of deaths caused by heart disease has been declining very slowly in recent years, but deaths from cerebrovascular disease have remained very constant.

The next two largest categories identified in Figure 9.2 are those of cancers and respiratory disease, which in 1990 accounted for 26 per cent and 11 per cent of all deaths respectively. The proportion of deaths caused by

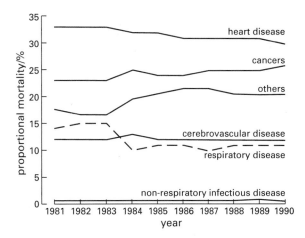

Figure 9.2 *Causes of death in England and Wales, 1981–90 (percentages of total for all males and females aged 28 days and over). (Data derived from Registrar-General, 1991 and 1992,* Annual Abstract of Statistics, *HMSO, London, Table 2.20, p. 37)*

cancers increased slightly throughout the 1980s, while deaths from respiratory disease (conditions affecting the lungs) fell. The main cause of death from non-malignant (i.e. not cancer-related) respiratory disease is pneumonia, and these deaths mostly occur in frail, elderly people who are already suffering from chronic lung conditions. Another cause of death in this respiratory group is influenza: deaths from influenza vary between a few hundred and 10 000 a year, reflecting the epidemic nature of this infection. In 1989, for example, there were over 2 000 deaths attributable to influenza, compared with fewer than 300 in the previous year. Finally, infectious diseases other than those affecting the lungs are responsible for less than half of one per cent of deaths, a fact that graphically illustrates the degree to which the health transition discussed in Chapter 6 has been accomplished in the United Kingdom. You should note that deaths from AIDS are classified under 'metabolic and immunity disorders' —which are grouped with the 'other' causes of death in Figure 9.2—and are not included in the infectious diseases category. To give some idea of the impact of this disease, it may be noted that, in the year ending April 1992, 1 220 deaths related to AIDS were reported in the United Kingdom.

The 'cancers' category includes a large number of cancers of different types and arising in different organs[2]. Figure 9.3 shows the age-standardised death rates for the commonest cancers among men and women.

In men the most common cancer is of the lung, followed by the prostate, stomach and colon (large intestine). The lung cancer rate has been falling steadily among men since the mid-1970s, and the stomach cancer rate has been falling for even longer, but cancers of the prostate show a long-term increase. In women the commonest cancer is of the breast, followed by lung cancer and then cancers of the ovary and stomach. The death rate from breast cancer has been rising among women in the United Kingdom, although this trend may have come to an end. There has been a sharp increase in lung cancer deaths, but the death rate from stomach cancer has been falling among women as among men. Across the population as a whole the top three cancers— of the lung, the female breast, and the stomach—account for around 40 per cent of all deaths from cancer.

[2]The biological differences are discussed in *The Biology of Health and Disease* (Open University Press, 1985, revised as *Human Biology and Health: An Evolutionary Approach*, 1994) and another book in this series, *Experiencing and Explaining Disease* (Open University Press, 1985, revised edition, 1995).

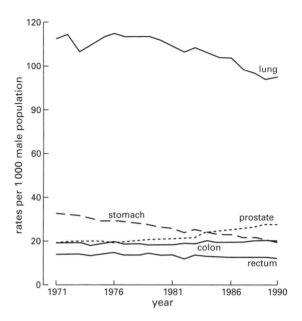

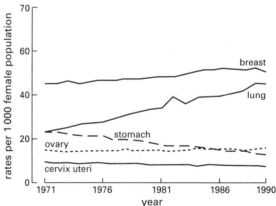

Figure 9.3 *Age-standardised mortality rates from cancers by sex and site, 1971–1990, United Kingdom. Note that 'cervix uteri' includes Fallopian tubes and broad ligaments. (Data from HMSO, 1992, Social Trends 22: 1991, HMSO, London, Figure 7.6, p. 125)*

The final category in Figure 9.2 is simply labelled 'others', which includes numerous causes of death. The actual number of deaths caused by some of these 'other' causes are shown in Figure 9.4. In 1990 they ranged from five deaths a year of women in labour or childbirth to 4 898 deaths in motor traffic accidents.

☐ Consider the following pairs of causes of death. In each pair, which cause is responsible for more deaths, and how much more common is it?

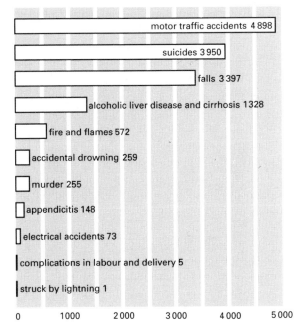

Figure 9.4 *Some examples of deaths from 'other causes' in England and Wales, 1990. (Data derived from OPCS, 1991, Mortality Statistics: Cause 1990, OPCS Series DH2, No. 17, HMSO, London, Table 2)*

(a) suicide and murder

(b) electrical accidents and burns (fire and flames)

(c) alcoholic liver disease including cirrhosis and deaths from falls

■ From Figure 9.4:

(a) Suicide is 15 times more common than murder.

(b) Burns cause eight times as many deaths as electrical accidents.

(c) Falls kill two and a half times as many people as do alcoholic diseases of the liver, including cirrhosis.

In summary, mortality in the United Kingdom population is dominated by a number of chronic and degenerative diseases, which have become the leading cause of death as the average expectation of life has increased. The largest groups are heart disease, cancers and cerebrovascular disease, which together account for around two-thirds of all deaths.

Morbidity

So far we have only considered mortality, but further information on the pattern of diseases can be obtained from studying morbidity. There are three commonly used methods of **measuring morbidity**.

□ Can you suggest what they are?

■ Measuring the use of health services (such as the number of people admitted to hospital with a particular disease); screening, in which the whole population or a sample are investigated in some way in order to identify those individuals who would benefit from treatment for a particular disease; and population surveys or self-assessment surveys in which people are examined or asked about their own state of health, but with no prior intention to treat.

Some sources of information, however, fall between these three categories: for example, certain infectious diseases must by law be reported to a central agency when they are detected, and the central agency (in England the Centre for Disease Surveillance and Control) is therefore an important source of information on these 'notifiable' diseases. Similarly, cancer registration schemes provide valuable data on the incidence of cancers.

Most of the routinely published information on morbidity is based on the use of health services. However, information derived in this way reflects not only the presence of ill-health and disease, but also such factors as the availability and accessibility of services, and people's knowledge, beliefs and attitudes about illness and health care. The influence of such factors on health service use will vary with the type of condition suffered: almost everyone with a fractured leg will attend a hospital, whereas only some people with low back-pain or influenza will see their doctor.

Another feature of morbidity measures that are based on health service use is that different patterns of morbidity will emerge depending on which part of the service is studied. This can be seen in Figure 9.5 (overleaf), which shows the top groups of conditions as measured by (i) the use of hospital beds; (ii) hospital admissions; and (iii) general practitioner (GP) consultations. You should note that mental handicap and pregnancy are not included in the figure, despite the fact that a great deal of health care is provided for both conditions, as they are not generally considered to be illnesses as such.

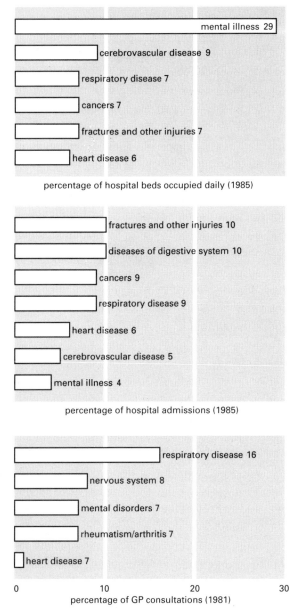

percentage of hospital beds occupied daily (1985)

percentage of hospital admissions (1985)

percentage of GP consultations (1981)

Figure 9.5 *Morbidity patterns for the commonest five groups of disorders/diseases in each category. (Data for hospital beds and admissions derived from HMSO, 1989, Health and Personal Social Services Statistics for England, 1989, HMSO, London, Tables 9.1, 9.2, 9.7 and 11.2; data for GP consultations from Royal College of General Practitioners/OPCS/DHSS, 1986, Morbidity Statistics from General Practice: Third National Study, OPCS Series MB5, No. 1, HMSO, London, Tables 12 and 13)*

□ By comparing Figures 9.2 and 9.5, what can you conclude about the contribution of cancers to mortality and morbidity rates?

■ In spite of being responsible for 25 per cent of all deaths, they account for only about 7 per cent of occupied hospital beds, 9 per cent of hospital admissions and do not figure as a major reason for GP consultations. This suggests that cancers are a disease category of high mortality, but of intermediate or low morbidity.

This is in contrast to a category such as rheumatism which is rarely fatal or requiring hospital admission, but is responsible for about 7 per cent of all GP consultations.

□ Now compare mental illness with fractures and other injuries in terms of hospital beds and admissions. What differences exist and how might you explain them?

■ The percentage of hospital beds occupied by people with a mental illness is much higher than the percentage of hospital admissions attributable to mental illness, whereas fractures and injuries are responsible for a much higher proportion of admissions than occupied beds. This suggests that patients with a mental illness tend to be in hospital for long periods, whereas patients with fractures and injuries have a fairly short length of stay in hospital.

These differences demonstrate the importance of examining a variety of measures of the impact of a disease or group of diseases when assessing its importance on the health of a population. Consider, for example, skin conditions, which, like rheumatism, cause few deaths or admissions to hospital, yet are a common source of distress, and sometimes discomfort, for people. Table 9.1 indicates how frequently these and other common conditions are encountered in one year in a general practice of fairly average size.

□ Which are the five most prevalent conditions seen in this general practice?

■ They are:

(i) upper respiratory infections (600): these include conditions such as tonsillitis and ear infections;

(ii) skin disorders (350), such as eczema and warts;

(iii) psycho-emotional problems (250);

(iv) high blood pressure (250);

(v) gastro-intestinal disorders (200), such as food poisoning, diarrhoea and vomiting.

Table 9.1 Annual prevalence of illness and other events in a primary care practice in a population of 2 500.

Condition	No. of sufferers
1 *Minor illness*	
upper respiratory infections	600
skin disorders	350
psychoemotional problems	250
gastro-intestinal conditions	200
2 *Chronic diseases*	
high blood pressure	250
chronic rheumatism	100
chronic psychiatric disorders	100
ischaemic heart disease	50
obesity	50
anaemia	30
cancers under care	30
asthma	30
diabetes	30
varicose veins	30
peptic ulcers	25
strokes	20
3 *Major acute diseases*	
acute bronchitis	100
pneumonia	20
severe depression	10
acute myocardial infarction (heart attack)	10
acute strokes	5
new cancers	5
acute appendicitis	5

Data derived from Fry, I. (1983) *Common Diseases*, M.T.P. Press, 3rd edn, Table 1.4, pp. 22–4.

These data reflect the everyday sorts of health problems which affect nearly all of us at some time or another: a general practitioner would only expect to see one new case of breast cancer and ten heart attacks (acute myocardial infarction in the table) in a year, compared with hundreds of people with emotional problems, skin disorders and chronic conditions.

However, as you have seen above, even data such as these from general practice may fail to reveal a considerable amount of ill-health and disability, such as foot-problems in the elderly which cause difficulty with walking and even complete immobility. Information on the prevalence of such 'minor' conditions has to be obtained from special surveys. One such survey that has been conducted on a number of occasions has focused on the dental health of adults, and some results are shown in Figure 9.6.

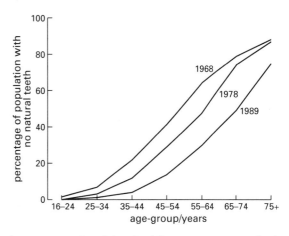

Figure 9.6 *Total tooth loss for different age-groups, England and Wales, 1989. (Data for 1968 and 1978 come from Adult Dental Health Surveys. The 1989 figures come from the OPCS, 1991,* General Household Survey 1989, *OPCS Series GHS, No. 20, HMSO, Table 4.41)*

☐ At what age had 50 per cent of the population lost all their natural teeth in 1968, 1978 and 1989, and what does this indicate about general standards of dental health?

■ By the age of 55–64 well over half the population in 1968 had lost all their natural teeth. By 1978 this age had risen to 65–74, and by 1989 it was only in the age group 75 and over that a majority of the population had no natural teeth. This suggests a substantial improvement in dental health.

In summary, different measurement methods suggest quite different patterns of morbidity. For example, data based on use of hospital beds show mental illness to predominate, whereas GP consultations also reflect distress and discomfort caused by upper respiratory infections and 'minor' conditions affecting the skin, muscles and joints.

Disability

Surveys of the prevalence of morbidity in the population sometimes attempt to define illness in terms of its impact on an individual's life. Thus a **physical impairment** may be said to exist if some bodily function is limited, such as having difficulty with breathing, as occurs with chronic bronchitis. If this impairment is sufficient to restrict the person's general physical functioning—for example if chronic bronchitis makes it impossible to walk to the shops or climb the stairs—it can be said to constitute a **disability**. Finally, it is sometimes argued that a **handicap** exists if the environment fails to accommodate a person's disability, with the effect that their social functioning is limited. The term 'environment' refers not only to physical structures, such as a lack of wheelchair access to a public building, but also society's attitude to disability which may either be welcoming and accommodating, or hostile and inflexible. In other words, disabled people may be handicapped by the able-bodied.

Some indication of the prevalence of disability from a wide range of causes among adults in Great Britain in 1986 is shown in Figure 9.7. The figure separates the population living at home from those in institutions.

It is often thought that disabilities are a consequence of either congenital conditions (those which a baby is born with) and birth trauma (e.g. spasticity), or of head and spinal injuries. But, as Figure 9.7 demonstrates, in the general population the commonest causes of disability in adults are musculoskeletal diseases such as arthritis, deafness and other ear complaints, and eye disorders. In institutions, mental disorders are the most prevalent, followed by musculoskeletal disorders and then diseases of the nervous system such as stroke.

☐ Is there a consistent relationship between the mortality (refer to Figure 9.2) and the disability (Figure 9.7) caused by a disease category?

■ No. Cancers cause a quarter of all deaths but are not a prevalent cause of disability. Circulatory disease results in both high mortality and high disability, whereas musculoskeletal diseases cause much disability but low mortality.

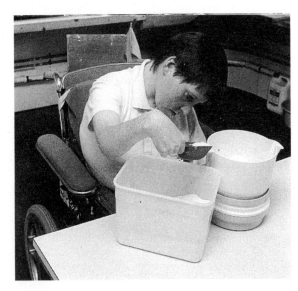

A disability need not be a handicap if the environment is sufficiently adapted. (Photo: Mike Levers)

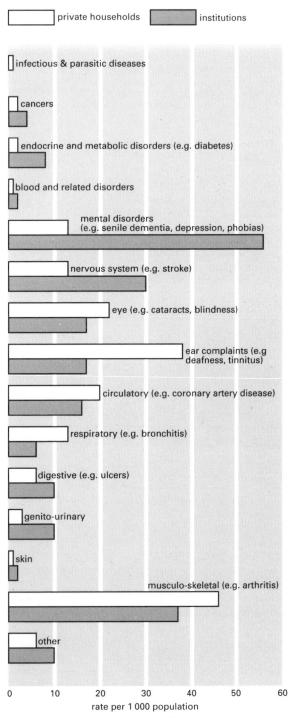

Figure 9.7 *The prevalence of disability among adults resulting from the causes shown, Great Britain, 1986. (Data from OPCS, 1988, The Prevalence of Disability among Adults, OPCS Report No. 1, HMSO, London, Tables 4.3 and 4.9)*

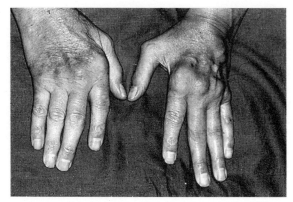

Hands affected by arthritis. Such musculoskeletal diseases are one of the commonest causes of disability in adults. (Photo: Maclean Hunter Ltd, Medical Division)

You should also note that some diseases, such as multiple sclerosis, are usually fatal after many years, but are rare enough to appear very low on the list of causes of death. In other words the population mortality from this disease is low, but the *case-fatality* is high.

Figure 9.7 shows very clearly the importance of diseases of the sense organs. Approximately 60 per cent of adult men and nearly 70 per cent of adult women in Britain wear glasses for at least some activities. In addition some of those not wearing glasses are thought to suffer from some visual difficulty. So although we tend to think of disabled people as a minority group, in reality there are few fully able-bodied adults.

To give some impression of how the prevalence of disability (and morbidity) may be changing over time, Figure 9.8 shows some data from the General Household Survey, an annual survey of **self-reported illness** in a sample of the British population which includes a number of questions concerning health. The figure shows

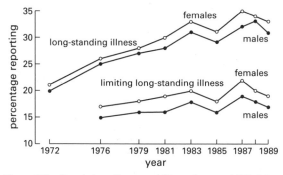

Figure 9.8 *Trends in self-reported illness by sex, 1972–89, Great Britain. (Data from OPCS, 1991,General Household Survey 1989, OPCS Series GHS, No. 20, HMSO, London, Figure 4a, p. 99, and Table 4.1, p. 104)*

the percentage of respondents who reported a long-standing illness, and of these, whether the illness limited their activities in any way. Data are shown separately for men and women.

It is clear that there has been a fairly substantial increase since the early 1970s (when this survey first began) in the proportion of men and women reporting some long-standing illness, and that this proportion now. stands at around one-third of the population. There has been a similar increase in the proportion who report that their activity is in some way restricted by a long-standing illness: around 12 per cent of the population claim to be restricted by illness.

□ What explanations can you think of for the increase over time in the proportion of people who report a long-standing illness?

■ One explanation may be that people's expectations, attitudes and assessments of their health have been changing: remember that these data are self-reported. Another possibility is that the increase simply reflects a changing population age structure: with more older people than in the past, there is likely to be more illness. A third possibility is that the increase is associated with rising life expectancy: people may be living longer, but these extra years of life may not be very healthy.

It seems almost certain that people's attitudes and expectations have changed over time, but there is no easy way to assess whether this has affected rates of self-reported illness: it might also be noted that such changes could have reduced or increased these rates. The second potential explanation, concerning changes in the age structure of the population, can easily be checked by age-standardising the data, and this does not in fact account for the increase.

This leaves the question of whether rising life expectancy has been accompanied by parallel improvements in health. One view, expressed for example by the American epidemiologist James Fries, is that, as life expectancy increases, so chronic illness will be restricted to the last few years of life, with the result that the healthy lifespan will also increase: Fries has described this essentially optimistic outlook as being characterised by the **compression of morbidity**. However, another more pessimistic view is that increases in life expectancy will not be free of illness, and will increase the proportion of life spent sick or disabled.

Figure 9.9 (overleaf) shows one attempt to address these questions. The figure shows how life expectancy changed for males and females between 1976 and 1988,

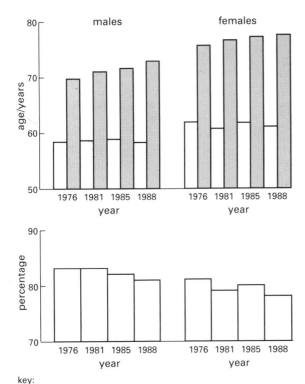

key:

☐ expectation of life without disability ▨ life expectancy ☐ percentage of life without disability

Figure 9.9 *Trends in life expectancy and expectation of life without disability, from birth, England and Wales, 1976–88. (Data from Bebbington, A. C., 1991, The expectation of life without disability in England and Wales: 1976–88,* Population Trends, **66** *(Winter), Table 1, p. 27)*

and also the expectation of life without disability (calculated from the General Household Survey's self-reported data).

The figure tends to bear out the view of the pessimists: overall life expectancy rose significantly, but expectation of life without disability appeared to increase hardly at all, so that the *proportion* of life spent without some form of disability if anything fell. Similar findings have been reported from the USA by a group led by Crimmins (1989).

This discussion prompts one final thought concerning the likely future trend in life expectancy. Although many of the initial gains in average life expectancy in countries such as the United Kingdom occurred because far more individuals survived infancy, in fact the expectation of life has been rising not just at birth but at every age: for example, a 60-year-old woman in the United Kingdom could expect to live for another 14.6 years in 1901, but by 1991 this had increased to almost 22 years. This trend is continuing for the present, but for how long? The demographer Bernard Benjamin has constructed

various projections based on different assumptions, some of which show life expectancy at birth of 88 years among men and 95 years among women. On these projections 10 per cent of males would survive to the age of 95 and 10 per cent of females would celebrate their 99th birthday. The underlying assumptions may seem far-fetched but, as Benjamin remarks:

> It is a fact that no individual has yet been observed credibly to exceed 114 years, but then no individual has yet lived in an environment that allows ageing unaffected by disease of external origin…. It seems at least plausible that there is no predetermined limit to the attainable lifespan. The only statistic we can depend upon is the longest life ever lived and every day the record grows longer. The fault lies not in our stars, but in ourselves that we are mortal. (Benjamin, 1989, p. 227)

Summary

To summarise: survival to middle and old age has led to a rise in the medical and social importance of chronic degenerative diseases (especially those affecting the cardiovascular and respiratory systems) and cancers. These conditions dominate the causes of mortality. Patterns of morbidity are dependent on how the measurements are made: for example, measuring the use of hospital services does not reflect the everyday experiences of distress and discomfort caused by upper respiratory infections, mental ill-health and emotional problems, and 'minor' conditions affecting the skin, muscles and joints. The causes of disability are primarily musculoskeletal disorders and diseases of the sense organs. The proportion of the population reporting some form of disabling disease appears to be rising, prompting questions about the proportion of life expectancy that is free of disability.

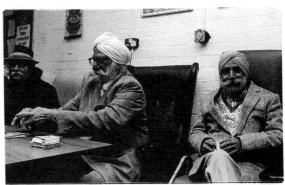

Rising life expectancy has resulted in many more old people in Britain, but it is not clear that life expectancy free of illness has increased. (Photo: Mike Levers)

Studying distributions of health and disease

A widely accepted definition of **epidemiology** is that it is concerned to interpret the health experience of human communities. More specifically, epidemiology addresses three types of questions.[3]

☐ Can you suggest what these questions are? And how might they be answered?

■ Three types of questions important to epidemiologists are:

(i)   Who gets ill?—answered by describing the distribution of health and disease in the population and how it changes over time.

(ii)   Why do they get ill?—addressed by investigating the aetiology (or cause) of disease, or establishing associations with other factors such as environment, life history, etc.

(iii)   What should the response be?—answered by evaluating the effectiveness of different treatments and other interventions such as prevention campaigns.

This chapter is primarily concerned with the first question, though by describing how particular conditions are distributed in the population, it is possible to suggest explanations for such patterns, that is, to start to answer the second question on the causality of disease.

Epidemiology is an eclectic science, which has borrowed many of its investigative methods from other areas. Consequently, the kinds of methodological problems that often arise, and which you will encounter at various points in this chapter, are not unique to epidemiology.

The first such problem is that the diseases or health conditions that are most feasible to study are, in general, those that have medical labels, definitions, and classifications attached to them. **Classification of diseases** has led to many advances in understanding illness, but it can also limit the scope of epidemiology, by encouraging epidemiologists to study those states of ill-health that are most easily identified and measured, and to neglect those that are not easily verified by a doctor or do not readily fit into the description of any disease. For example, feeling 'under the weather' is a common condition but is not usually given a specific disease-label, and does not attract much serious research effort. Too rigid an adherence to the current classification of diseases may also limit advances in knowledge. For instance, it is possible that our understanding of the causes of coronary heart disease

is being impeded because the current disease definition actually comprises several different diseases, each with its own cause (or causes). In practice one of the roles of epidemiology should be to challenge such definitions and help to redefine diseases in more useful ways.

A second set of problems concerns the factors that may contribute to disease patterns. Studying these often requires **population stratification**: that is, sections of the population are grouped in accordance with the characteristic of interest. This is fairly straightforward for factors such as age and sex, but it may present considerable difficulties with factors such as social class, which cannot be measured directly. One solution is to develop 'proxy' or indirect measures, for example, by using country of origin as a measure of ethnic background, or occupation as a measure of social class. Going beyond these practical difficulties, there is the question of selecting which factors or types of factor to study. For instance, most studies of gastroenteritis (diarrhoea and vomiting) in infants have been concerned with biological factors such as whether or not the mother breast-fed her infant, rather than with social variables such as housing conditions and income. If the conclusion is that gastroenteritis is caused by mothers failing to breast-feed their infants, the recommended change might be to encourage mothers to breast-feed. But an investigation embracing social factors may draw attention to circumstances that discourage some mothers from breast-feeding, such as insufficient advice and support, and so recommend that more breast-feeding counsellors be trained. Policy implications are, therefore, very much dependent on the factors chosen to be studied, and that choice is influenced not only by practical considerations, but also the interests and values of the investigator or the funding body behind the research.

A third problem concerns **interaction between different factors**. A study of the effectiveness of a drug may attempt to simplify the issues by looking separately at two factors: age and sex. It may then show that the drug's effectiveness declines in older age groups and that it is less effective among men than women. But for biological or other reasons the effect of age and sex may not be independent: effectiveness may decline more rapidly in older men than older women, so that the *combined* influence of age and sex is not the same as the separate influence of each factor: there is an interaction between them. Although sophisticated statistical methods exist to cope with the interaction of factors, many epidemiological studies (especially much of the routine descriptive data) make no such attempt.

Finally, it is often very difficult to establish whether an association between, for example, a disease and a factor such as age, is *causal*, or whether some other possible explanation exists. There are many **levels of causality**: explanations of the cause of a disease may be offered in terms of chemicals and cells at one extreme,

[3]Epidemiological methods are discussed in *Studying Health and Disease* (Open University Press, 1985, revised edition, 1994).

and in terms of politics and economics at the other. In theory, a causal relationship can only be assumed after an exhaustive analysis has considered and rejected all other possible explanations—causal and non-causal—of the association. For instance, in our infant feeding/gastroenteritis example we cannot be certain that the colour of the mother's hair, her astrological sign or her relationship with the infant's father are not relevant unless these are also studied. In practice, epidemiologists have to decide which factors to study on the basis of a wide range of criteria including clinical, biological, demographic or social plausibility. But they may have a prior inclination to emphasise one group of factors, for example biomedical (or clinical), or social factors, and neglect others.

These methodological difficulties, which as noted earlier are not unique to epidemiology, can be and often are overcome in collaboration with other disciplines, and the result has been a major contribution to the study of health and disease. The rest of this chapter is devoted to describing this contribution in the case of the United Kingdom and discussing some of the explanations epidemiological work has suggested. Each of the six main characteristics (sex and gender, age, marital status, ethnicity, geographical location and social class as defined by occupation) is discussed below in terms of the following: (i) the distribution of mortality; (ii) the distribution of morbidity (and disability where appropriate); and (iii) a discussion of possible explanations of such patterns, considering biological and social elements and the influence of personal life-histories.

Sex and gender

Figure 9.9 showed a feature of the average expectation of life that should now be familiar to you: female lives in the United Kingdom are on average around 6 years longer than male lives. As Figure 9.10 shows, this advantage is present throughout life.

☐ Is there any age-group in which the male mortality rate is lower than that for females?

■ No. In England and Wales the male mortality rate is higher at all ages.

☐ Can you recall from previous chapters any exceptions to this finding in other places or times?

■ In some Third World countries the female mortality rate exceeds the male rate (Chapter 2), and this was also true of industrialised countries until the nineteenth century.

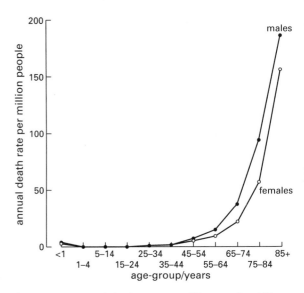

Figure 9.10 *Annual death rates per million people within each age-group for 1990, England and Wales. (Data derived from OPCS, 1991, Mortality Statistics: Cause 1990, OPCS Series DH2, No. 17, HMSO, London, Table 3)*

About 40 per cent of the sex difference in overall mortality is accounted for by deaths from coronary heart disease. The higher rate of deaths among men from coronary heart disease occurs all at ages, but is greatest in late middle age when it accounts for 40 per cent of all male deaths, but less than 15 per cent in females. Although there are several problems concerning the diagnosis and definition of deaths due to this cause, there is no doubt that both the incidence of myocardial infarction (heart attack) and the prevalence of coronary atherosclerosis (degeneration of arteries supplying the heart muscle) are higher in men than in women of the same age. The overall cancer mortality rate is also around 10 per cent higher in males than in females. Referring back to Figure 9.3, for example, you will see that lung cancer rates are much higher in men than women, and that males also suffer higher rates of stomach cancer. In fact the only specific sites in which the female mortality rate exceeds that of males (apart from exclusively female sites such as the uterus) are the breast (a few cases do occur in men), pancreas and skin.

The consistently higher overall death rates for males in the United Kingdom are not reflected in higher overall morbidity rates. Although the morbidity rates for many major chronic diseases are higher in males (e.g. coronary heart disease), for others there either does not appear to be any substantial difference or the female rate is higher. Studies have shown that the incidence of acute conditions, days of restricted activity because of illness, and visits to GPs tend to be higher in women than men. In Figure 9.8 you saw that the proportion reporting long-standing illnesses was consistently higher among women than men. One disease that illustrates this difference in morbidity is rheumatoid arthritis, a chronic disease of the joints resulting in stiffness, pain and loss of mobility. Not only is it more prevalent in women than in men but, in addition, the disease appears to advance more rapidly in women.

How can these male : female differences in mortality and morbidity be explained? What is the relative contribution of biological sex and socially constructed gender? This question has given rise to considerable debate and speculation. Several biological explanations have been suggested for the lower mortality rate in females, including differences in the genetic material between males and females.[4] It has been suggested that this may result in greater resistance to infections in females. Females may also benefit from hormonal differences from males. The higher levels of oestrogens in females may exert some protective effect, particularly against cardiovascular disease. In support of this view, it has been suggested that the reason the female mortality rate from coronary heart disease increases sharply after the age of 50 years is because of the fall in the level of oestrogens around the time of the menopause. Finally, it has been suggested that the biological hazards associated with pregnancy may underlie the higher female mortality rate noted in some Third World countries and in the past in the United Kingdom. Widely available contraception and improvements in the safety of childbirth in industrialised countries may have nullified this disadvantage, leading to a fall in female mortality rates.

In addition to these biological theories, a number of social explanations for the *gender* difference in mortality have been suggested. First, there are increased risks to men stemming from their higher rates of employment outside the home and in more physically hazardous jobs. Second, there are systematic differences in behaviour between the sexes, which are in part biological but may also result from social pressures operating from childhood or be related to gender differences in the access to resources.[5] These are then manifested in, for example,

[4]The biological determinants of greater female longevity are discussed in *Human Biology and Health: An Evolutionary Approach* (Open University Press, 1994).

[5]See another book in this series, *Birth to Old Age: Health in Transition* (Open University Press, 1985, revised edition 1995).

higher risk-taking behaviour among men: greater use of dangerous drugs, faster driving, or higher smoking rates. In turn this behaviour feeds through to mortality: for example the higher prevalence of smoking in men is reflected in the higher incidence of cancers of the lung, as shown in Figure 9.3, as well as higher rates of coronary heart disease and of other cancers including those of the mouth and pharynx, oesophagus and bladder.

Other behavioural differences, apart from smoking, that may contribute to the excess of male mortality include the higher consumption of alcohol by men which contributes to the higher incidence of cancer of the larynx and oesophagus, and cirrhosis of the liver. The transmission pattern of HIV in the early stages of the United Kingdom AIDS epidemic has also primarily affected men, especially homosexuals and intravenous drug users; in the ten years up to 1992 only 6 per cent of the almost 6 000 people with AIDS in the United Kingdom were female. However, the proportion of women appears to be rising as the epidemic progresses, and is much higher in other affected areas, notably in Africa, where transmission has occurred mainly via heterosexual intercourse.

Gender differences in behaviour have also been suggested as part of the explanation for the higher mortality from coronary heart disease in men, such as a higher prevalence among men of a so-called 'coronary-prone personality' characterised by aggressive and competitive behavioural traits. However, despite a considerable amount of research in this area, the influence of personality types on the distribution of coronary heart disease (or any other disease) is still unclear.

How might the apparently paradoxical observation of higher *morbidity* rates for some diseases in women be explained? This finding may partly result from the method of measuring morbidity (based on health service use) and partly from gender differences in attitudes to health care.

□ Can you suggest how these two factors might explain some of the gender difference in morbidity rates?

■ The difference might be explained as follows:

(i)   Methodological problems in the measurement of women's visits to a GP may arise as a result of the inclusion of consultations for contraception, antenatal, and post-natal care.

(ii)   Women may be more predisposed to care for their health. This would contribute to their higher consultation rate and might also lower their mortality rate. They may also have greater access to health services, because they are less likely to be in full-time employment. In addition, women have traditionally cared for the health of other members of the family. This may have lowered the consultation rate of men while raising women's own rate, especially if they consult on their own behalf while, for example, taking children to the GP.

Gender differences in psychiatric morbidity provide an example of how health-care factors may partly account for such differences. General practitioners report that many more women than men consult them for anxiety and depression. However there is also good evidence that doctors are readier to diagnose women as suffering from psychiatric disturbance than men. Both may be true.

The patterns of gender and disease illustrate well the complex interaction between biological, social and life-history factors in determining health status, and as you progress through this chapter you will see gender differences reappearing in many different contexts. To summarise, you should note the following:

1   Male mortality rates exceed those for females at all ages.

2   Male : female differences in morbidity vary between different conditions.

3   Biological factors, such as genetic and hormonal differences, are thought to account for some of the relative health advantages of females (although post-menopausal disorders are a source of morbidity among women that men do not experience).

4   Social relations and structures, on average, place males in more hazardous work, and appear to influence their adoption of more health-damaging behaviour.

5   Some of the apparent differences in morbidity between the sexes may result from systematic differences in measurement or in the use of health services, or perhaps because of inconsistent social attitudes towards women compared with men who report themselves as ill.

Age

In Chapter 2 you saw how, in industrialised countries, mortality rates typically increase with increasing age after early childhood. Though this pattern is true for almost all causes of death in the United Kingdom as in other industrialised countries, there are a few interesting exceptions. For example, deaths from road traffic accidents among males have a peak at 15–24 years of age. This fits the image many people have of reckless young men in fast cars and motorbikes, although we will suggest shortly that this may not be the whole picture. However, there is a second peak in road traffic accidents—among

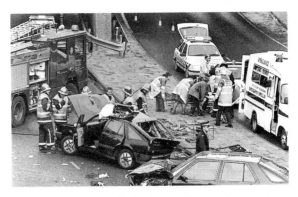

Unlike most causes of death, the mortality rate from road traffic accidents peaks among males aged 15–24. (Source White and Reed, Reading)

elderly people—which is seldom considered. These deaths are the result mainly of pedestrians being injured by vehicles. Another exception to the general pattern is AIDS: three-quarters of AIDS-related deaths in the United Kingdom have occurred between the ages of 25 and 44.

For most conditions, the association of morbidity with age follows a similar pattern to that of mortality—the older we become, the more ill-health we experience. This can be seen in the increasing incidence of most cancers with age (Figure 9.11).

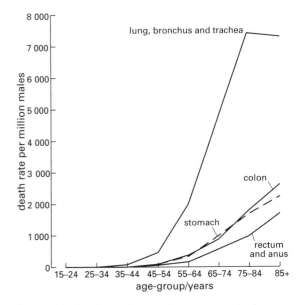

Figure 9.11 *Incidence of selected cancers in males by age, England and Wales, 1990. (Data from OPCS, 1991, Mortality Statistics: Cause 1990, OPCS Series DH2, No. 17, HMSO, London, Table 3)*

☐ From Figure 9.11, what is the rather surprising exception to this association?

■ The incidence of lung cancer declines after the age of 84.

☐ Approximately 90 per cent of lung cancers are thought to be due to smoking tobacco. How might you explain the apparent fall in the incidence of the disease after the age of 84?

■ There are three possibilities you may have considered:

(i)   Some men may have survived to later ages because of some form of resistance to the disease.

(ii)   All the men who are at risk from smoking all their lives die of lung cancer (and other smoking-related diseases) by the age of 84, leaving few lifetime smokers surviving.

(iii)   All the men born more than 84 years ago have some common experiences that make them less likely to develop lung cancer than younger men.

The third explanation, which commands most support, is known as a **birth cohort effect.** A cohort is a group of people who all share a common experience. In the case of a birth cohort the common factor is their year of birth. Such a group tends to share similar life experiences from birth to death. It is known that the prevalence of smoking has varied during this century. Suppose that men who were born during or after the First World War smoked more heavily throughout their lives than men born earlier. In 1990 (when the data in Figure 9.11 were collected) these heavy smokers would have been represented in the birth cohorts of up to ages 75–84 but not older, and would be expected to be suffering from higher lung cancer rates than the older group who had smoked less. The importance of the cohort effect is that it can distort the appearance of the relationship between mortality and age and lead to misinterpretation of that association. You should bear this in mind when you meet further examples.

Much of the reason for the observed age distribution of disease is the biological ageing of the cells, tissues and organs of the body.[6] However, social factors are also thought to influence the pattern. As you will see in the

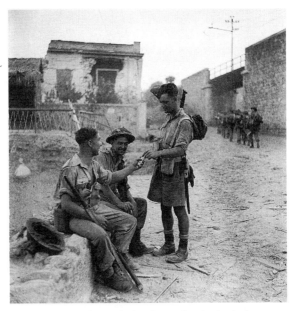

World War II soldiers in Italy taking a break. The high prevalence of smoking during this period was reflected in rising lung cancer rates several decades later. (Photo: Imperial War Museum)

next chapter, the social position of some age-groups (particularly the elderly) means that they are more likely to be exposed to poorer, health-damaging conditions. This may be reinforced by ageist attitudes in society. Apart from biological and social causes, the influence of a person's life history—that is, the influence of past events on the present state of health—is particularly important in the context of age. The birth-cohort effect on the incidence of lung cancer illustrates the importance of considering this influence: in that example it was men's tobacco consumption. This is not to suggest that the decision to smoke was an entirely personal choice. In fact, many biological and social factors can influence our 'personal' behaviour. Another example of such influences may lie behind the high mortality rates in young men caused by road traffic accidents. As we noted earlier, this is often ascribed to the high risk-taking behaviour of young adult males—in particular by those on motorbikes. However, additional factors include their social position which may preclude them financially from car ownership, and the behaviour of other road users towards motor cyclists. Filmed research has suggested that part of the explanation for their high mortality rate may be aggressive driving behaviour by car and lorry drivers in response to motorcyclists' risk-taking behaviour.

[6]This process is discussed more fully in *The Biology of Health and Disease* (Open University Press, 1985, revised as *Human Biology and Health: An Evolutionary Approach*, 1994).

In summary, you should note the following points:

1   Mortality rates increase with age. This is true for almost all causes of death.

2   Morbidity rates also increase with increasing age.

3   Biological factors (cell and tissue ageing) are largely responsible for this pattern.

4   The health of some age-groups (such as the elderly) is adversely affected by their relative social disadvantage.

5   Health status at any age will be influenced by a person's social circumstances and by their personal life history (their experiences and the past events in their life), as well as their current behaviour (such as risk-taking).

Marital status

Like gender and age, **marital status** forms another pervasive personal and social characteristic.

> Marital state is a socially, and generally legally, defined condition, and serves to distinguish between currently married, never married (single) and formerly married (widowed and divorced) people. Although marital state is defined in terms of the presence or absence of a marital partner, it involves more than a personal relationship, for each marital condition is associated with socially sanctioned rights and obligations with regard to children, sexuality, kinship ties, property and domestic and economic services. (Morgan, 1980, p. 633)

This quote from Myfanwy Morgan, a contemporary British sociologist, highlights the social importance of marital status but also the difficulties of determining precisely how to interpret its relationship to health status. By studying marital status, we are in fact attempting to investigate both the effect of a personal relationship on health status and the social consequences in terms of rights, obligations and resources such as income and housing.

☐ What two assumptions do you think there are in using a person's marital status in such investigations?

■ It assumes that people who are married enjoy the benefits of a close personal relationship; and it assumes that single and formerly married people are not experiencing such a relationship.[7]

An association between marital status and mortality was first demonstrated in the nineteenth century, when it was shown that mortality rates were lowest for the married, higher for the single and highest for those widowed or divorced. This has been consistently found ever since. Married people experience lower mortality rates than non-married for all causes of death. The overall **standardised mortality ratios (SMRs)** for men and women are shown in Table 9.2. SMRs express the actual deaths in a group as a ratio of the number of deaths that would be expected if that group experienced the age-specific death rates of the population as a whole, or of some specified comparitor population. In this case, the comparitor population for each group is the entire population of England irrespective of marital status[8].

Table 9.2   Standardised mortality ratios (SMRs) for men and women by marital status in 1971–5, using the population of England as the standard population (i.e. = 100)

	SMR by marital status			
	Single	Married	Widowed	Divorced
women	99	97	103	117
men	117	96	109	123

Data from Fox, J. and Goldblatt, P. O. (1982) *OPCS Longitudinal Study, 1971–5, Socio-Demographic Mortality Differentials*, Series LS, No. 1, HMSO, London, Table 4.2)

☐ Which sex appears to suffer higher mortality from being single?

■ Men. The SMR for single men (117) is much higher than that for married men (96), whereas the difference between the equivalent figures for women is much less: 99 among single women, 97 among married women.

A *change* in marital status has also been found to be strongly associated with changes in health status. A number of studies over several decades have looked at what happens to the surviving partner after their spouse dies, and have identified a small 'peak' of excess mortality among widows and widowers in the first year after their bereavement. One of the first and perhaps the best known of these studies, published by Colin Murray Parkes and colleagues in 1969, reported that the death rate among widowers during the first six months of bereavement was

[7]The use of marital status and social class in social research are discussed in detail in *Studying Health and Disease* (Open University Press, 1985; revised edition 1994).

[8]Standardised mortality ratios are examined in detail in *Studying Health and Disease* (Open University Press, 1985, revised edition 1994).

40 per cent greater than would be expected among married men of that age. The principal cause of death was cardiovascular disease: the authors suggested that the widowers were quite literally dying of a broken heart. However, more recent work has been less clear-cut: for example, one analysis based on the OPCS Longitudinal Study (Fox and Goldblatt, 1982) did find a small but statistically significant increase in deaths among widowers from heart disease (in agreement with the Parkes study) but no increase in mortality among widows. More recently, another analysis, also based on data from the Longitudinal Study, found that both widows and widowers suffered about 10 per cent more deaths after bereavement than would be expected, but there was no conclusive evidence that they were dying from heart disease (Jones, 1987). Perhaps the health consequences of bereavement are changing over time.

Divorce can have a similar effect, though usually during the later stages of marital breakdown rather than at the time of the divorce action. As with single status, divorce appears to have a greater adverse effect on men than on women—compare for instance, the mortality experiences of divorced men and women in Table 9.2. But, although both bereavement and divorce certainly have an adverse effect on health, there are some circumstances when they could have a positive effect: for example if they follow a period of stress such as a spouse's long terminal illness, or in cases of domestic violence.

The pattern of morbidity in relation to marital status does not follow that of mortality. Figure 9.12, which shows general practice consultation rates by marital sta-

tus, indicates that, whereas widowed and divorced people appear to experience the *most* morbidity (consistent with their position regarding mortality), single people appear to suffer *less* morbidity than married people.

The figure also shows that the relatively small differences between groups when all consultations are lumped together conceal much more striking associations at the level of specific diseases: consultation rates for mental disorders, musculoskeletal disorders (rheumatism, arthritis), and accidents are generally substantially higher among widowed and divorced people than among the married, whereas rates among the single can be quite markedly lower. Rates of self-reported illness (that is, rates obtained from household surveys, for example, rather than rates derived from the use of the health service) show similar patterns.

How can we explain these differences in the mortality and morbidity rates of different marital states? Biological explanations may play some role: some of the 'protective' effect of marriage on women's mortality could be due to differential rates of reproductive system cancer—such as cancers of the breast, uterus or cervix—which are related to sexual or reproductive history to some degree. Several social factors have also been suggested, and these will be discussed in a moment. First, though, it is necessary to consider the process of *marital selection*. In all the discussions in this chapter, it is assumed that health status is a consequence of the biological and social factor under investigation. However, it is possible that the reverse may be true, that is, states of health may influence social status.

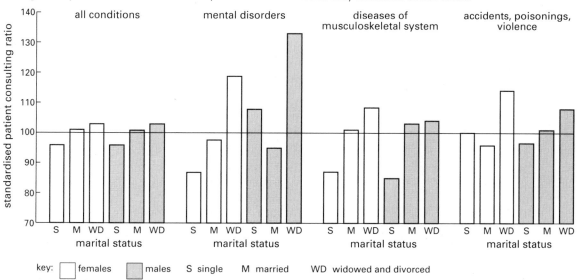

Figure 9.12 *Standardised patient consulting ratios by marital status, men and women aged 16+, England and Wales, 1980–81. (All marital states = 100.) (Data derived from Royal College of General Practitioners/OPCS/DHSS, 1986, Morbidity Statistics from General Practice: Third National Study: Socio-economic analysis, OPCS Series MB5 No. 2, HMSO, London, Table 3.1)*

☐ Can you suggest how health may affect marital status?

■ People suffering from poor health may be more likely to remain single, and those bereaved or divorced who suffer poor health may be less likely to remarry than people enjoying good health. Divorce may also be more likely in a marriage in which one partner is often ill.

Although this is probably a contributory rather than a major factor, it is one worth bearing in mind and considering for each of the factors discussed in this chapter.

There are several possible social explanations of ways in which the pattern of health may be influenced by marital status. The social conditions and position enjoyed by different groups will affect their health status: for example, widowed and divorced people will tend to be less well off financially than the other groups, whereas couples have certain advantages such as work-sharing.

Emile Durkheim, one of the founders of empirical sociology, concluded in 1897 in *Suicide: A Study in Sociology* that marriage reduced the chances of suicide by almost one-half, owing to the greater social integration of married people. In contrast, the anomalous social position of the single (whether never married or divorced or widowed) may serve as a source of stress. Just as was seen with age and gender, some groups are discriminated against. In those instances we recognise the existence of ageist and sexist attitudes. Although it is less well recognised, those not married may suffer in similar ways. However, as more and more households fail to conform to the nuclear 'ideal', the power of discrimination may wane, just as it has for couples who live together without marrying.[9]

Systematic differences in *health service use* by people of different marital status also need to be considered.

☐ Why is it important to do this?

■ As has been discussed previously in this chapter, differences in morbidity rates derived from health service usage may reflect systematic differences in illness behaviour (how people respond to ill-health) within different marital states, and in the response people receive from doctors.

The highest consulting ratios for mental disorders, for example, are by divorced people, and the lowest by single people. This is true of both men and women. These

may reflect, first, a real difference in the prevalence of morbidity between the groups; second, widowed and divorced people may be more likely to consult their doctor when depressed, anxious, etc., because they have no partner to confide in; or third, doctors may be more willing to label patients' problems as being psychological rather than physical in the knowledge of their marital status, particularly if the person is widowed or divorced.

Finally, the *lifestyles* associated with different marital conditions may contribute to the observed differences. Married people may have a stronger motivation to guard their health for the sake of their partner and dependants. The high mortality rates for road accidents and alcohol-induced cirrhosis of the liver among single men would support this theory. The existence of several equally plausible hypotheses underlines the need for more empirical evidence on the clearly important subject of marital status and health, and in particular the different experiences of men and women. However, the key points to remember are:

1   Mortality rates are lowest for married, higher for single and highest for those widowed or divorced.

2   Being unmarried has a greater adverse effect on male than on female mortality. Similarly, divorce appears to be more health-damaging to men than to women.

3   Several social explanations of the apparent 'protective' effects of marriage have been suggested.

4   Unlike mortality differences, the single appear to suffer less morbidity than the married, though the reasons for this observation are unclear.

Ethnicity and race

Another way in which the population can be stratified is on the basis of **ethnicity** or race. Many people have objected to the term **'race'** as its use in the past has suggested a primarily biological or genetic basis for cultural differences between groups—an assertion that genetic studies do not support. Others have argued that using the term 'ethnicity' implies that health differences arise primarily from cultural variations, and thereby encourages 'victim-blaming'. The term ethnicity is used here, but without prior assumptions about the causes of health differences between different ethnic or racial groups.

There are many difficulties in defining and using the concept of ethnicity: for example, is a person's own country of birth, or their parents' country of birth, of more relevance?[10] Despite the multi-racial nature of British

[9]This is discussed in *Birth to Old Age: Health in Transition* (Open University Press, 1985; revised edition 1995).

[10]See *Studying Health and Disease* (Open University Press, 1985; revised edition 1994).

society, both now and in the past, many routinely collected statistics on health and disease do not provide information on different ethnic groups. However, let us begin by looking at mortality in England and Wales by sex and country of birth (Table 9.3).

The table shows that the excess mortality in 1979–83 was highest among migrants to England and Wales who were born in Ireland or Scotland (between 18 per cent and 28 per cent higher). There was a much smaller excess for Indian and African born men (6–9 per cent higher), whereas among men born in European countries such as France, old Commonwealth countries such as Australia, and the Caribbean, mortality levels were 15–21 per cent *lower* than the prevailing levels in England and Wales as a whole. A broadly similar pattern existed for women.

Table 9.3 also contains comparable information on the mortality of these groups for the earlier period 1970–2.

□ What changes occurred between 1970–2 and 1979–83 in the mortality experience of different ethnic groups by country of birth?

■ Excess mortality in the African, Caribbean and Indian groups fell substantially, but there was much less improvement among migrants from Ireland or Scotland.

Table 9.3 Mortality at ages 20–69, from all causes by sex and country of birth, of migrants to England and Wales, 1970–2 and 1979–83

| Country of birth | Standardised mortality ratios (England and Wales 1979–83 = 100) | | | |
	Males, 1970–2	Females, 1970–2	Males, 1979–83	Females, 1979–83
England and Wales	114	110	100	100
All Ireland (Republic and Northern)	139	129	128	120
Scotland	128	119	118	118
Indian sub-continent	114	124	106	105
Caribbean Commonwealth	110	150	79	105
African Commonwealth	152	167	109	114
Australia	n.a.	n.a.	85	83
France	98	98	80	75

n.a. = not available. (Data from OPCS, 1990, *Mortality and Geography: a Review in the mid-1980s; England and Wales*, HMSO, London, p. 107, Table 9.4)

At this point you should note that the ethnic groups in Table 9.3 are defined by *country of birth*.

□ What influence might this definition have on the patterns of mortality observed?

■ There are at least three possible influences:

(i) Members of minority ethnic groups born in England and Wales are excluded.

(ii) It is difficult to know how long these immigrants spent in England and Wales prior to death, and therefore how much their health experience may have been influenced by their life in England and Wales.

(iii) It is possible that the decision to migrate may have been influenced by a person's existing state of health.

All these factors must be born in mind. For example, the first Immigrant Mortality Study in England and Wales, published in 1984 (Marmot *et al.,* 1984), showed that almost all immigrant groups had lower rates of mortality (all causes combined) than prevailed in their country of birth, suggesting that individuals of above average health tended to migrate.

For these and other reasons it is extremely difficult to explain the variations in mortality that are observed between different ethnic groups. However, some clues can be found among the main causes of death. In comparison with death rates for England and Wales as a whole, African and Caribbean immigrants tend to have high death rates from hypertension (high blood pressure) and stroke, whereas immigrants from the whole of the Indian sub-continent suffer unusually high rates of cardiovascular disease, regardless of their country of origin, religion and language. Other patterns emerge when specific ethnic groups are studied: for example, the large Bangladeshi community in east London also has high rates of diabetes, but lower than average mortality from cancers of the bowel. All immigrant groups tend to have higher death rates from tuberculosis and from accidents and violence. But death rates among immigrants tend to be lower from most forms of cancer, especially lung cancer, and from bronchitis.

Turning to morbidity, Table 9.4 (overleaf) gives an indication of the health concerns of a predominantly Asian community living in London: these data were obtained from a phone-in counselling service for health problems.

Table 9.4 Reasons for phoning the counselling service

Reason given	No. of questions	Percentage of total
asthma, hay fever, breathlessness	479	13
family planning, fertility, infertility, psychosexual problems	408	11
diabetes	391	11
general nutrition and slimming (not rickets)	288	8
all mental health problems (ranging from mild depression to those receiving hospital treatment)	282	8
homeopathic treaments/herbal treatments	271	7
skin complaints	252	7
back pain	138	4
child care	100	3
eye complaints	87	2
specific gynaecological problems	83	2
arthritis	82	2
queries concerning pregnancy	80	2
mild gastric problems	79	2
second opinions	79	2
minor ailments	67	2
headaches	59	2
others	323	12
total	**3 679**	**100**

Data from Webb, P. (1981) Health problems of London's Asians and Afro-Caribbeans, *Health Visitor,* **54** (April), p.144.

☐ Comparing Table 9.4 with the data in Table 9.1 for a general practice serving a predominantly white population in Kent, what pattern do you detect?

■ The main health concerns of the two groups were broadly similar: respiratory problems, mental health and skin complaints.

Only 7 of the 3 679 callers from the Asian community were concerned about rickets and only 45 about tuberculosis, although these are the main health concerns often perceived by the medical world. On this evidence, the majority of health problems experienced by minority ethnic groups in the United Kingdom are different in degree, but not in kind, from the majority.

Finally, Figure 9.13 provides some information on general practitioner consultation rates by sex and ethnicity.

☐ Look first at the columns for all complaints grouped together. What pattern exists?

■ The differences between the different ethnic groups are fairly minor, although the consultation rate for Indian males appears to be substantially above average.

☐ Now compare this with consultations for serious complaints. What differences emerge?

■ Males and females of Indian or Caribbean ethnicity, and Irish males, have much higher consultation rates for serious complaints.

What could account for the differences in mortality, morbidity and health service use outlined above? As in the previous sections on age, gender and marital status, we shall first consider biological explanations. There is a considerable amount of information on the tiny minority of diseases specific to certain ethnic or racial groups. This reflects the dominant biological interest of scientific medicine. These diseases are *genetic* in origin and arise in specific ethnic groups because of a higher frequency of a particular gene. Two of the commonest and most important of these conditions are *thalassaemia* and *sickle-cell disease* (which was discussed in Chapter 3).

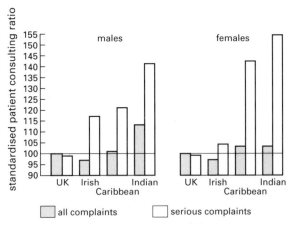

Figure 9.13 *Standardised patient consulting ratios in general practice by sex and ethnicity, 1981–2. (All ethnic groups = 100.) (Data derived from Royal College of General Practitioners/OPCS/DHSS, 1986, Morbidity Statistics from General Practice: Third National Study: Socio-economic Analysis, OPCS Series MB5, No. 2, HMSO, London, Table 3.6)*

Another example is called *Tay–Sachs disease* (a very rare disease which causes progressive blindness and brain degeneration in childhood). Although found in most populations, 90 per cent of cases occur in Jews and in particular in those of Ashkenazi descent whose ancestors lived around the Polish–Lithuanian border at the end of the nineteenth century.

A final example is *cystic fibrosis*, a common condition in which mucus produced by several organs in the body, particularly the lungs and pancreas, is abnormally viscid (sticky) causing blockage and obstruction to the normal functioning of these organs. Cystic fibrosis, which is the commonest disease associated with a single gene defect in the United Kingdom, mainly affects white people: in the USA 98 per cent of patients are white.[11]

These particular inherited conditions account for only a small proportion of the ill-health suffered by different ethnic groups. For instance, although there is a significant excess mortality among American blacks compared with white Americans, a calculation in 1977 suggested that sickle-cell anaemia and thalassaemia accounted for only 0.3 per cent of this excess. However, advances in biological science may well find other examples of ethnic differences with a biological component. For example, during the early 1990s biochemical differences were described which probably account for the high rates of *diabetes* among Bangladeshis in east London mentioned earlier.

Apart from these biological differences, what other factors could help to explain the health differences between ethnic groups? *Cultural differences* are a frequently cited possibility. For example, there are significant differences between ethnic groups in terms of diet. A study of Asian immigrants in England and Wales, published in 1985 by Michael Marmot and colleagues (McKeigue *et al.*, 1985), found that Asians consumed less saturated fats and cholesterol and more polyunsaturated fats and vegetable fibre than the British population. This dietary difference is consistent with theories about a possible protective effect of high-fibre diets on cancers of the bowel, which have a low incidence in Asian immigrants, but it runs counter to theories about the protective effects of low-cholesterol diets on cardiovascular disease, which causes unusually high mortality among this same ethnic group. There are also well-documented differences in smoking behaviour and consumption of alcohol: men and women born in the Indian sub-continent generally smoke and drink much less than the average for England and Wales, but there are variations between Muslims and Hindus with, for example, very high rates of smoking found among Bangladeshi men living in the United Kingdom.

These differences may reflect in part religious adherence, but this cannot explain why immigrant men born in Ireland drink more than average, and Irish and Scottish male immigrants smoke more than average. So cultural differences do explain some of the health differences observed, but many other differences remain unexplained.

□ Comparing the causes of death among ethnic groups mentioned earlier with these patterns of smoking and drinking, can you identify any anomalies?

■ One puzzle is that people born in the Indian sub-continent have high rates of heart disease but low rates of smoking and alcohol consumption, both of which are considered to be risk factors.

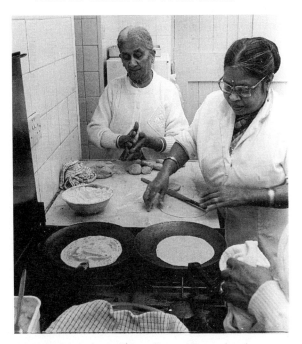

Asians in Britain have distinct dietary patterns, but the relationship between these and their health is not clear. (Photo: Mike Levers)

[11]The mechanisms by which single gene defects can cause disease are discussed in greater detail in *The Biology of Health and Disease* (Open University Press, 1985, revised as *Human Biology and Health: An Evolutionary Approach*, 1994).

Finally, therefore, we come to the influence of *social and life history factors*. Members of minority ethnic groups in the United Kingdom tend to be concentrated in lower social classes and are therefore subject to the poorer health status associated with relative disadvantages such as lower income, poor housing, and inadequate health care. For instance, it is likely that the higher incidence of tuberculosis in Asians results in part because they are over-represented among people living in conditions of domestic over-crowding associated with poor inner city housing and poverty. These disadvantages are exacerbated by **racism** which may, for instance, limit employment and housing opportunities. In addition, racist attacks are likely to result not only in physical injury, but also fear and anxiety.

Racism can affect not only health status but also the care that members of black and Asian communities receive from health services. In this context, the term 'institutional racism' is usually used. What this means is that racist beliefs are accepted as factual evidence for differences between ethnic groups. The beliefs therefore become normalised, that is, they become incorporated into the belief system that is a feature of any society (or section of society). These views then come to influence and determine the behaviour of the members of that society. In health care this is most obvious in psychiatric practice,[12] some examples of which are given by Roland Littlewood and Maurice Lipsedge in their book *Aliens and Alienists: Ethnic Minorities and The Psychiatrist* (1982). The institutionalisation of prejudiced beliefs is not of course confined to racial views, but occurs with views of gender, age and the other factors being discussed in this chapter.

Finally, it should be noted that social and cultural influences are not independent, and in fact are a good illustration of the kinds of *interaction* discussed earlier in this chapter. For example, the pattern of general practitioner consultations shown in Figure 9.13 could plausibly be interpreted as showing that minority ethnic groups do in general experience higher levels of morbidity, but are deterred by a range of cultural barriers, institutionalised racism and social/economic disadvantages from seeking medical advice from general practitioners in all save the most serious of cases.

In summary the main points to note are:

1   Despite the lack of meaningful routine statistics on the health status of different ethnic groups, there is sufficient evidence to demonstrate the poorer health suffered by certain minorities. But these minorities do generally have lower rates of mortality than do people in their country of origin.

2   Biological factors are known to account for a small proportion of observed differences, but in the main they are probably due to a mixture of social and cultural factors, reinforced by the existence of racism.

Geography

Variations in mortality rates between different regions of Britain have been noted since at least the last century. Figure 9.14 shows the standardised mortality ratios for males for 1989.

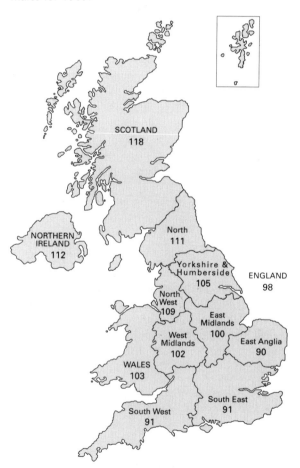

Figure 9.14 *Geographical variations in mortality in the United Kingdom, 1989. (Data derived from Central Statistical Office, 1991, Regional Trends No. 26, HMSO, London, Table 4.13, HMSO, London.)*

[12]This is discussed in *Experiencing and Explaining Disease* (Open University Press, 1985, revised edition 1995).

□ How would you describe the regional pattern of mortality?

■ The highest rates are experienced in Scotland (18 per cent higher than might be expected on United Kingdom age-specific death rates), Northern Ireland (12 per cent higher), and the North and North West of England (respectively 11 per cent and 9 per cent higher). The lowest rates are in the area of England south of the line between the Severn and the Wash.

Similar geographical variations exist among morbidity rates for a wide range of diseases. Figure 9.15, for example, shows data for the same standard regions as shown in Figure 9.14 on tooth loss and long-standing illness.

□ How consistent are these differences in morbidity with the mortality differences shown in Figure 9.14?

■ In general, regions with an excess mortality also have higher morbidity—for example the North and North West of England and Scotland—while areas of comparatively low mortality such as the South East also have lower morbidity.

What are the possible explanations for regional differences in mortality and morbidity rates? First, it should be noted that the information on morbidity in Figure 9.15 was not standardised in order to eliminate differences in the age- and sex-structure of the population of each region, but doing so would remove only a small proportion of the differences.

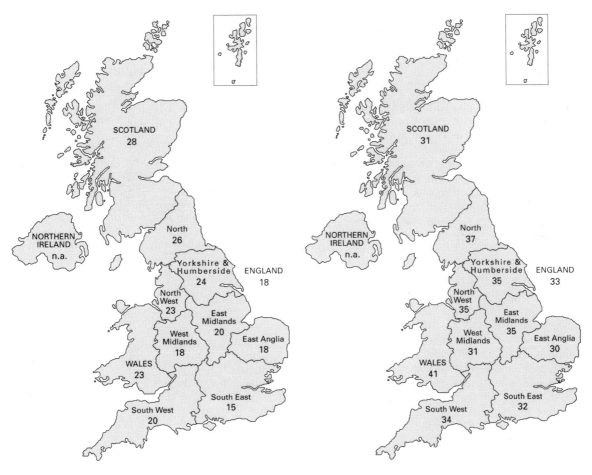

(a) United Kingdom (=20)

(b) United Kingdom (=33)

Figure 9.15 *Geographical variations in morbidity in Great Britain: (a) percentage of adults with no natural teeth, 1989; (b) percentage of persons reporting a long-standing illness, 1987. (Data on tooth loss from OPCS, 1991,* General Household Survey 1989, *OPCS Series GHS, No. 20, HMSO, London, Tables 4.44 and 4.45; on long-standing illness from Central Statistical Office, 1989,* Regional Trends No. 24, *HMSO, London, Table 7.2)*

Climatic and *environmental factors* such as hours of sunshine, humidity and water hardness have been suggested as explanations for some regional variations. For example, it has been shown that the standardised mortality ratios for malignant melanoma of the skin (skin cancer) are significantly higher in the south of the country than the north: a reversal of the usual pattern. This type of cancer is associated with exposure to ultraviolet light, which is the greater in the south because on average it receives more sunshine of higher intensity (Swerdlow, 1979). Another environmental feature long held to be beneficial to health is residence by the seaside with its fresh air and absence of heavy pollution. However, detailed studies of this indicate very little difference: in 1979–83 the SMR for coastal areas in England and Wales was 98 for both males and females, compared with 100 for males and 101 for females in inland areas (OPCS, 1990b). Even this slight difference may be an artefact in that older people retiring to seaside areas may be healthier than their peers who do not move on retirement.

Another environmental feature to have attracted attention in recent years is *water quality*. It has been established that deaths from cardiovascular disease are partly associated with 'soft' water (containing low concentrations of calcium salts), although whether this association has any causal significance is still uncertain.

Another feature of the environment with long-established links to the pattern of mortality is the degree of *urbanisation*. The standard regions shown in Figure 9.14 cover huge and disparate areas of country which include urban and rural areas, and in order to measure the degree of urbanisation it is necessary to look at smaller areas such as local districts or health authorities (these measurement problems have already been encountered in the discussion of Third World countries in Chapter 3). When local authorities with excess mortality from particular causes are ranked by SMR, it has been demonstrated that those with the greatest excess mortality are predominantly inner-city urban areas[13]. This is true of cardiovascular disease—a leading cause of death. It is also true for deaths from lung cancer, pneumonia, bronchitis and stomach ulcer.

Of course, the reasons for these differences vary: many studies around the world have shown a highly significant association in inner cities between the levels of air pollution, particularly from vehicle exhaust emissions, and the incidence of lung problems ranging from

[13]Patterns of health and disease within cities are the subject of a TV programme, 'A Tale of Four Cities', for Open University students.

persistent cough and phlegm production and severe breathlessness, to mortality from asthma attacks, bronchitis and pneumonia. Excess deaths from lung cancer in urban areas may have some connection with air pollution, but 90 per cent of lung cancer is caused by smoking, and smoking is more prevalent in urban areas. This in turn may reflect the *social class* composition of inner city urban areas. And again it should be noted that the urban–rural pattern of mortality is not uniform across all causes of death: there is excess mortality in rural areas for a number of diseases including prostate cancer—an important cause of death among men; some rural areas appear to have fairly high mortality rates from female breast cancer; and rural areas also experience excess mortality from motor vehicle accidents.

At a more localised level, the *geological structure* of different parts of the United Kingdom can also have an influence on patterns of disease, particularly on the incidence of those cancers associated with radiation. Houses built above granite, or constructed from granite blocks, expose their occupants to higher than normal background levels of radiation, and where naturally-occurring radon gas seeps into houses from the underlying rock the radiation levels may pose a serious threat to health.

Rather more attention has been focused in recent years on the environmental hazards of living near a nuclear power station, in particular the Sellafield nuclear plant in Cumbria. A number of epidemiological analyses of the health of the local population established that there was a small increase in deaths from leukaemia and lymphoma (cancers of white blood cells) among children living around the plant, many of whom had fathers employed at Sellafield. In 1990, a controversial study by M. J. Gardner and colleagues claimed that these cancers were associated with exposure of the children's *fathers* to high doses of radiation at work in the period before the child was conceived. One possibility is that damage to the genetic material in developing sperm was responsible for cancer in the men's offspring. This would suggest an occupational rather than an environmental explanation of the resultant disease. However, at the time of writing, in 1992, these findings are hotly contested, partly on the basis that no such effect has been detected in the children of men exposed to radiation during the nuclear explosions at Hiroshima and Nagasaki.

Despite all these well-documented influences of environment on mortality, there is *no* evidence that they are the *main* reason for the striking regional variations shown in Figure 9.14. And there is considerable evidence that socio-economic factors are closely related to many of the differences. For instance, it is known that the social class composition of the population varies significantly

Table 9.5 Standardised mortality ratios, males, 1979–83 (England and Wales = 100) by region and social class

Region	Regional male SMR	SMRs for local authorities where: less than 20% of heads of household are in Social Class I or II	SMRs for local authorities where: over 25% of heads of household are in Social Class I or II	Percentage of local authorities where: less than 20% of heads of household are in Social Class I or II	Percentage of local authorities where: over 25% of heads of household are in Social Class I or II
North	112	115	103	59	14
North West	111	117	103	41	30
Wales	107	112	100	49	27
Yorkshire and Humberside	106	109	107	39	31
West Midlands	104	110	96	31	50
England and Wales	100	109	91	27	46
East Midlands	99	105	93	25	40
South East	94	106	90	12	66
South West	90	98	87	13	49
East Anglia	88	90	86	30	50

Data derived from OPCS (1990) *Mortality and Geography: a review in the mid-1980s; England and Wales*, OPCS Series DS, No. 9, HMSO, London, Table 6.1.

between regions, and also that social class is closely associated with health and disease. Table 9.5 shows some features of this.

The first two columns shows the regions of England and Wales ranked according to their male SMR in 1979–83. The next two columns show for each region the SMR in local authority areas where (a) fewer than 20 per cent of heads of household, and (b) more than 25 per cent of heads of household, are in Social Class I or II. In the first row, for example, the SMR in all local authorities in the Northern region where more than 25 per cent of heads of household are in the upper social classes is 103. The final two columns show the actual proportions of local authorities in each Region with (a) fewer than 20 per cent and (b) more than 25 per cent of heads of household, in Social Class I or II. Again to illustrate, in row 1 the proportion of all local authorities in the Northern region where more than 25 per cent of heads of household are in the upper social classes is 14 per cent.

☐ First study the SMRs carefully in the table. What strikes you about them?

■ Within each region, SMRs are lower in the local authorities where the proportion of household heads in the upper social classes is high, and vice versa.

This is as expected. But when a comparison is made across regions, there are clear and consistent differences in SMRs even when social class characteristics are similar.

☐ Now look at the final two columns. How do these data relate to the SMR data in the table?

■ Regions with low SMRs have a higher *proportion* of household heads in Social Classes I or II.

☐ Putting these observations together, what conclusion do you reach?

■ Differences in the social class composition of the population explain some of the regional differences in mortality, but even when the social class composition of the population is taken into account regional differences remain.

An analysis of other social variables such as *housing tenure* would reveal similar patterns and lead to similar conclusions: there are regional variations in housing tenure (for example a higher proportion of houses are owner-occupied in the South than in the North), and housing tenure is associated with mortality, but some regions exhibit higher levels of mortality within each type of housing tenure than others.

A final possible explanation of regional differences in mortality is that healthy people are attracted from some areas such as the North of England to other regions such as South East England with better employment or other opportunities, leaving behind a relatively less healthy population. The little research conducted on this topic (for example the first report of the OPCS Longitudinal Study; Fox and Goldbatt, 1982) suggests that migration has indeed tended to widen regional differences, but that the effect has been small. It might also be noted that in some cases people with particular health problems will be attracted to areas of the country where treatment opportunities may be better: for example, between 1982 and 1992 over 70 per cent of all diagnoses of AIDS occurred in one of the four Regional Health Authorities covering London and the South East of England, a proportion far in excess of the population covered by these health authorities. One explanation is that some people moved to London from other areas of the United Kingdom to obtain treatment in recognised centres, and perhaps also to get more help from support organisations.

In summary, you should note the following:

1   Mortality and morbidity rates are highest in Scotland, Northern Ireland and Northern England and lowest in South East England.

2   Many of the regional variations in mortality appear to be associated with environmental and social factors (the degree of urbanisation; differences in social class structure; the effect of geographical mobility), but these factors still leave some regional variations unaccounted for.

Occupation and social class

You have seen that differences in social class structure are one of the factors explaining regional variations in health. Let us now look in more detail at the association between health and occupation or social class. Although occupation and social class are closely related, they are not interchangeable: **occupational mortality** attempts to measure workplace hazards and other health risks that are *intrinsic* to a person's occupation, whereas **social class mortality** attempts to embrace a wide range of additional factors *extrinsic* to occupation—such as environment, social position or lifestyle—that may influence mortality[14].

[14]A full discussion of these methods of classification, and the problems associated with them, can be found in *Studying Health and Disease*, (Open University Press, 1985; revised edition 1994).

Some illustrations of differences in occupational mortality for the period 1979–83 are given in Table 9.6.

Table 9.6   Standardised mortality ratios for men aged 15 and over, and women aged 15–59, by type of occupation, 1976–81; England and Wales = 100.

Occupation	SMRs	
	Men	Women
glass and ceramic makers	134	–
textile workers	118	103
labourers	118	–
miners and quarrymen	113	–
engineering and allied trades	100	135
clerical workers	93	77
administrators and managers	79	55
professional and technical workers	68	80
all	**100**	**100**

Data from OPCS (1990) *Longitudinal Study 1971–81 England and Wales: Mortality and Social Organisation*, OPCS Series LS, No. 6, HMSO, London, Tables 7.2 and 8.2.

As the table indicates, there are substantial variations in the SMR for people in different occupations and, as expected, people in manual occupations tend to experience excess mortality. This may arise from direct risks to health and physical well-being in many manual jobs, which may result in direct loss of life, either suddenly in the form of accidents, or in an attenuated manner through exposure to damaging substances in the workplace over a long period. You may be aware of some examples, such as pneumoconiosis, a chronic lung condition suffered by coal miners.

In addition to specific occupational hazards, many health risks associated with work are of a non-specific nature and arise from *stress*. Stress may arise in a number of ways but tends to originate from how work is organised. Some examples include low pay (leading to excessive overtime work), incentive payment schemes (speeding up potentially dangerous processes), shift-work (disrupting biological, psychological and social functioning), poor job design (producing boredom, and little satisfaction), and bad industrial relations. The effects of stress on health have been demonstrated in terms of accident and sickness absence rates associated with different work practices.

However, it is possible that the relatively high mortality of men in, for example, the glass and ceramic industries is a result not only of health hazards directly associated with their occupation, but also the areas they tend to live in, the size and standard of their housing, the quality of their diet, or many other aspects of their lifestyle and environment. One way of separating out the direct effects of occupation from those due to factors extrinsic to the workplace is by relating the mortality or morbidity of the workers in that occupation to that of their spouses. This process has suggested, for example, that leather workers are at increased risk of suffering from tuberculosis, chronic rheumatic heart disease, and bronchitis—all as a direct consequence of their occupation.

☐ Why do you think spouses are a good control group?

■ Spouses share most of the same social conditions as the worker (housing, income, etc.) and the same residential hazards (such as environmental pollutants), but not the working environment.

☐ For what factors can spouses not act as controls?

■ Biological factors relating to sex and social factors relating to gender cannot be controlled for.

Care needs to be taken in making comparisons based on worker–spouse differences. This is well illustrated in studies of the dangers of asbestos. Not only were the male workers at risk of inhaling asbestos fibres, but so were their wives. This was because men took their contaminated clothes home to be laundered by their wives.

In general, and despite the examples given above, it is not thought that occupation as such can explain more than a small part of mortality differences such as those shown in Table 9.6. One calculation has estimated the proportion of all cancers that can be related to occupational exposures as no more than 5 per cent (Davies, 1982). Because risks to health intrinsic to the workplace are only one of many influences on health, it has become common to group people into social classes based on groupings of broadly similar occupations. One of the most frequently used classifications in the United Kingdom is the **Registrar-General's classification of occupations**; this groups all occupations into six categories (although they are sometimes combined in various permutations):

I	Professional (for example, a doctor or accountant)
II	Intermediate (for example, a nurse or teacher)
IIIN	Skilled non-manual (for example, a typist)
IIIM	Skilled manual (for example, a butcher or electrician)

| IV | Partly skilled manual (for example, a postman) |
| V | Unskilled (for example, a labourer) |

It is generally the case that these *occupational* classes are also referred to as *social* classes I to V in research publications, as in this chapter. You will also encounter other classifications in this book, for instance that used by the General Household Survey.

When using these classifications, it has generally been found that the social class of a married woman in employment is less predictive of her mortality than is her husband's class, and so it is conventional to assign women their own class if they are single but their husband's if they are married: this is the basis on which the following tables and graphs have been constructed.

Figure 9.16 shows separately for males and females at different ages the SMR for each social class in 1979–83.

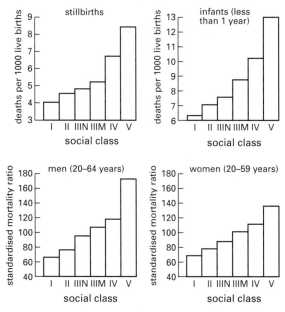

Figure 9.16 *Mortality by social class, infants, England and Wales, 1984, and adults, Great Britain, 1979–83, using the Registrar-General's classification of occupations. Note: It is not necessary to age-standardise the data for stillbirths and infant deaths, as both categories refer to small age-ranges. (Data from OPCS, 1986, Mortality Statistics, Perinatal and Infant: Social and Biological Factors for 1984, Series DH3, No. 17, HMSO, London; OPCS, 1988, Occupational Mortality:Childhood Supplement, OPCS Series DS, No. 8, HMSO, London, Table 2.12; and OPCS, 1986, Registrar-General's Decennial Supplement on Occupational Mortality, 1979–83, HMSO, London, Tables GD28 and GD34)*

A clear gradient across social classes is evident both in infancy and adulthood and for both sexes. At birth and during the first year of life the risk of death in social class V is approximately double that in social class I, and differences in adult mortality are of a similar order.

Table 9.7 concentrates on differences in adulthood. In addition to showing death rates by social class for men and women separately, it also shows (a) the ratio between men and women for each social class (the right-hand column), and (b) the ratio between social classes V and I for each sex (the bottom row). If there were no differences, the ratio would be 1.0. The ratio of social classes V to I, for men, of 2.5 means that the death rate for social class V (944 per 100 000) is two and a half times higher than that for social class I (375 per 100 000).

☐ Does the association between sex and mortality vary with social class?

■ The difference between male and female mortality rates is large across all social classes but, although smallest in social class I and greatest in social class V, the ratios (far right-hand column in Table 9.7) vary only slightly from 2.31 to 2.70.

Similarly the association between social class and mortality does not appear to be much influenced by gender (the ratio of social class V to social class I is 2.5 for males and 2.2 for females). Taken together, this evidence suggests that the 'protective' effect of being female persists almost independently of social class.

Next, Figure 9.17 looks at social class differences in mortality according to some major causes of death.

Table 9.7 Adult death rates per 100 000 population by sex and social class, Great Britain, 1979–83

| Social class | Death rate per 100 000 | | Ratio of male : female death rate |
	Males aged 20–64	Females (married) aged 20–59	
I	375	162	2.31
II	425	180	2.36
IIIN	529	201	2.63
IIIM	597	240	2.49
IV	651	270	2.41
V	944	350	2.70
Ratio V/I	2.5	2.2	

Data from OPCS (1986) *Registrar-General's Decennial Supplement on Occupational Mortality 1979–83*, HMSO, London, Tables GD16 and GD24.

☐ In the figure, what categories of disease show the steepest social class gradient, and for which sex?

■ The strongest class association is shown by injuries and poisonings (men), diseases of the nervous system (men); and circulatory disease (men and women). For some diseases, the class gradient is much steeper in one sex than the other. For example, the gradient for cancers is much steeper among men than women.

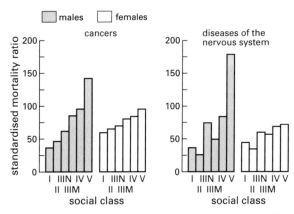

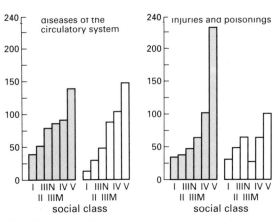

Figure 9.17 *Standardised mortality ratios by major cause and social class for men aged 20–64 years and women aged 20–59 years, Great Britain, 1979–83 (all causes combined = 100). (Data from OPCS, 1986,* Registrar-General's Decennial Supplement on Occupational Mortality 1979–83, *HMSO, London, Tables GD28 and GD34)*

However, when the focus is moved down to specific cancers rather than the whole group, as in Figure 9.18, some interesting patterns emerge.

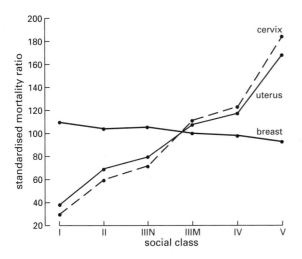

Figure 9.18 *Standardised mortality ratios for cancers of the female reproductive system, by social class (women aged 20–59), Great Britain 1979–83. (Data from OPCS, 1986, Registrar-General's Decennial Supplement on Occupational Mortality 1979–83, HMSO, London, Table GD34)*

☐ What is the social class gradient in mortality from breast cancer?

■ It departs from the norm in that mortality is higher in the higher social classes.

☐ How much greater is the risk of death from cervical cancer in women in social class V than to those in social class I?

■ Six times greater (SMR of 186 compared with 29).

This staggering social class difference in mortality from cervical cancer has given rise to several explanations, which also illustrate how the interpretation of epidemiological data can be influenced by the views and values of researchers. An early explanation to be proposed was that cervical cancer is caused by a sexually-transmitted viral infection of the cervix, that women in lower social classes are younger at the time of first intercourse, have more sexual partners and a poorer standard of personal hygiene, and therefore experience a higher incidence of the disease. Though all these aspects of women's behaviour would increase their likelihood of contracting a sexually transmitted infection, such an explanation failed to consider several other possibilities.

First, if cervical cancer was caused by a sexually transmitted infection, then the sexual experience of *men* was equally important. Second, the assumption about social class differences in sexual experience lacked any reliable supporting data. And, third, as evidence accumulated on the epidemiology of the disease, so it became apparent that the highest risks of disease were to be found in the wives of men working in dirty occupations such as steel erecting and metal working. This prompted a revised view that the disease might have a viral component but also be related to a carcinogen (cancer-causing substance) carried home from work. There are still a number of poorly understood aspects of cancer of the cervix (a strong association with smoking has emerged as another possible explanation of the social class gradient), but the point to note here is that the competing explanations proposed can reflect the biases and assumptions of the investigators.

Population surveys of morbidity reinforce the finding from mortality data, that people in lower social classes suffer from poorer health than those in higher social classes. An example is total tooth loss. You have already seen its association with age (Figure 9.6); in Figure 9.19 you can see the additional effect of social class.

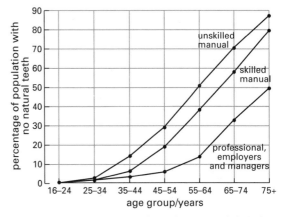

Figure 9.19 *Percentage of adults with no natural teeth, by age and socio-economic group, Great Britain, 1989. (Data from OPCS, 1991, General Household Survey 1989, OPCS Series GHS, No. 20, HMSO, London, Table 4.50)*

☐ At what age is there the greatest difference in the percentage of toothless people between the professional classes and the unskilled manual class? Look first at *absolute differences* between the three groups at each age (that is, subtract the lowest from the highest percentage). Then look at *relative differences* (that is, divide the highest by the lowest percentage).

■ In *absolute* terms, the difference is greatest in the oldest age-groups (for example, 88 minus 50 equals a difference of 38 per cent after age 75). In *relative* terms, the difference is greatest among those aged 45–54 years of age, when the percentage of unskilled manual workers with no natural teeth is almost five times higher than the percentage among the professional classes (29 ÷ 6 = 4.83).

Another example of social class and morbidity comes from the General Household Survey in which, as noted earlier, people are asked to report on their own health status. Figure 9.20 shows rates of limiting long-standing illness for males and females by social class (note that slightly different class categories are used in this survey from those you have seen already in this section).

There is a clear association between self-assessment of limiting long-standing illness and social class. There also appears to be a large gender difference among the semi-skilled and unskilled manual classes, with women reporting much more illness than men. This may have surprised you, given the much lower rates of mortality

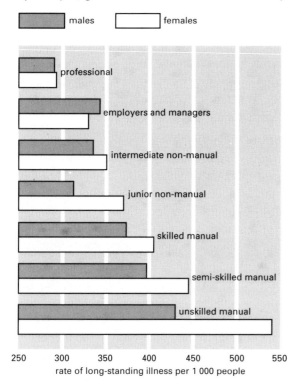

Figure 9.20 *Persons who reported a limiting long-standing illness by sex and social class, all ages, Great Britain, 1989. (Data from OPCS, 1991,* General Household Survey 1989, *OPCS Series GHS No. 20, HMSO, London, Table 4.2)*

among women, but recall our earlier discussion of the reasons why this may be so.

How can the social class differences in mortality and morbidity observed in this chapter be explained? A number of explanations have been put forward and they will be discussed in detail in Chapter 10, where some further examples of the mortality and morbidity associated with various occupations and with social class will be given. The consequences for health of unemployment will also be considered. However, the strength of the association between health and social class is not in doubt, and is best summed up by a quote from the 1980 report, *Inequalities in Health*, which was referred to in the introduction to this chapter:

> If the mortality rate of class I had applied to classes IV and V during 1970–72...74 000 lives of people aged under 75 would not have been lost. This estimate includes nearly 10 000 children, and 32 000 men of working age. (DHSS, 1980, p. 356)

In summary, the main points you should note are:

1   Mortality and morbidity rates in lower social classes are higher than in upper social classes. The magnitude of this difference varies with age, being greatest in infancy and childhood, and least in old age.

2   The association between social class and mortality and morbidity varies with different diseases. For some diseases there is no association; for many the incidence and prevalence is highest in lower social classes, and for a very few the rates are highest in upper social classes.

3   Health risks associated with different occupations account only for some of the social class differences described. (Other explanations are discussed in Chapter 10.)

Conclusion

In this chapter, the contemporary patterns of health and disease in the United Kingdom have been described in terms of the main biological and social factors. The patterns that emerge can contribute to our understanding and explanation of the causes of ill-health. Thus, although biological factors may explain much of the age-related pattern, they appear to make a less significant contribution to the patterns associated with the other forms of stratification, such as sex and gender and social class. In comparison, environmental and social conditions account for much of the observed differences between population groups, with much of the remainder resulting from variations in life histories (or culture). The importance and impact of social factors on these patterns is probably best illustrated by the example of inequalities in the health of different social classes, and consequently these form the subject of the following chapter.

OBJECTIVES FOR CHAPTER 9

When you have studied this chapter, you should be able to:

9.1 Identify the main diseases responsible for the overall patterns of mortality, morbidity and disability in the United Kingdom in recent years.

9.2 Describe the association of both age and sex or gender with disease, and review the explanations for these patterns.

9.3 Describe the association between marital status and both mortality and morbidity; the different effects of marital status on men and women; and the social explanations for these differences.

9.4 Outline the main patterns of mortality and morbidity in different ethnic groups, and some possible reasons for these differences.

9.5 Describe the main regional differences in health status in Britain and suggest factors that would explain some of the differences.

9.6 Describe the association between lower social class and higher mortality and morbidity rates, and discuss the contribution of occupational factors to this association.

9.7 Use appropriate examples to illustrate interactions between the factors discussed in this chapter and the need to take account of such interactions when constructing explanations.

QUESTIONS FOR CHAPTER 9

Question 1 (*Objective 9.1*)

How serious for the health of the population are skin diseases? To answer this, you will need to consider Figures 9.5 and 9.7, and Tables 9.1 and 9.4.

Question 2 (*Objective 9.2*)

In 1989, 75 per cent of people aged 75 or over had no teeth, while this was true of only 4 per cent of those aged 35–44 years (see Figure 9.6). Does this mean a further 70 per cent of the younger age group will lose all their remaining teeth over the next 30 years?

Question 3 (*Objective 9.3*)

Divorce appears to have a more health-damaging effect on men (SMR of 123) than on women (SMR of 117), as judged by mortality. Is the same true for morbidity, as measured by consultations in general practice (see Figure 9.12)? Is the gender difference the same for mental disorders as it is for diseases of the musculoskeletal system?

Question 4 (*Objective 9.4*)

How different are minority ethnic groups from the population as a whole in terms of morbidity and mortality?

Question 5 (*Objective 9.5*)

Suggest (a) biological, (b) social, and (c) life-history explanations for the regional variation in SMRs seen in Figure 9.14.

Question 6 (*Objective 9.6*)

Overall mortality rates are higher in social class V than in social class I at all ages and for both sexes. Is the same class difference in mortality true for all conditions and for measures of morbidity and disability?

Question 7 (*Objective 9.7*)

A major cause of days lost from work is low-back pain. Suggest how age and social class may interact in causing this condition. What might be the limitations of analysing the distribution of low-back pain in relation to only *one* of these dimensions of population structure?

10

Explaining inequalities in health in the United Kingdom

During this chapter you will be asked to read an extract from a report by the Medical Services Study Group of the Royal College of Physicians contained in Health and Disease: A Reader[1]—'Deaths under 50'. *A television programme ('A Tale of Four Cities') and an audiotape sequence on women and smoking are associated with this chapter. They look at the impact of the living and working environment on health in the United Kingdom and examine the interaction of social factors such as poverty with 'lifestyle' factors. Details of these can be found in the Broadcast and Audiocassette Notes.*

Chapter 9 explored some of the many ways in which mortality and morbidity vary across the population of the United Kingdom. In this chapter we look in more detail at how these variations might be explained. We shall refer to many of the dimensions of variation discussed in the previous chapter, such as gender or ethnic group, but will devote particular attention to *socio-economic characteristics* such as social class, occupation, income and housing. There are two main reasons for this. First, partly in consequence of the significance attached to these characteristics, an extensive body of data exists. Second, these factors receive more attention here because other factors such as gender or age are discussed in greater detail in other books in this series.

This chapter considers explanations for inequalities in health under four main headings. It begins by examining the argument that they are mainly an *artefact*, a consequence of the ways in which data are collected and analysed rather than a reflection of a social reality. The second type of explanation is that people move between social classes on a *selective* basis according to whether they are sick or healthy, thus magnifying any differences that exist. Third, it is sometimes argued that health inequalities arise largely from the *behaviour* of individuals. Finally, a set of arguments are grouped around the idea that health inequalities are primarily a reflection of inequalities in the *life circumstances* and *material conditions* of the population.

Inequalities in health: fact or artefact?

Artefact explanations dominated much of the discussion of inequalities in health during the 1980s. Figure 10.1 shows trends in mortality by social class defined by occupation between 1931 and 1981.

☐ What is the trend over time in social class mortality differences is revealed in Figure 10.1?

■ The differences appear to have widened substantially since 1931. The SMRs for the professional and managerial classes (social classes I and II respectively) have fallen very substantially, while the SMR for the unskilled class (social class V) has risen. Thus in 1931 the gap separating the SMRs of the top and bottom classes was 21 (111 − 90), but by 1981 this had risen to 100 (166 − 66).

This evidence that social class differences in mortality were apparently widening has been challenged on a number of grounds. Four arguments in particular have

[1]*Health and Disease: a Reader* (Open University Press, 1984; revised edition 1994).

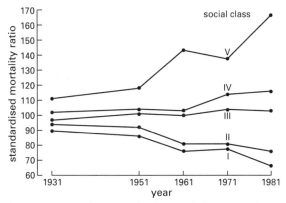

Figure 10.1 *Trends in mortality by social class, using the Registrar-General's classifications, men aged 15–64, England and Wales. (All social classes = 100.) (Data from Wilkinson, 1986, Socio-economic differences in mortality: interpreting the data on their size and trends, in Wilkinson, R. G. (ed.), Class and Health: Research and Longitudiinal Data, Tavistock, London, Table 1.1)*

been used to suggest that the trend, and to some extent the inequalities themselves, are an artefact:

1   The information on deaths and the information on the numbers in each class come from different sources, and errors in either can lead to a **numerator/denominator problem** (explained below);

2   Occupations have been re-classified over time into different social classes, making comparisons over time difficult to perform;

3   Published statistics are often based on narrow age-groups containing a small proportion of total deaths, which may not be typical of the entire spectrum of ages;

4   The size of social classes has been changing, and the proportions of the population at either extreme of the social class spectrum are quite small, so that the widest mortality differences affect relatively small numbers.

Let us examine these in turn, beginning with the numerator/denominator problem.

The numerator/denominator problem

The main source of information on health inequalities by social class in England and Wales has traditionally been the **Decennial Supplements on Occupational Mortality**, which have been published since the nineteenth century. Every ten years, cross-sectional information from the census on the social class composition of the population, measured using occupation as a 'proxy', is combined with information about deaths by social class during the period around the census. So the 1981 census was combined with data on deaths for 1979–80 and 1982–3 to create the Decennial Supplement on Occupational Mortality. Putting together information from different

sources in this way carries a number of problems, but one in particular is that to calculate a *rate*, for example a death rate among women in social class V, it is necessary to divide the number of such women who died (the numerator in the fraction) by the number of such women in total (the denominator), e.g.

$$\frac{\text{no. of women in social class V who died (numerator)}}{\text{total no. of women in social class V (denominator)}}$$

Errors in the number above *or* below the line in such a fraction can produce misleading results. When the results of the 1979–83 Decennial Supplement on Occupational Mortality were published, they were accompanied by a warning that some of the data were subject to serious bias from this and other sources.

One way of avoiding the 'numerator/denominator' problem is to measure mortality not as a rate, but instead in terms of a **proportional mortality ratio**: that is, the percentage of *actual* deaths from a particular cause in a population group as a ratio of the percentage of deaths that would be *expected* in a standard population. Thus, if in Great Britain as a whole 25 per cent of deaths are caused by cancers, but in social class V cancers cause 37.5 per cent of deaths, the proportional mortality ratio for cancers in social class V would be 150 (that is, 37.5/25 = 1.5 × 100 = 150). Figure 10.2 (overleaf) shows a comparison of SMRs and proportional mortality ratios for deaths from diseases of the respiratory system.

☐ How in general terms would you describe the differences between SMRs and PMRs shown in the figure?

■ When PMRs are used, the gradient of mortality between social classes is less steep, but is still very clear for both males and females.

However, although PMRs do avoid the possibility of a numerator/denominator problem, they also have limitations. In particular, if a particular disease causes an unusually high proportion of deaths, this will necessarily *lower* the proportions dying from *other* causes, and vice versa.

Another way of avoiding the problems potentially inherent in the cross-sectional Decennial Supplements is to follow a cohort of individuals over time. Since 1971 this has been done by the **OPCS Longitudinal Study**, in which a one per cent sample of the population is being followed over time, and any vital events such as deaths are recorded alongside information on employment and other characteristics. The Longitudinal Study has the limitation that, because it is based on relatively small numbers, there may be insufficient information to make sub-classifications such as deaths by age, sex, cause of

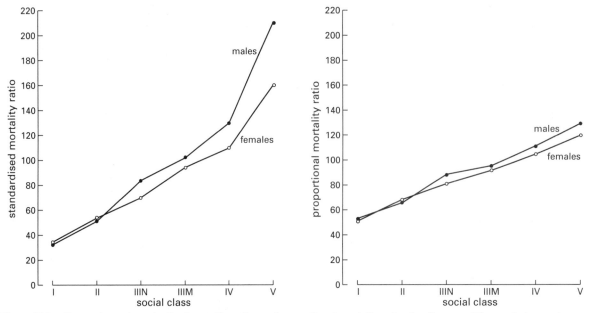

Figure 10.2 *Comparison of standardised mortality ratios and proportional mortality ratios for diseases of the respiratory system, by sex and social class, 1979–83, Great Britain. (Data from OPCS, 1986,* Registrar General's Decennial Supplement on Occupational Mortality 1979–83, *HMSO, London,Table GD34)*

death and occupation. However, it has already produced a vast amount of useful information, and as time goes on is likely to be an increasingly valuable data source for social scientists, epidemiologists and others. You will encounter the Longitudinal Study regularly in this chapter!

Table 10.1 Trends in mortality (standardised mortality ratios) among men aged 15–64 at death in 1971–5 or 1981–5 by social class, based on Longitudinal Study data, England and Wales. (All social classes = 100.)

Social class at 1971 Census	SMR based on deaths during	
	1971–5	**1981–5**
I	79	72
II	80	80
IIN	91	96
IIIM	90	100
IV	97	110
V	111	129
all men aged 15–64	**100**	**100**

Data from Goldblatt, P. (1989) Mortality by social class, 1971–85, *Population Trends*, **56** (Summer), pp. 6–15.

Table 10.1 shows some information taken from the Longitudinal Study, which compares mortality by social class

between 1971–75 and 1981–85. There is no possibility of a numerator/denominator problem here, and yet there is clearly a widening of social class mortality differences.

Reclassification of occupations

A second potential artefact explanation for mortality differences arises from the reclassification of occupations that takes place between censuses. For example, between 1951 and 1961 the SMR for men in social class V increased from 118 to 143, as shown in Figure 10.1, but a reclassification of occupations took place between these two dates, potentially distorting any comparison. This problem however, has long been recognised by official statisticians, and is normally dealt with by presenting figures on the basis of the old as well as the new classification. Thus, when the 1961 mortality was calculated on the same basis as in 1951, the SMR for social class V men was still found to have increased, to 127, while the SMR for social class I remained the same.

Another way of assessing the effect of reclassification on social class inequalities is to follow the mortality experience of specific occupations over time. One researcher managed to track mortality in no less than 143 occupations drawn from all social classes over the period 1921 to 1971, and found that trends towards a widening gap in mortality inequalities were very similar whether measured between social classes or between occupations representing each social class (Pamuk, 1985).

Small proportion of deaths

The argument that evidence for health inequalities is sometimes based on a relatively small proportion of deaths occurring in certain age-groups can easily be addressed by looking at differences across a wider range of age-groups. You have already seen in the previous chapter (Figure 9.16) that a social class gradient already exists at birth and in infancy. Figure 10.3, again derived from the Longitudinal Study, shows mortality differences between males of working age and at older ages, and thus includes a high proportion of all male deaths.

This shows that the mortality gradient across the social classes continues into the oldest age-groups, so that even for men aged 75 and over the death rate in social class V is around 50 per cent higher than in social class I. Thus mortality differences can be observed across all age-groups from birth to old age.

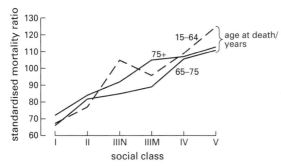

Figure 10.3 *Standardised mortality ratios for males in 1976–81 by social class in 1971 and age at death. (All social classes = 100.) (Data from Fox, J. et al., 1990, Social class mortality differentials: artifact, selection or life circumstances? in OCPS, 1990,* Longitudinal Study: Mortality and Social Organisation, *HMSO, London, Table 6.2)*

Changes in size of social classes

Finally we turn to the argument that observed inequalities in health may be influenced by changes in the size of different social classes. This argument has two elements: first, that the lowest social classes, which suffer the highest mortality rates, are declining as a proportion of the population, and that some allowance should therefore be made for the falling numbers involved; and, second, that the sizes of the social classes at the top and bottom extremes are relatively small. Table 10.2 shows the percentage of economically active men in each social class between 1931 and 1981.

Table 10.2 Percentage of economically active men in different classes, 1931–81, England and Wales

Social class	Percentage of economically active men in different classes				
	1931	**1951**	**1961**	**1971**	**1981**
I	2	3	4	5	5
II	12	13	15	18	19
III	48	51	52	51	51
IV	25	23	21	18	17
V	13	10	9	8	8

Data from Townsend, P. *et al.* (1990) *Inequalities in Health,* Penguin, London, Table 1, p. 208, and OPCS (1984), *Census 1981: Economic Activity in Great Britain,* CEN 81 EA, HMSO, London, p. xvii.

☐ What changes occurred over this period in the size of the different social classes?

■ A falling proportion of the population was classified as being in social classes IV and V (from 38 per cent to 25 per cent), and an increasing proportion in the top two classes (from 14 per cent to 24 per cent).

Debate tends to focus on the decline in the relative size of the lowest groups, but the expansion of the top social classes with *lower* than average mortality is also relevant to this discussion, whereas the group in the middle with a mortality experience close to average has hardly changed in size. This important point, that measures of inequality have to take into account those with lower than average mortality as well as those with above average mortality, is often neglected. Moreover, some of the reduction in the proportion of the population in the lowest social classes has come about, not because of people moving up into higher classes, but as a result of people moving *downwards* off the social class scale into the ranks of the unemployed or permanently sick: the information in Table 10.2 relates only to the male *economically active* population, and so excludes these groups. So the effect of changes in the class distribution of the population on observed mortality differences is far from obvious.

One way of addressing the fact that the proportion of the population at the extremes of the social class spectrum is relatively small has been suggested by researchers working on the Longitudinal Study. Table 10.3 (overleaf) outlines their approach and findings.

First they noted that the SMRs they were reporting for men of working age at the two extremes of the social class spectrum—67 in social class I and 125 in social class V—were based on just 12 per cent of all expected male deaths in the age-group 15–64 (in effect, they contained 12 per cent of all men aged 15–64). By combining social classes I and II and comparing them with social classes IV and V combined, the coverage increased to almost 50 per cent, while the disparity in SMRs was reduced, to 75 compared with 114. If all the non-manual classes were combined and compared with all the manual classes combined, 96 per cent of men of working age would be covered, while the difference in SMRs would again be reduced, to 84 compared with 103.

The researchers then examined alternative social classifications to see if a similar pattern emerged. They focused on type of **housing tenure** (defined in Table 10.3) and access to car transport, both of which indicate income and way of life. When men were classified according to either criterion a clear mortality gradient emerged, as Table 10.3 shows: for example the SMR in relation to car access varied from 77 to 122, and these two extremes contained 48 per cent of men in the age-group 15–64. So although in each case the SMRs at the top and bottom extremes were not so far apart as in the classification by the six strata of occupational social class, the actual size of the groups at the extremes was substantially larger. Finally, when tenure and car access were combined, the analysis showed that the group of men in owner-occupied housing with access to a car contained 40 per cent of the age-group and had an SMR of just 77, whereas the men in privately rented or local authority housing with no car access had an SMR of 129 and contained 22 per cent of the age-group.

These findings indicate very clearly that there are indeed large differences in mortality between very sizeable social groups, and contradict the argument that mortality differences are an artefact based on small and diminishing numbers at the extremes of the spectrum. When classified according to housing tenure and car access rather than social class as defined by occupation, a far higher proportion of men aged 15–64 have either very high or very low mortality. This suggests that social class groupings based on occupation are not a very accurate way of identifying people with either very high or very low mortality, which in turn implies that within social classes there is considerable variation in terms of mortality experience. This has also been confirmed using data from the Longitudinal Study: *within* the largest social class—III Manual—the SMRs of men of working age were found to vary from 75 among those in owner-occupied housing with one or more cars to 122 among those in rented accommodation with no car. In other words, the mortality differences within this social group were almost as great as those between social classes I and V.

Table 10.3 Mortality in 1976–81 of men at ages 15–64 years by alternative social classifications

Social classification	SMR	% of expected deaths (% of age-group in classification)
Social class		
I	67	5
II	77	20
IIIN	105	10
IIIM	96	37
IV	109	17
V	125	7
other	189	4
Household-based		
Tenure		
owner occupied	85	51
privately rented	108	16
local authority	117	31
Car access		
two or more	77	15
one	90	50
none	122	33
owner-occupier with access to car	78	40
privately rented or local authority housing, no car access	129	22
all men aged 15–64	**100**	**100**

*Occupation inadequately described to be classified. (Data from Goldblatt, P., 1990, Mortality and alternative social classifications, in OPCS, 1990, *1971–1981 Longitudinal Study: Mortality and Social Organisation*, HMSO, London, Table 10.1, p. 166)

Summary

This section has examined four main ways in which observed social class differences in health might be statistically misleading. In each case the evidence indicates that dealing with the statistical problem does not remove the social class differences in health:

1 The numerator/denominator problem can be avoided by using longitudinal data or proportional mortality ratios: both methods indicate social class differences in mortality.

2 Problems arising from the re-classification of occupations into different social classes can be avoided by making comparisons over time using the same classification, or by tracking individual occupations: both

methods confirm the existence of social class differences in mortality.

3   Published statistics are often based on narrow age-groups containing a small proportion of total deaths, but social class differences in mortality are found in all age-groups from birth to old age.

4   The proportions of the population at either extreme of the social class spectrum are quite small, but equally great mortality differences can be found between large groups defined on other socio-economic criteria such as housing tenure or car access. We shall return to these alternative social classifications later in the chapter.

Social selection on the basis of health

At the heart of the theory of **health-related social selection** is the idea that moves made by individuals into or out of occupations, social classes, or employment are partly determined by a process of 'selection' on health grounds. For example, people in poor health might move into lower, less skilled occupations if their health poses problems to themselves or their employers. Conversely, people in good health may be more likely to move into higher status and more skilled occupations. Note that the theory assumes **social mobility**, i.e. that people can change their social class during their lifetime.

If social mobility were influenced by health, then the lower occupational classes would have a growing proportion of members in poor health and the SMRs for these classes would be pushed *up*, whereas in the higher occupational classes SMRs would be pushed *down* by new class entrants in good health and class leavers in bad health. Thus health differences between occupational classes would exist, not because class position influenced health, but because health influenced class position.

Evidence for social selection

Evidence of health-related social selection has come from a number of studies. For example, one study conducted in the United Kingdom in the 1950s examined the distribution of men with schizophrenia by social class on admission to hospital.

☐ How might you test the hypothesis that the social class distribution of these men was the same as in the population as a whole?

■ One way would be to compare the social class distribution of males of the same ages among the patients and in the population as a whole.

In fact, the observed number of patients in social class V was roughly twice as high as would have been predicted using this method. In addition, the social class distribution of the patients was quite different from the social class distribution of the *fathers* of the patients (their class of origin). One explanation might be that these males had fallen to the bottom social class *because* they had developed schizophrenia.

Another well-known study conducted over a period of years, by the medical sociologist Raymond Illsley on a sample of women in Aberdeen, found that when women were classified according to the social class of their father, the proportion of those who originated in social classes I or II who were over 5 ft 4 inches tall was 15 per cent greater than among those originating in social classes IV and V. But when they were classified according to the social class of their husband (the class into which they moved) this difference increased to 18 per cent. The likely interpretation of these findings is that women who were taller than other women in their class of origin were more likely to marry into a higher social class. As height is influenced not only by genetic inheritance but by health in the early years of life, this suggested that health was indeed a factor influencing the social mobility of these women.

Illsley was able to pursue this issue by using the longitudinal Aberdeen Maternity and Neonatal Data Bank to examine the perinatal mortality rate of (first-born) babies of women (a measure of the **reproductive efficiency** of these women) again classified according to the social class of their father (their class of origin), and the social class of their husband (the class into which they moved). Table 10.4 shows some results from this study.

Table 10.4 Perinatal mortality rate (per 1 000 births) in relation to the social class of the husbands or fathers of the mothers

Social class of woman's father	Perinatal mortality rate Social class of woman's husband			
	I–IIINM	IIIM	IV and V	All classes
I–IIINM	17	18	31	19
IIIM	19	26	29	26
IV and V	17	26	33	27
All classes	18	24	31	24

Data from research by Raymond Illsley on the Aberdeen Maternity and Neonatal Data Bank, reported in Wilkinson, R. G. (1986), Socio-economic differences in mortality: interpreting the data on their size and trends, in Wilkinson, R. G. (ed.) *Class and Health: Research and Logitudinal Data*, Tavistock, London, Table 1.2.

☐ What does the table reveal about the health of women (measured by their reproductive efficiency) who were *upwardly* mobile compared with those who were *downwardly* mobile?

■ The health of women who moved up the social class structure was markedly better than the health of women who moved down. For example, the perinatal mortality rate for babies born to upwardly mobile women from social class III Manual (that is, who had married men in social classes I–III Non-manual), was 19 per 1 000, compared with 29 per 1 000 for babies born to women from the same social class of origin who were downwardly mobile (that is, who had married men in social classes IV or V).

However, the study was unable to estimate how much of these differences in perinatal mortality could be attributed to the influence of social mobility. On the one hand, it is known that perinatal mortality is influenced by environmental circumstances during early pregnancy: these would be associated with the class women married into and no information on social mobility would be necessary. On the other hand, it is known that maternal height is another factor influencing perinatal outcome, although the association is not straightforward. Further-more, although social selection increased the differences in height between social classes, they already existed: only 3 per cent of the 18 per cent difference in height noted above in Illsley's Aberdeen study—that is, 17 per cent of the total inequality—could be attributed to social selection, leaving 83 per cent unaccounted for. If the same reasoning were applied to perinatal mortality, less than one-fifth of the social class differences shown in Table 10.4 could be attributed to social selection.

Social selection and unemployment

Another group in which the potential contribution of health-related social selection has attracted much atten-tion has been the unemployed. There seems to be little doubt that **unemployment and health** are in some way associated—ill-health, in fact, seems to be a feature of unemployment. For example, the OPCS Longitudinal Study found that between 1971 and 1981 the mortality of men aged 15–64 seeking employment was 37 per cent in excess of that of all men in that age-group and, even allowing for the higher proportions of lower social classes among the unemployed, was 23 per cent in excess. With respect to morbidity, the General Household Survey reported in 1989 that 34 per cent of unemployed men and 35 per cent of unemployed women reported long-stand-ing illness, compared with 26 cent of employed men and

women. The differences between employed and unem-ployed people for long-standing illnesses causing a limi-tation to normal life were even greater.

Similarly, it is known that psychological disturbance and mental distress are more prevalent among unem-ployed people than employed (Warr, 1987). In a follow-up study of a sample of men made redundant from a Wiltshire meat products factory in the 1980s, those who remained unemployed for four years after compulsory redundancy in comparison with those who had got replacement jobs consulted their general practitioners 57 per cent more often about 13 per cent more illnesses, and were referred to hospital out-patient departments 63 per cent more frequently. A number of studies have shown small increases in the incidence of suicide and parasui-cide (known colloquially as a 'cry for help' suicide attempt, i.e. one that would be unlikely to succeed) among long-term unemployed men (Platt and Dyer, 1987).

☐ What alternative interpretations could you place on this evidence that ill-health and mortality are higher among unemployed people than among those in employment?

■ It could be that unemployment causes ill-health and mortality. However, it could also be that poor health leads to unemployment. Finally, there could be some other explanation in which both unemploy-ment and poor health are independently related to some third factor or factors.

The final point is illustrated by the fact that unemploy-ment is concentrated among certain social groups that are known more generally to experience poorer than average health. For example, unemployment is proportionately higher among non-professional and less-skilled workers: the General Household Survey in 1989 classified 19 per cent of all men aged 15–64 as semi-skilled or unskilled manual, but no fewer than 39 per cent of unemployed men were in these classes. Single, widowed and divorced people, who, as seen in Chapter 9, generally have a poorer health record than married people, are also over-represented among the unemployed. And geographi-cally, unemployment is most pronounced in areas that have a poorer health status than the national average.

One way of seeing how much of the health differ-ence between employed and unemployed people might be attributable to health-related social selection is to follow individuals over time. If selection due to ill-health were a major reason for the observed difference in health between unemployed and employed people at the beginning of the study period, this difference should *decrease* over time as increasing numbers of the originally healthy become ill, while a proportion of those made unemployed because of ill-health either died or recovered.

To test this, using information from the OPCS Longitudinal Study, researchers tracked a group of men who in 1971 were seeking work; they had possibly been made redundant on health grounds, but they were not at the time recorded as temporarily or permanently sick. However, rather than finding that the differences between this group and those in employment in 1981 narrowed over time, they found that they increased: between 1971 and 1976 the SMR of the group seeking work was 129 compared with 85 among the employed (all men = 100), but by 1976–81 the SMR of the group seeking work had increased to 146, compared with 92 among the employed group (Moser *et al.*, 1990).

☐ How would you interpret these data?

■ They suggest that as time passed the health of the group who were out of work in 1971 deteriorated. This evidence strongly suggests that health-related social selection was not a major reason for the increased mortality among those seeking work.

As with differences between unemployed and employed, so with differences between social classes: if a major reason for the existence of health inequalities is health-related social selection, then by following a group of individuals over time the original differences should become less pronounced as those who were originally ill recover or die, while those who were originally healthy become sick. And again the OPCS Longitudinal Study has provided an opportunity to examine this. Turn back to Table 10.1, which shows the SMRs in 1971–5 and 1981–5 of men aged 15–64, by their social class in 1971.

☐ Does the table indicate a narrowing or widening of mortality differences between these groups over time, and what does this suggest in relation to health-related social selection?

■ The table suggests a widening of mortality differences over time, indicating that the influence of social selection on the observed differences between social classes must be minor.

Summary

Social class differences in health could in theory exist for no other reason than health-related social selection: upward mobility among the more healthy and downward mobility among the less healthy. In practice, it is difficult to estimate the proportion of observed social class differences that could be attributed to social selection, but comparisons of groups by class of origin versus class of attainment, and longitudinal research, indicate that this proportion must be small. The major explanations for health inequalities between social groups must lie elsewhere.

Lifestyle and behaviour: a case of self-destruction?

We can now turn to the third possible explanation for health inequalities between social classes: that they arise because there are differences in the health-promoting or health-damaging behaviour of individuals in different social classes. This view is well exemplified by a report from the Medical Services Study Group of the Royal College of Physicians, 'Deaths under 50', which is reprinted in the Reader[2] and which you should now read.

☐ The Study Group paid particular attention to 98 cases from a sample of 250 patients who died. How did they label the cases, and why?

■ The 98 cases were described as cases of 'self-destruction' because, according to the Study Group, 'the patients contributed in large measure to their own deaths'.

☐ In attempting to explain the 'causes' of these deaths, what factors did the Study Group emphasise?

■ In the article they emphasise self-poisoning, excessive smoking, drinking and eating, non-compliance with medical treatment, and failure to seek medical help.

☐ How did the Study Group seek to explain these aspects of individual behaviour?

■ They did this primarily by discussing existing mental illness, reckless or uncooperative attitudes, and a failure to heed health education in general and doctors' advice in particular.

To examine this argument in more detail, let us first look at some of the factors cited by the Study Group.

[2]*Health and Disease: A Reader* (Open University Press, 1984; revised edition 1994)

Evidence for 'self-destructive' behaviour

Smoking may contribute to the patterns of mortality and morbidity with which we are concerned and which are frequently described as aspects of lifestyle or behaviour. Table 10.5 shows patterns of cigarette smoking in the United Kingdom in 1980 and 1990.

Table 10.5 Prevalence of cigarette smoking among men and women aged 16+ in manual and non-manual classes, Great Britain, 1980 and 1990

Socio-economic group*	Percentage smoking cigarettes in		Percentage reduction, 1980–90
	1980	1990	
Men			
Manual	49	38	22
Non-manual	33	23	30
Women			
Manual	41	34	17
Non-manual	32	25	22

*Married women were classified according to husband's present or last occupation. (Data from OPCS, 1990, *General Household Survey 1988*, HMSO, London, Table 5.36, and OPCS, 1991, *OPCS Monitor*, No. ss91/3, HMSO, London, p. 4)

☐ What has been happening to cigarette smoking among men and women in non-manual classes compared with those in manual classes between 1980 and 1990?

■ Cigarette smoking has fallen among men and women in both classes, but by different amounts. The fall among men in non-manual classes was 30 per cent compared with a smaller decline of 22 per cent among men in manual classes. Among women the differences were less marked, with a fall of 22 per cent in the number of women smoking in non-manual classes compared with a fall of 17 per cent among women in manual classes.

The relationship between cigarette smoking and many diseases, especially lung cancers and other respiratory diseases, is now well-established and it is therefore predictable that the different smoking habits illustrated in Table 10.5 will contribute to social class differences in mortality and morbidity.[3] It is also clear from these data that the higher rate of cigarette smoking among men may help to explain some of the gender differences in the incidence of specific diseases.

[3]The factors underlying the social class gradient in smoking among women are discussed in an audiotape 'Smoking and women's health', for Open University students.

But the narrowing differences between the sexes in smoking prevalence will also have important consequences for gender-related mortality patterns. For example, between 1982 and 1989 the mortality rate for lung cancer among men fell by 17 per cent, but that among women *rose* by 14 per cent. This pattern of falling smoking rates but rising lung cancer rates is due to a cohort effect, as discussed in Chapter 9: lung cancer is caused by smoking *in the past*, and the increase in lung cancer now reflects an increase in smoking among women in the past.

Another example of 'self-destructive' behaviour mentioned by the Medical Services Study Group was excessive drinking. As with smoking, there is strong evidence that excessive alcohol consumption has a number of detrimental health consequences, including digestive cancers, cirrhosis of the liver, fatal road traffic accidents, and psychiatric disorders. Figure 10.4 shows the proportion of men and women by socio-economic group whose alcohol consumption would be classified as fairly high, high, or very high.

☐ How would you describe the social class and gender differences in high alcohol consumption?

■ The proportion of men who drink heavily is between two and three times that for women. Among men there is no clear gradient across social classes, but among women heavy drinking is more common among the higher social classes.

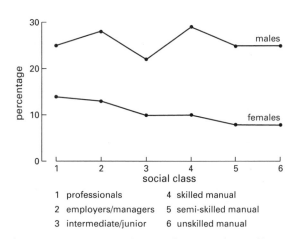

1 professionals   4 skilled manual
2 employers/managers   5 semi-skilled manual
3 intermediate/junior   6 unskilled manual

Figure 10.4 *Percentage of men and women whose self-reported alcohol consumption is classified as fairly high, high or very high, by socio-economic group, Great Britain, 1988. (Data derived from OPCS, 1990,* General Household Survey 1988, *HMSO, London, Table 6.18)*

Thus, in contrast to smoking, we cannot look to alcohol consumption to explain systematic mortality gradients across social classes: the relationship between drinking behaviour and social class is not clear-cut.

Another aspect of behaviour that may have health consequences is voluntary participation in physical activities. Figure 10.5 provides some information on participation rates in a sample of such activities in 1986 by social class, and shows that in each case participation is higher in higher social classes.

Many other aspects of the lifestyle or the behaviour of individuals could be discussed in the present context: for example, aggressive risk-taking behaviour among young people; differences in the use of contraception; or differences in the lifestyles of many ethnic groups or in diet.

Studies of *vaccination* rates also show clear social class gradients. Failure to immunise children appears to be particularly high among groups defined as 'especially disadvantaged' according to 'composite' indicators

which include such factors as housing amenities and parental education. Social class differences in the use of health services are also apparent in relation to other preventive services, such as those for ante-natal care and child health. The effectiveness of some aspects of health care is hotly disputed, but if we assume at this point that these preventive services do make a positive contribution to health, then the lower use of such services among the socially disadvantaged is a factor that must be considered when trying to explain differences in mortality and morbidity.

So, although the relationship between behaviour and health and disease is often far from straightforward, enough information exists to indicate that differences in health-influencing behaviour do contribute to social class differences in mortality and morbidity. This raises a number of questions: first, how much do they contribute; second, why do such differences in health-influencing behaviour exist; and third, what other factors should be considered?

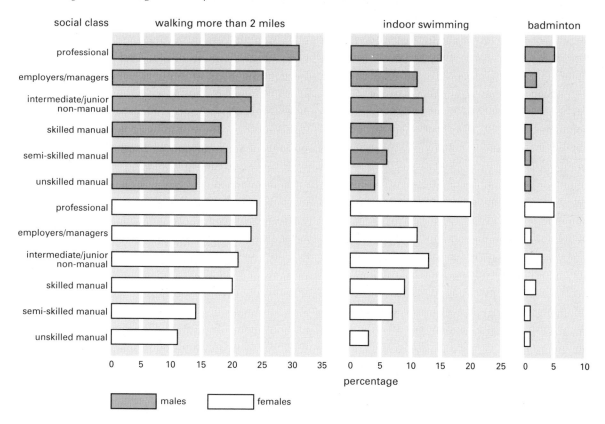

Figure 10.5 *Participation rates of adults in voluntary physical activity, by social class and sex, Great Britain, 1986. (Data from OPCS, 1989, General Household Survey 1986, HMSO, London, Table 13.13)*

Estimating the contribution of behaviour

One attempt to answer the first question has been made in a cohort study begun in 1967 of almost 18 000 civil servants working in London (the 'Whitehall Study'). This study found that for almost every cause of death the lower employment grades had higher mortality rates than the higher employment grades. The gradient was particularly steep for lung cancer and other smoking-related diseases such as bronchitis, and smoking was also much more prevalent in the lower employment grades. This suggested that at least some of the difference between the grades was due to smoking behaviour. However, even after all smoking-related causes of death were put aside, the excess mortality among the lowest grades compared with the professional and executive grades remained, being reduced from a 110 per cent excess to an 80 per cent excess.

The researchers also looked in detail at coronary heart disease, and found a 70 per cent excess mortality among the lowest grades compared with the professional and executive grades. They then adjusted these figures to make allowance for all factors known to increase the risk of coronary heart disease, including smoking, high blood pressure, high levels of cholesterol and blood sugar, and lower than average height—almost all of which were again more prevalent in the lowest grades. These adjustments did reduce the excess mortality, but still left unexplained an excess mortality in the lowest grades of almost 40 per cent. Thus, men in the lowest employment grades had 40 per cent higher mortality than men in the top grades, *even* when all known risk factors were excluded (Marmot, 1986). Comparing these findings with the initial results from a study begun in 1985–88 of a second cohort of over 10 000 civil servants (the Whitehall II Study), the researchers found no diminution in social class differences over time (Marmot *et al.*, 1991).

Similar findings have been found in studies of unemployed people in the United Kingdom and of American families with low income: known risk factors and behavioural differences do explain a part of the observed inequalities in health between social groups, but no matter how many such factors are taken into account, substantial inequalities in health remain.

Where does self-damaging behaviour originate?

The second question raised by behavioural explanations of health inequalities is where such differences in behaviour originate. It has been suggested that certain behavioural traits and attitudes, which may adversely affect health, are passed on from generation to generation, for example, through child-rearing practices. In this way, health disadvantage may persist despite considerable improvements in education, living standards,

and other factors. Figure 10.6 illustrates this with reference to patterns of dental attendance.

The upper part of the figure shows the percentage of adults attending a dentist for regular check-ups, by social class. A clear and strong gradient exists, with 62 per cent for adults in the professional class making regular attendances, compared with 29 per cent in' the unskilled manual class.

☐ The lower part of the figure shows how the attendance pattern of a mother may be passed on to her children. Summarise the pattern shown by the figure.

■ If the mother is a regular attender, then the likelihood that her children have *never* attended a dentist is quite low: between 13 per cent and 17 per cent. But if the mother does not regularly attend the dentist for a check-up and only goes because of some kind of trouble, there is a much higher likelihood that her children will never have been to the dentist: over one in three will never have done so. But most interesting of all, the differences between the manual and non-manual classes is small or non-existent: the mother's behaviour and attitude seems to be the most important thing.

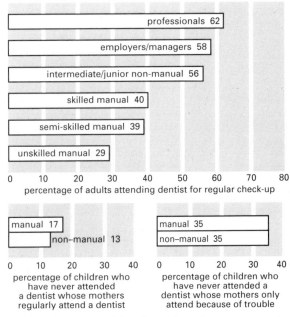

Figure 10.6 *Patterns of dental attendance by socio-economic group, Great Britain, 1989. (Data from OPCS, 1991,* General Household Survey 1989, *OPCS Series GHS, No. 20, HMSO, London, Tables 4.54 and 4.59.)*

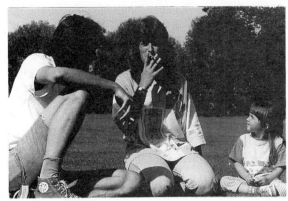

Health-damaging parental behaviour: children of smokers are more likely to become smokers. (Photo: Mike Levers)

A great deal of research has focused on the mechanisms by which disadvantage may be passed from generation to generation—a process often referred to as the **cycle of deprivation**. As one might expect, this suggests that, although there are some relationships between the attitudes and behaviour of parents and those of their children, they are far from straightforward. However, even acknowledging that parental influences play some part, this would only provide part of a transmission mechanism from one generation to another, not an explanation of why these differences exist and are related to social class in the first place. Returning to Figure 10.6, for example, the question of why dental attendance patterns are so strongly related to social class is clearly still of fundamental importance. This raises a particular criticism of explanations of health inequality based on the behaviour of *individuals*: namely that it is unrealistic to examine the behaviour of individuals in isolation from their social and material circumstances. If income, education, housing, access to transport, work environment and other factors all vary across social groups, can individual behaviour be assumed to be unrelated to them? The next section examines these factors and attempts to reach some conclusions.

Summary

It has been argued that higher mortality in some social groups may be related to health-damaging behaviour. It is clear that health-damaging activities such as smoking are more prevalent in social groups with higher mortality, and that potentially health-improving activities such as physical exercise are more prevalent in social groups with lower mortality, although some factors such as high alcohol consumption do not fit this pattern so neatly. There is firm evidence that these behavioural differences do explain part of the differences in mortality between social classes, but that at least 40 per cent of the difference cannot be explained by behavioural differences. More

important, however, it is not clear that the behaviour of individuals can be isolated from their social and material environment. This environment forms the subject of the next section.

Material circumstances

The social and material environment may affect the distribution of health and disease in broadly three ways. First, factors such as housing conditions or employment may have a direct effect on the state of someone's health: for example, damp housing may lead to chest disease, employment hazards to accidents. Second, there may be indirect effects: the income associated with an occupation may constrain a person's ability to purchase good housing, adequate nutrition, and so on, or may lead to stresses that in turn make it more likely that a person will smoke or drink to relieve inescapable tensions. Or, the social context of an occupation or a particular social status may encourage or discourage certain types of health-related social behaviour such as smoking or risk-taking. Third, the social and material environment may affect a person's use of health services, which may in turn affect their health (this point has already been discussed in the previous chapter in the context of interpreting morbidity statistics derived from health-service use). Evidence of the effect of health care on health is considered elsewhere[4]; here we are primarily concerned to examine the evidence on the direct and indirect effects of social and material circumstances on health.

Occupational hazards

Let us begin with the working environment and health. The different risks to health associated with different occupations are reflected in *occupational mortality rates*, some examples of which were given in Table 9.6 in the previous chapter. These reflect not only the more obvious work hazards, but other aspects of occupation that are likely to be related to health and safety at work. For example, manual workers are much more likely to work out of doors, to spend most of the day standing, to have insecure jobs with a high risk of unemployment, to have shorter holidays and much less access to 'fringe benefits', first-aid facilities or toilets.

Occupations involve their own specific hazards to health. Industrial accidents and disease, for example, still take a considerable toll. In 1988 almost 600 deaths and 35 000 major injuries at work were officially notified to government agencies in the United Kingdom. In addition to these, 160 000 injuries were reported in which the

[4]See *Caring for Health: History and Diversity*, Open University Press (1985, revised edition 1993)

person involved had to take more than three days off work to recover. It is known that some accidents and injuries which should be reported to the official health and safety agencies in fact go unreported, and that this under-reporting is especially prevalent in relation to less serious accidents. Yet even these 'non-major' accidents might involve the loss of a joint from a finger for example, or concussion resulting in a hospital stay of up to 24 hours. You might like to consider whether you would regard losing a piece of a finger at work as serious or not!

In 1991 the Health and Safety Executive attempted to uncover the likely degree of under-reporting in the official injury figures by commissioning a survey of 40 000 households in which questions were asked about workplace accidents and ill-health. This indicated that on average more than two-thirds of injuries go unreported in breach of the law, but that the problem is especially bad in some industries: in agriculture, for example, the study found that 83 per cent of accidents which should have been reported went unreported. On the basis of these findings, the number of reported injuries at work should be around 680 000 per annum, rather than the 200 000 actually reported in 1991.

Figure 10.7 shows injuries to employees reported to enforcement authorities in 1989–90 by industry. All fatal, non-fatal and 'over 3-day' injuries are included, and the figure also shows the actual numbers of injuries in each industry. In total, there were over 80 000 such injuries in 1989–90.

The patterns are not always what might be expected: the injury rate is higher in the food, drink and tobacco industry than in the construction industry; higher in the water supply industry than in nuclear fuel production; almost five times higher in air transport than in sea transport; higher in postal services than in the chemical industry, and almost as high in the health services as in agriculture, forestry and fishing.

However, if the less serious injuries are excluded, then the most dangerous sector by far is the construction industry, where on average 20 workers are seriously injured every day, one worker dies every three days, and a member of the public is killed every month.

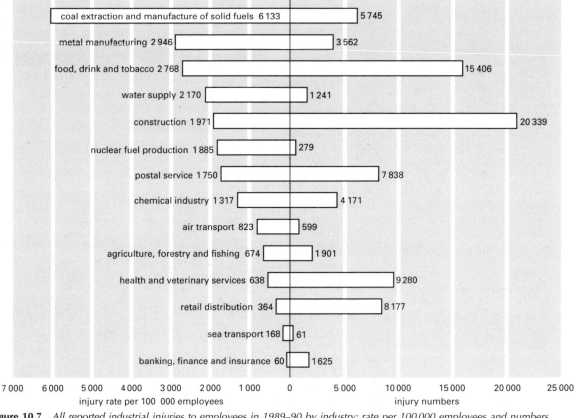

Figure 10.7 *All reported industrial injuries to employees in 1989–90 by industry: rate per 100 000 employees and numbers (total = 80 224). (Data from Health and Safety Commission, 1991, Annual Report 1989/90, HMSO, London, Table 1)*

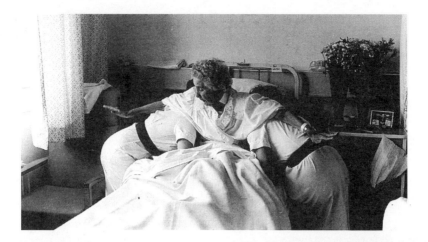

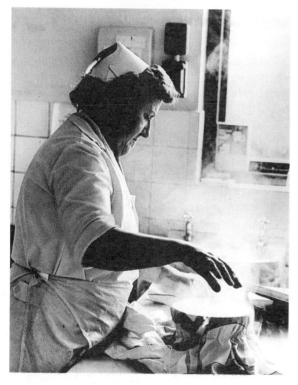

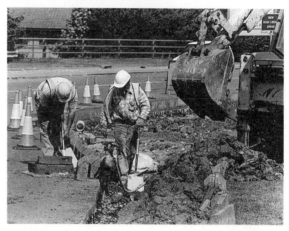

Occupational injuries: Among nurses back injury is a major problem. In the construction industry, 20 workers in the United Kingdom are seriously injured every day. Catering workers are exposed to injury from scalds and burns. (Photos: Mike Levers)

Well over one-half of fatal injuries are the consequence of falls from a height or of being struck by a moving object or vehicle, but major injuries are most often caused by slips, trips and falls on the same level, which account for 28 per cent of such injuries. This is one reason why postal workers have a fairly high injury rate, especially in winter when paths and steps may be icy. And one-third of all 'over 3-day' injuries are caused by handling, lifting or carrying: this commonly occurs in areas such as retail distribution, but also in health care, where back injuries resulting from the handling of patients are a well-known problem.

It is clear, therefore, that the likelihood of having an accident at work varies enormously depending on occupation, but that many different types of occupations have quite high injury and accident rates associated with them. Who is responsible for industrial accidents? Opinion varies, and the debate may now be familiar to you. One approach emphasises individual responsibility and carelessness much as the Medical Services Study Group did:

Accidents do not happen, they are caused; horseplay and tomfoolery, carelessness and thoughtlessness, lack of concentration, lack of

respect for oneself and others, familiarity, drinking, fatigue, haste, working conditions, irrita-
bility and boredom. (From a Royal Society for
the Prevention of Accidents booklet, quoted by
Kinnersley, 1974, p. l97)

Another approach stresses the influence of the actual
conditions at work and the way work is organised:

The 'attitude of the worker to safety' is no more
the cause of industrial accidents today than it
was in the days when little children were man-
gled in unguarded machinery in the cotton
mills. Machines, buildings, and arrangements
of work are still designed to the cheapest speci-
fications that will produce goods at the greatest
profits. Engineering design concentrates on the
product and excludes the operator until the last
moment. Safety, health and last of all comfort
are treated as bolt-on goodies. (Kinnersley,
1974, p. l95)

Here we see an illustration of the point made in the
previous section, that behaviour is relevant, but cannot
be divorced from social and material circumstances.

In addition to injury, we must also consider industrial
disease resulting from exposure to toxic substances such
as chemicals, dust, gases or fumes, or to hazards due to
excessive heat, noise or vibration. The main source of
information on occupational disease in the United Kingdom is the Industrial Injuries Scheme administered by the
Department of Social Security, under which individuals
are examined to see whether they are sufficiently disabled by the disease in question to qualify for a disability
allowance. Benefits may be paid in respect of around 50
'prescribed' diseases or conditions, and Table 10.6 shows
the number of new cases diagnosed under this scheme in
1989.

Some of these cases involve poisoning from a variety
of substances still found in certain industries. *Pneumoconiosis*, the chronic lung condition suffered by many
miners, is included. So is *asbestosis*, a disease caused by
inhalation of asbestos fibres, and *byssinosis*, a lung disease found among textile workers and caused by inhaling
cotton fibres. Other prescribed conditions include
tenosynovitis (inflammation of the tendons) due to frequent or repeated movement of the hand and wrist, as on
an assembly line for instance; *dermatitis* (inflammation of
the skin) resulting from contact with substances such as
mineral oil, soot or tar; *'beat' conditions*, where the hand,
elbow or knee may swell as a result of prolonged or
severe pressure on the affected area; and *occupational
deafness*.

Table 10.6 New cases of occupational disease diagnosed
under the Industrial Injuries Scheme, 1989, United Kingdom

Occupational disease	New cases in 1989
occupational deafness	1 506
vibration white finger	1 056
mesothelioma	441
pneumoconiosis	437
tenosynovitis	294
dermatitis	285
asbestosis	280
occupational asthma	214
beat conditions	112
byssinosis	15
farmer's lung	13
other diseases	253
total	**4 906**

Data from Health and Safety Commission (1991), *Annual
Report 1989/90*, HMSO, London, Table 15.

Once again, however, these figures do not tell the whole
story. First, many people suffer from an occupational
disease which is not recognised as being severe enough
to qualify for benefit. For example, a survey of GPs in
1989 suggested that around 60 000 people consulted
their GPs with occupational dermatitis, although, as
Table 10.6 indicates, fewer than 300 were recognised as
qualifying for benefit. Another survey of work-related
occupational respiratory disease in 1989 showed that for
asthma, infections and 'farmer's lung' substantially more
cases were detected than appear in the official statistics as
qualifying for benefit. Second, many conditions related to
occupations are not on the official list of prescribed diseases. One such is *emphysema*, a respiratory disease
common among people working in dusty conditions. The
difficulty is that diseases such as emphysema may be
caused or aggravated by atmospheric pollution or smoking. One detailed survey carried out for the Royal Commission on Civil Liabilities and Compensation for
Personal Injury (the 'Pearson Report'), which reported in
1978, suggested that 'illness believed to have arisen at
work but not presently prescribed may be of the order of
five times as numerous as those which are prescribed',
and more recent research confirms this.

Another problem in assessing the scale of occupational disease is that the effects of exposure to industrial
hazards may take many years to become apparent. The

story of *mesothelioma* (a cancer of the chest lining caused by exposure to asbestos) illustrates this point. Between 1968 and 1989 the number of cases of the disease recorded on death certificates rose from 154 to over 800 and they are still rising. New regulations to control asbestos were introduced in 1969, but as this type of cancer may take up to forty years to develop, it will be many years before these improvements are reflected in lower mortality rates. Since the worst exposures occurred between 1935 and 1970 (many of them during the lagging of ships with blue and brown asbestos in the early years of the Second World War, and its removal when the hazards became known after the war), the peak of cases is probably still to come. Some estimates have suggested that at least 50 000 more asbestos-related deaths may occur between 1990 and 2020. Similarly, regulations to control noise levels in the workplace have gradually been tightened, with new controls introduced in 1990, but the legacy of laxer controls will be apparent in the occupational deafness figures for many years into the future.

One way to separate out the direct contribution of occupational hazards to observed health inequalities between social classes is to examine differences in death rates between occupations, and then to standardise these rates for the social class of the people in the occupation and see how much difference this makes. One exercise along these lines indicated that standardising for social class removed about 80 per cent of the difference between the occupations compared, suggesting that *direct* occupational hazards were responsible for the remaining 20 per cent of the health inequalities between occupations (Fox and Adelstein, 1978). These findings are therefore an appropriate place at which to turn to the *indirect* effects of occupation on health inequalities.

Income

The most likely way in which occupation will indirectly exert an influence on health is through earnings, which help to determine the living standards of individuals and other members of their families. Before looking at the evidence linking income to health, it is worth looking at the distribution of income in the United Kingdom.

There are wide differences in average weekly earnings before tax between manual and non-manual, male and female full-time workers, and substantial disparities of income also exist within these categories. Figure 10.8 shows a broader picture: the percentage of total income taken by each quintile (20 per cent group) of households in 1979 and again in 1987.

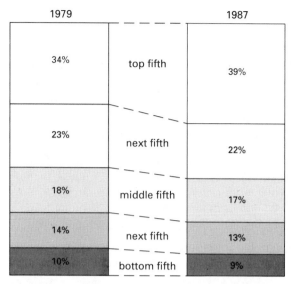

Figure 10.8 *Percentage of total income (after tax) taken by quintile groups of households, Great Britain, 1979 and 1987 (data rounded to nearest whole number). Note: Income here includes salaries, social security benefits, rents, interest and dividends. (Data from HMSO, 1992,* Social Trends 22: 1991, *HMSO, London, Table 5.16)*

☐ How would you describe the distribution of income in 1987, and how has it changed since 1979?

■ In 1987 the top 20 per cent of the population received almost 40 per cent of all income in the United Kingdom. In contrast, the bottom 20 per cent of the population received only 10 per cent. Since 1979 the top 20 per cent has increased its share of income, while all other groups have seen their share decline.

An alternative way of examining income and its distribution is to attempt to draw a line defining the number of people who are in **poverty**. Poverty can be conceptualised in relative terms, as:

...the absence or inadequacy of those diets, amenities, standards, services and activities which are common or customary in society. People are deprived of the conditions of life which ordinarily define membership of society. (Townsend, 1979, p. 915)

However, this approach does not escape the necessity of defining the level of resources that is necessary to allow people to live 'as is common and customary in society'.

Another approach adopted in many studies of poverty is to lay down a set of minimum necessities in nutrition, clothing, household goods and so on, then assess whether families or individuals have sufficient income to obtain these minimum necessities.

This **subsistence approach** was pioneered in York in 1899 by Seebohm Rowntree, a member of the Rowntree family whose chocolate firm is still based in York. Subsequent studies in this and other countries have been deeply influenced by the concept of subsistence standards, which has also formed the basis for recommending minimum state social security benefits and minimum earnings in a number of countries. In the United Kingdom, social security benefits are still implicitly based on a subsistence view, and Parliamentary Regulations define the items of normal day-to-day living that families are expected to meet once they are in receipt of Income Support.

Using benefit levels to define poverty has been criticised on a number of grounds, but in particular that increases in benefit levels have the effect of increasing the numbers of people classified as being in poverty. How-ever, this method does give some rough indication of the number of people on income levels that restrict them to basic necessities. Table 10.7 indicates the numbers of people in Britain in 1987 who were receiving Supplementary Benefit or Housing Benefit, and the numbers with incomes below the Supplementary Benefit or Housing Benefit level who did not qualify for or take up these benefits for a number of reasons.

Looking along the first row of the table, you will see that an estimated 10.2 million people were living in 1987 at or below the income levels that are often considered to be the poverty level. (This is around 20 per cent of the population of Britain.) The next three rows of the table, which relate to families over pension age, show that 28 per cent of people below the poverty line are pensioners, especially single pensioners. Single persons with or without children (rows 7 and 9 of the table) also figure large among those below pension age who are in poverty, and their numbers have been growing quite rapidly in recent years. Many families with children (row 6) exist at these income levels, and in fact around 2.5 million of the 10 million people in the table are children.

Table 10.7 Estimated number of persons receiving benefits or with incomes below the benefit levels, Great Britain, 1987.

Row	Type of family to which person belongs	No. of persons receiving Supplementary Benefit or Housing Benefit Supplement/thousands	No. of persons not receiving these benefits but with incomes below the qualifying level /thousands	Total no. of persons living below the poverty line /thousands (and percentage of those in poverty)		Percentage of total population of Britain in the same type of family
1	all	7 310	2 890	10 200	(100)	100
2	*Families over pension age:*	1 870	930	2 800	(28)	17
3	married couples	520	280	800	(8)	9
4	single persons	1 350	650	2 000	(20)	8
5	*Families under pension age:*	5 440	1 960	7 400	(72)	83
6	married couples with children	1 780	880	2 660	(26)	40
7	single persons with children	1 700	90	1 790	(17)	5
8	married couples without children	600	260	860	(8)	18
9	single persons without children	1 360	740	2 100	(21)	20
10	families in rows 6 and 7 under pension age with three or more children	1 240	350	1 590	(16)	10
11	*By economic status:*					
12	full-time work and self-employed	—	940	940	(9)	60
13	sick/disabled	390	100	490	(5)	3
14	unemployed/other	5 050	910	5 960	(58)	19

Data derived from Johnson, P. and Webb, S. (1990), *Poverty in Official Statistics: Two Reports*, Institute for Fiscal Studies Commentary No. 24, IFS, London, Tables 3, 4 and 8.

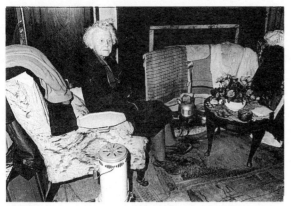

Elderly person alone at home in Ladbroke Grove, London. 28 per cent of those below the poverty line in the United Kingdom are pensioners. (Photo: Shelter Photographic Library: Nigel Dickinson)

☐ Comparing the percentages of the poor in different family types with the percentages of the total population in different family types (that is, the two columns on the far right of the table), which groups seem to be most (a) under-represented, and (b) over-represented in the ranks of the poor?

■ Pensioners, especially if single, are much more likely to be poor than their total numbers in the population would suggest, as are single persons with children (row 7), large families (row 10) and unemployed people (row 14). Married couples with or without children (rows 6 and 8) and those in full-time work (row 12) are less likely to be poor.

Comparisons over time in the numbers of the poor are complicated by the many changes that have taken place in the social security system: in 1988, for example, Supplementary Benefit was abolished and replaced by an Income Support scheme, making before-and-after comparisons difficult. However, if the figures in Table 10.7 were to be compared with identical information for 1979, we would see that the numbers living on the income provided by these benefit safety nets rose by two-thirds, while the numbers with incomes below these levels had also risen, by around 20 per cent. And because the value of state benefits grew much more slowly than did real earnings during the 1980s, the *relative* position of the poor deteriorated: between 1979 and 1988 the real income of those living on benefits probably rose by around 5 per cent while the real income of the population as a whole rose by 33 per cent (Johnson and Webb, 1991). Indeed, between 1979 and 1991 the *absolute* position of the poorest 10 per cent of the population deteriorated, as their real income fell. So there is little doubt that the

numbers of poor people on almost any definition increased significantly during the 1980s.

Even among those receiving benefits, however, there are substantial variations in living standards, which are reflected in surveys showing that 70 per cent of couples with children on Supplementary Benefit reported real anxiety about money, most had bad debts and a majority ran out of money almost every week; whereas among pensioners far fewer claimed to be anxious about money (18 per cent), and fewer than one in ten had bad debts or ran out of money (Berthoud, 1986).

Housing and the built environment

One way in which income may influence living standards is shown in Figure 10.9, which contains information on the relation between level of household income and **standard of housing** from a survey conducted in 1986: those with low household incomes were much more likely than those with high household incomes to be in a house which lacked basic amenities, was in poor repair, or was unfit for human habitation.

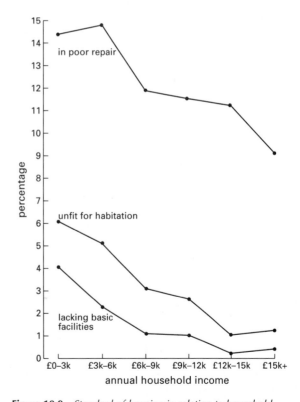

Figure 10.9 *Standard of housing in relation to household income (£1k = £1 000), England, 1986. (Data from Department of the Environment, 1988,* English House Condition Survey 1986, *HMSO, London, Table A6.6)*

Concern about the relationship between housing conditions and health goes back many years. T. H. C. Stevenson, a key figure in the development of the Registrar-General's classification of occupations, looked in the 1920s at the relationship between infant and child mortality and tenement size, and found clear associations between the child mortality rate and the number of available rooms, which he used as the index of overcrowded conditions. These are illustrated in Figure 10.10, Stevenson's original hand-drawn graph. The different lines on the graph relate to duration of marriage: the greater the duration of marriage (and therefore presumably the older the mother and/or larger the family), the higher the child death rate in that tenement size.

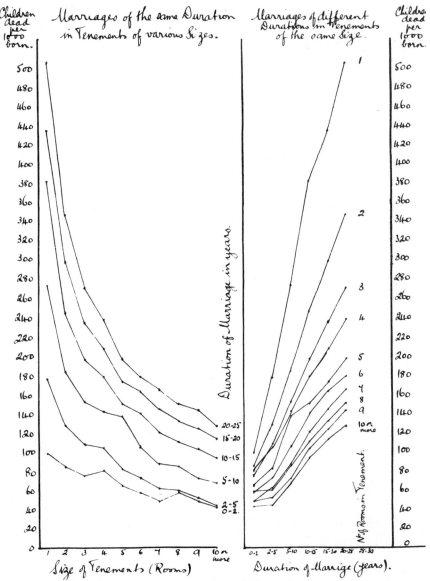

Figure 10.10 *Diagram drawn by Stevenson to show child mortality, tenement size and duration of marriage, based on data from the 1911 Census (from Fox, J. and Goldblatt, P. O.,1982, OPCS Longitudinal Study 1971–5, Socio-Demographic Mortality Differentials, Series LS, No. 1, HMSO, London, Figure 5.1. p. 65)*

Since Stevenson drew his graph, housing standards have been immensely improved. Millions of homes have been demolished in slum clearances, and half of today's housing stock was built after 1948, although some of these are alienating and sometimes uninhabitable houses and flats. However, our knowledge about the relationship between housing and health is still limited. Attention has focused on aspects such as lack of amenities and overcrowding, the latter being presumed to be associated with an increased risk of infection among children, for example, and the former with accidents when children have no protected place to play. Damp housing has been suggested as a cause or exacerbating factor in respiratory diseases. Structural defects such as poor wiring may put children at particular risk. The psychological and practical difficulties associated with high-rise flats or isolated housing estates may also adversely affect the health of those who live in them, particularly women or children at home or elderly people.

One factor that is related to the state of repair, amenities and habitability of housing is the type of *housing tenure*, and the OPCS Longitudinal Study has been used to examine mortality in relation to housing tenure. Some evidence on this was presented in Table 10.3, and the expected gradients were found. However, when the researchers looked at these mortality patterns by cause of death, they found that the gradient existed for almost all causes and not just the kinds of diseases mentioned above that might be directly related to housing conditions; in fact they were steepest for smoking-related diseases.

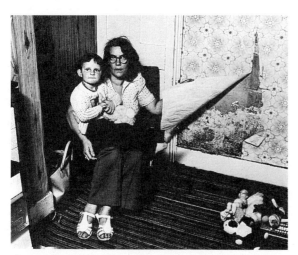

Chronic damp affects this house, occupied by this woman and her son. (Photo: Shelter Photographic Library)

Although it would clearly be desirable to be able to measure housing conditions more accurately than by the type of tenure, these findings do suggest that housing is essentially an indicator of a more general way of life that may influence mortality, rather than being an important influence on mortality in its own right. However, there is one group that has grown substantially during the 1980s in which the connection may be more direct: the *homeless*.

In 1992 around 90 000 families were classified as homeless, equivalent to perhaps a quarter of a million people. Mostly they were accommodated in temporary accommodation, such as bed and breakfast hotels or hostels, although a study by the Audit Commission in 1992 found that in London the average time spent in such 'temporary' accommodation was just under a year. The number of homeless people actually sleeping on the streets is extremely hard to measure, but on most reckonings this also increased during the 1980s; by 1992 several thousand people were probably sleeping rough in the United Kingdom.

It is known that homelessness is associated with many forms of ill-health. Homeless women are three times as likely to be admitted to hospital with problems while pregnant, and their babies are three times as likely to be of low birth weight, compared with those of other women. Children are much more likely to miss immunisations and routine health checks, and are more likely to be involved in accidents.

From a research perspective, it is often hard to prove that homelessness *causes* ill-health, as many other factors may be involved. For example, some surveys have found a high prevalence of mental disorders among the homeless, but this is partly because a growing number of homeless people are from mental hospitals which have been run down and closed. Despite these difficulties, the association between homelessness and health is sufficiently strong to have made housing a growing public health issue in the 1990s.

So far, the discussion of housing has focused primarily on the health consequences of houses and their physical condition. There is also some evidence that the configuration of houses, street layouts and so on can have health implications: for example, a detailed study of differences in health between Middlesborough and Sunderland found that children's mortality from road traffic accidents in housing estates in Middlesborough was over three times higher than in the comparable areas of Sunderland, suggesting that layout of estates in Sunderland was safer and more sympathetic to the lives of the residents (Phillimore and Morris, 1991).[5]

However, the same research has emphasised that these fairly obvious differences in housing and other conditions are not the whole story, and that people in apparently identical circumstances can experience quite different health outcomes. One possibility is that these are related to the constant changes in local economies, the rise and fall of industries, employment, prosperity, confidence and uncertainty, and the ways in which people respond to these changes. The health consequences of these responses would be subtle but might be far-reaching.

To illustrate the kind of mechanisms that might be involved, it is worth considering studies of severe threats to survival such as famines, when all the informal arrangements for mutual insurance and social support are thrown into doubt:

> ...their failure in times of widespread calamity is in fact well documented: in times of famine the ordinary rules of patronage, credit, charity, reciprocity, and even family support tend to undergo severe strain and can hardly be relied upon to ensure the survival of vulnerable groups (Drèze and Sen, 1989, p. 74).

This is sometimes referred to as the breakdown of the **moral economy**, and the group researching the health differences between Sunderland and Middlesborough seem to be suggesting that it is in this moral economy of informal social ties, habits and values that some clues may be found to the health differences between apparently very similar communities. This may be so, although the evidence also suggests that, although the moral economy may be strained to breaking point in the advanced stages of famines, it may well be *reinforced* in the earlier stages or in the face of less severe stresses.

Food and fuel

Families living on different incomes display many clear differences in addition to housing in their patterns of expenditure. In 1990 the average household in the United Kingdom devoted less than 5 per cent of its total expenditure to fuel, light and power, and about 18 per cent to food. However, those on lower incomes devoted a much higher proportion of their income to food and fuel: for example, retired households mainly dependent on state pensions devoted 11 per cent of their expenditure to

fuel, light and power, and a further 31 per cent to food (Central Statistical Office, 1992).

Some research has suggested that poor families who experience a further reduction in income—for example if a wage-earner has to go onto short-time working or a member of the household loses a benefit—will try to make ends meet by cutting back on these items. This can pose a threat to health, which is reflected in part by the 500 or so annual deaths from causes associated with hypothermia. However, one detailed study of a small sample of victims of hypothermia indicated that they had usually collapsed at home as a result of serious disease and had cooled as a result of the illness and immobility, although they were often in heated rooms (Woodhouse *et al.*, 1989).

Cutting back on food expenditure can have severe effects on diet. One study of the meals eaten by parents and their children in eight families on low incomes over the course of one day found that the meals were monotonous and not nutritionally balanced, with a complete lack of fruit and vegetables of any form—fresh, tinned or frozen. The possible health consequences of such a diet are not easy to predict, however, as Chapter 11 will show.

Income: cause or proxy?

Many of the studies surveyed in this chapter suggest a relationship between income and health, but there have been very few attempts to measure the association directly: the usual approach, as noted earlier, is to use social class as a proxy for income, despite the great variations in income levels within social classes. One attempt to do so identified 22 specific occupations for which data on income *and* on mortality were available for the years 1951 and 1971 (Wilkinson, 1986). The occupations were mainly skilled or semi-skilled manual and contained about 2.5 million men. The analysis then examined the relationship between changes in occupation-specific death rates and changes in occupational incomes over this 20-year period.

The results indicated that there was an inverse relationship, as would be expected: men in occupations in which incomes rose faster than average appeared to have a lower than average death rate, and vice versa. However, the results were weak. This is perhaps not surprising given that those on the lowest income levels, where detrimental health effects are likely to be strongest, are seldom in an occupation at all: as Table 10.7 showed, fewer than one in ten of the poor in Britain in 1987 were in full-time work. Again, this leads to the conclusion that although income, occupation or groupings by housing tenure and car access may be more refined ways of classifying a population than social class alone, they are

---

[5]This research is featured in a TV programme for Open University students, 'A Tale of Four Cities'.

essentially indicators of a way of life that influences health in a multitude of different ways, rather than being important influences on health in their own right.

The 'programming' hypothesis

It seems clear that many of the factors we have considered in this chapter, such as smoking, housing conditions or unemployment, might have health effects which would not become apparent for many years. Thus attempts to intervene to reduce cardiovascular disease, which is predominantly a disease of late-middle and old age, have increasingly concentrated on getting young adults to change aspects of their lifestyle, for example by taking more exercise, altering their diet, or stopping smoking.

However, since the late 1980s a group of epidemiologists from Southampton have produced a series of research findings which challenge this view of the origins of cardiovascular disease, suggesting instead that the risk of dying in adult life from cardiovascular disease is profoundly affected by factors in infancy and even in fetal life.

The group began with the observation that differences in mortality from heart disease in different parts of England were too great to be explained by differences in adult lifestyle such as smoking, diet or exercise. But they noted that areas *currently* with high rates of mortality from cardiovascular diseases had in the past had above average rates of *infant* mortality, suggesting that their might be some relation between early influences and later disease.

To test this hypothesis, the group managed to track down the birth records of almost 6 000 men who had been born in Hertfordshire between 1911 and 1930, containing information on their birth weight, whether they were breast- or bottle-fed, when they were weaned, and so on. They then traced the history of these men, to see if they had died, and medically examined those who were still alive. The initial results were surprising but clear: men who had had a low birth weight or were small at the age of one year ran a much higher risk of serious heart disease in adult life (Barker *et al.*, 1989).

A second set of detailed birth records compiled in Preston in the 1930s and 1940s allowed the group to refine their analysis, and to establish that the events in early life that influenced later mortality and morbidity occurred at very precise points or 'windows' in time: for example, the risk of stroke in adult life seemed to be related to the period at and immediately after birth, whereas the risk of chronic bronchitis seemed to be related more to events in a slightly later period of infancy. It appeared that events during one of these critical periods, for example the method of infant feeding, could

'program' a life-long influence on that individual—a view that has been called the **programming hypothesis**.

How do these findings tie in with the evidence of social class differences in morbidity and mortality? There is known to be a clear relationship between social class and birth weight, and the Southampton group found that, within each socio-economic group, the link between early weight and the adult risk of cardiovascular diseases was similar. This suggests that the early life experiences they identified exert an influence which to some extent transcends the socio-economic factors that continue through life.

The 'programming' hypothesis is still the subject of much debate, but has also been applied in other areas. As you will see in Chapter 11, for example, it seems that illness early in life can have a long-term effect on the height an individual is likely to attain as an adult. If the hypothesis continues to gain ground then we can expect to see, for example, interventions against cardiovascular and perhaps other diseases redirected from early adult life to the nutrition and care of pregnant women and infants right at the beginning of life.

Conclusion

A theme running through this chapter, and indeed the book as a whole, is that by exploring the social and economic system and its patterns of inequality, the distribution of health and disease becomes more readily understandable. The material in this chapter has shown that although artefact and social selection explanations do account for a small proportion of the observed inequalities, recurring patterns of social and economic inequality in Britain are systematically associated with inequalities in mortality and morbidity. Cumulatively, these social and economic inequalities are an important part of the explanation for the observable inequalities in health. However, it seems clear that health differences may be present when social and economic circumstances seem very similar, and there can be very long lags between a factor exerting an influence and the health outcome, as the 'programming' discussion indicated.

In apportioning relative weights to factors associated with ill-health, emphasis is too often placed on one particular type of variable rather than acknowledging the interactions between them. Many of the 'behavioural' explanations for health inequalities are influenced by environment and social context, diet is influenced by low income, and so on. Attitudes to health-influencing activities such as regular dental care may reflect individual outlook, which may be influenced by parental attitudes, all of which may be related to availability, accessibility or quality of care. The same variety of explanations are seen in public perceptions of why people are poor. Some suggest individual characteristics such as laziness and lack of will-power as the reason, whereas others suggest social injustice and the abstract workings of society.

Chapter 11 concludes this book with a detailed study of the relation between nutrition and health, which exemplifies and explores many of these themes. But perhaps an appropriate point on which to finish this chapter is to note that concern with how inequalities can be explained is not just idle academic curiosity: different explanations have very different implications for policies to reduce inequalities in health[6]. Picking an informed route through these various explanations is therefore central to choosing and designing effective policies.

[6]Strategies to reduce inequalities in health are considered in another book in this series, *Dilemmas in Health Care* (Open University Press, 1993) Chapter 11.

OBJECTIVES FOR CHAPTER 10

When you have studied this chapter, you should be able to:

10.1 Identify different ways in which inequalities in health can be measured across social classifications, and comment on trends over time in social class composition and health inequalities between social classes.

10.2 Outline and evaluate the various artefact explanations of health inequalities in the United Kingdom.

10.3 Discuss the potential contribution of individual behaviour to contemporary patterns of health and disease in the United Kingdom, and describe methods by which this contribution has been evaluated.

10.4 Outline ways in which the social and material environment may affect the distribution of health and disease, stressing interactions between factors.

QUESTIONS FOR CHAPTER 10

Question 1 (*Objective 10.1*)

Drawing on data presented in this chapter, summarise recent trends in health inequalities between social classes.

Question 2 (*Objective 10.2*)

The proportion of the population in the lowest social classes with the poorest health experience has been declining. Does this not suggest that health inequalities must have declined also?

Question 3 (*Objective 10.3*)

To what extent might patterns of smoking and drinking contribute to social class inequalities in health?

Question 4 (*Objective 10.4*)

When examining health inequalities, occupations are often used to define different social classes. Is this because different occupations have different health consequences?

11

Food, health and disease: a case study

Introduction

By now, you will have built up a general picture of the improved health and chances of survival experienced by virtually all human populations during the past century. These have been reflected in increases in longevity, growth and body size. However, it will also have become clear that these improvements have been more rapid and extensive in some countries than in others during the past few decades, with the result that there are now quite substantial differences in health between human populations alive today in different parts of the world.

One response to this might be to say that such disparities are just a reflection of countries being at different stages of economic and social development and that they will disappear again, as the poorer countries acquire more wealth and distribute that wealth among their populations more equitably. Although there is undoubtedly some truth in this view, it sets aside a number of important issues.

The first, which was raised in the introduction to this book and has been a recurrent theme throughout, is that it is not easy to distinguish the relative impact on the health of populations of the introduction of techniques for the control and cure of disease, as compared to the effects of improvements in the more general material and social conditions of life. Clearly, a better understanding of this is important if the investment of money and human resources in developing countries is to be directed into areas where it can have most effect. The choice may be between different aspects of public health, but may also be between health interventions as a whole and other areas such as industrial investment or road building.

Second, few people now believe in the rather simple picture of global development as a more or less inevitable procession, in which nations pass independently in sequence along a common pathway, each one repeating the same stages on their way to the same goal. Instead, it is now understood that the development process itself is shaped by **interdependencies** between countries. For example, the movements of people across national boundaries can nullify the effect of local programmes for

the control of infectious disease agents or their vectors. Even more serious for the future, it is becoming increasingly clear that countries are interdependent in their effect on the global environment: one country's pollution may be to the detriment of all. What if those at the rear of the development 'procession' never reach the goal because those in the van have 'trampled the ground'?

It now seems unlikely that either the industrialised countries or the countries of the Third World can continue indefinitely along development paths broadly similar to those of the past. A continued improvement of health in the Third World—and even maintaining the levels already achieved in the industrialised countries— may be critically dependent upon a better understanding of the ways in which economic, social and environmental factors interact to sustain not only the health of the human population, but also the integrity of the environment itself.

In Chapter 4, we introduced the case study technique, as a way of enhancing our understanding of processes in which the 'cause' of change is a 'web' of interconnected factors. This final chapter is also a case study, but this time the focus of the 'case' will be a particular aspect of the health environment, namely the food we eat and how this interacts with other disease factors to determine health and performance.

It is important to emphasise that the intention of this case study is not to try to implicate food supply as the single or even principle cause of the differences in health status between the populations of the Third World and those of the more industrialised countries. As in the case of Bangladesh in Chapter 4, it is the *interconnectedness* between nutrition and other factors that determines the outcome. Indeed, we could have chosen a quite different starting point, for example a particular kind of disease pathogen, or social class, or housing, or public sanitation, or gender. In any of those cases, the end result would have been a description of the same web of causes.

An important consequence of thinking in terms of interconnectedness, rather than of linear sequences of cause and effect, is that the direction of causality between particular factors may be reversed in specific circumstances or at particular times. For example, the focus of this chapter is the changing nature of food production and distribution in societies, and the implications for health of the knowledge about nutrition that has been gained during this century. But the conclusion is not that the causes of the different health 'problems' of the industrialised countries and Third World are simply mirror images—over-eating in the one and hunger in the other. As you will see, it makes no more sense to say that people in the Third World are generally smaller in size than those of the industrialised countries *because* they have been unable to eat as much food all their lives, than it does to say that they eat less food because they are smaller. Neither proposition, taken on its own, helps us to understand how the differences arose: moreover, as a basis for intervening in that process, such simplistic diagnoses have so far led only to frustration.

Diet and disease

Many nutritional diseases caused by deficiencies of **micronutrients** (i.e. substances essential for life but needed in very small quantities, like the vitamins and some mineral elements) were common in the United Kingdom before this present century, though not understood as such.

☐ Can you recall some examples of these?

■ Scurvy, which is caused by a lack of vitamin C; anaemia due to iron deficiency; rickets, a result either of insufficient vitamin D in the food or of insufficient exposure to sunlight (which promotes the synthesis of vitamin D in the skin).

Today, such **deficiency diseases** are very uncommon in industrialised countries, but not primarily because we can cure or prevent them by taking tablets (although many people do nonetheless choose to 'dose' themselves in this way). These conditions have disappeared simply because a sufficiently diverse range of foods, both fresh and well preserved, are continuously available *and affordable* by the vast majority of British people.

Nutritional deficiency diseases are still common in much of the Third World, and nutritionists often advise that governments in those countries should take a short cut to better health by using technical means such as tablets, injections or food supplements to prevent them. Others argue that, although these substances themselves are cheap, the same cannot be said of the resources needed for the transport, distribution management and supervision of such mass interventions. These 'human

resources' are very scarce in poor countries. Indeed, their scarcity is as much a part of the poverty of a nation as is a lack of money. Programmes for distributing micronutrients may therefore be at the expense of doing other things, some of which might contribute as much or more to social or economic improvement in the longer term. On this, as on many other 'magic bullet' recipes, there is still much disagreement.

In countries such as Britain, where the health and demographic transitions are already well advanced, there is now much less general fear of infectious disease. However, this has been replaced by an increase in anxiety about **degenerative diseases**—any kind of progressive or catastrophic loss of bodily function, which might prematurely rob us of the quality of living, or of life itself. The belief has been encouraged that some causes of death might be avoided, or at least postponed, by changes of 'lifestyle'. In particular, the popular imagination has been captured by the idea that what we eat is an important determinant of how long we are likely to live.

Food is suspected as being connected with degenerative diseases in at least three major ways.

☐ Can you suggest what these are?

■ You might have thought of the following:

1 In addition to the good things, food can carry harmful substances: naturally present toxins that plants and bacteria produce as a means of defence against animals (including humans) or insects that might eat them, or of offence against competitors. Other potentially harmful substances are accidentally or deliberately introduced by people: residual amounts of insecticides, herbicides and fertilisers used in the production process; additives to act as preservatives during storage, to modify flavour or appearance, or as extenders, to increase profit.

2 Some substances, for example fibre, although not essential for life in the way that the vitamins are, are believed to have protective activity against diseases: they help to sustain and sometimes reinforce the functions and mechanisms of the body which are responsible for fighting both infectious and degenerative diseases.

3 During the past few years there has been great interest in the possibly harmful effects of *overconsumption*—either of total energy, or of particular kinds of foods, such as some kinds of fats or oils or refined sugar.

The words and phrases used above such as 'may be', 'believed to be' and 'possibly' are not intended to engender total scepticism about the scientific basis of contemporary ideas about the connections between health and food. Rather, this is to emphasise the different degrees of confidence we can attach to them as compared to the much more specific knowledge about the micronutrients responsible for particular deficiency diseases. In addition, the likely benefits to the individual of dietary change are both less certain and less dramatic than, for example, the curing of scurvy, rickets or anaemia.

Over the past thirty or so years we have come to know more precisely the smallest amounts of the vitamins and other nutrients that are sufficient to maintain health, and to understand that, provided those minimal amounts are available, the body has a remarkable capacity for adjusting successfully to a wide range of different patterns of diet. This has led to greater confidence that few people in the United Kingdom are at risk of nutritional deficiency diseases. Thus the advice which used to emphasise getting 'enough' sources of vitamins and protein, cutting down on starches and maintaining a 'good mixed' diet of animal and vegetable foods, has given way to a much more cautious advocacy of the benefits of a moderate or **prudent diet**.

The prudent diet is based on a rather loose consensus between nutritionists about what kind of diet might minimise the lifetime risk of coronary or arterial disease, obesity, intestinal problems, tooth decay, etc. Not surprisingly, the consensus shifts from time to time according to both public and professional views about what is fashionable, important, researchable, or provable. At the time of writing (1992), the 'official' (i.e. Department of Health) view of a prudent diet is that people should aim to get no more than 30 per cent of their energy from animal fat, and should minimise their intakes of 'free' or refined sugars. (It is now deemed all right to eat starch, which is made of joined-up sugar molecules.) For their protective effects, more should be eaten of certain kinds of fat (such as fish oil), more vegetable fibre and fresh fruit.

Whether or not a prudent diet of this kind would make us healthier and longer-lived, it is now widely assumed that developed countries need food policies to maximise health, just as poor countries need them to minimise hunger. One of the objectives of this chapter is to ask how we have reached this position. We also need to ask what might be the instruments of such food policies, especially now that the collapse of the European central command economies has left most countries increasingly reliant on the free market as a basis for the management of both supply and effective demand.

Hunger and malnutrition: the normal lot of humans?

In Chapter 5 we traced the changes which have taken place in the human population from prehistory up to present times. Table 11.1 attempts to summarise the consequences for lifespan and body size of the human species' increasingly effective exploitation of the environment. An 'archaic' society represents a major part of human evolutionary history—the past 1 million years perhaps—during which the physiological and biochemical adaptations to our present omnivorous dietary pattern took place. Members of such a society would have been hunters and gatherers of food, certainly, but also making use of the very early phases of agriculture. Such people exist today in only a few very small groups, for example the Yanomani of South America or some tribes in New Guinea. 'Transitional' societies refer to people currently in the midst of the demographic and health transition. This includes most Asian and African countries, for example, which have predominantly young, fast-growing populations, even though birth and death rates are now falling. 'Modern' refers to societies such as that in the United Kingdom which have largely passed through the transition and are once more approaching stability of numbers and of age structure.

Table 11.1 Characteristics of average representatives of different types of societies

Average individual	Archaic	Transitional	Industrial
life expectancy	31 years	51 years	76 years
age	19 years	23 years	38 years
height	118 cm	135 cm	153 cm
weight	27 kg	33 kg	55 kg
daily energy requirement*	1 500 kcal	1 830 kcal	2 200 kcal

*These are the amounts of food individuals would need, expressed as energy (kcal is defined on p.44). (Data for the 'archaic' group are based on a a synthesis of forest-living tribes in Brazil and Papua New Guinea from Velazquez, A. and Bourges, H.(eds), 1984, *Genetic Factors in Nutrition*, Academic Press, London and New York; Malcolm, L. A., 1974, Ecological factors relating to child growth and nutritional status, in Roche, A. F. and Falkner, F. (eds) *Nutrition and Malnutrition*, Plenum, New York; and Rappoport, R. A., 1968, *Pigs for the Ancestors: Ritual in the Ecology of a New Guinea People*, Yale University Press, New Haven. The transitional and industrial data are based on those for Bangladesh and the United Kingdom respectively.)

It is to be hoped that both transitional and industrial societies will go on to achieve again a long-term equilibrium with their environments. If this happens, the period of time over which a rough balance between high birth and death rates was transformed into a rough balance between low birth and death rates will seem—from a distant future perspective—a singularity in human history.

The morphological characteristics in the table are intended to give an impression of the age, size and life expectancy at birth, of a member of each type of society selected at random. The heights and weights therefore are not necessarily those of fully grown adults: in the case of the archaic and transitional populations, they are of the somewhat younger individuals, who are average representatives of each population.

Energy expenditure would in practice have varied quite widely in archaic societies, according to the ecology of their habitat and the amounts of energy expended in hunting, gathering, or exploiting it in other ways for food. The figure in the table is chosen to represent the needs of hunter-gatherers living in an 'easy' situation, similar to that of contemporary coastal tribes in New Guinea. Only an hour or so of gardening work a day is necessary, so that food energy needs are determined mainly by the average body size. The value for the 'transitionals' assumes a fairly high work load typical of a highly organised, but non-mechanised agriculture, such as Bangladesh. Even if some animal power is used, a substantial part of the daily food needs of such people has to be directly re-invested in the form of work done on the soil and the crops, much of which—shifting, lifting, carrying—is independent of the body weight of the workers themselves. The industrial population is that of the United Kingdom: highly mechanised and therefore similar to the archaic people in having food needs which are largely a reflection of their (greater) average body size.

Although it is clear that the maximum amount of food energy that could be extracted from the environment must have had some influence on the numbers, ages, body sizes and food consumption levels of the population, there is nothing to suggest that those characteristics were entirely dominated by the amount of food available. Rather, the daily rates at which food energy are expended by an average individual in each stage can be seen as the outcome of an equilibrium exchange between the species itself and the ecology of the food system of which it forms a part. You will remember from the discussion in Chapter 5 that, in addition to Malthus's idea of 'positive checks', there are several biological/evolutionary theories about the regulation of population size. Many animal species regulate their numbers at a level below the maximum

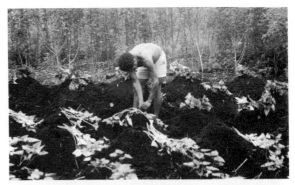

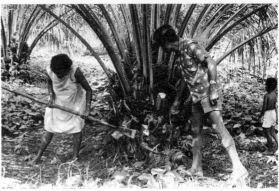

Gardening in New Guinea. Food energy needs can be met in an hour or so of gardening work a day. (Photo: Papua New Guinea Church Partnership)

which food supply could sustain. This ecological perspective, however, leaves us with an account that differs markedly from many descriptions of the contemporary world, in which much of the existing population is said to be constantly beset by hunger.

Is it correct that two-thirds of the world's present population suffer throughout their lives some degree of hunger or deprivation, as John Boyd Orr said when he became the first Director General of the UN Food and Agriculture Organisation in 1947? Or is it only one-quarter, as that same organisation suggested in 1984? Or is it less still? And if one of these is true of the present, was it always so in the past?

These apparently straightforward questions turn out to be quite difficult to answer. Perhaps the first thing to say is that, if hunger and malnutrition are the normal lot of humankind, then in terms of *biological fitness* the human species has nonetheless up to now been outstandingly successful. We now have a larger total **biomass** (i.e. the sum of the body weights of all people now alive) than that of any other mammal with the possible exception of the cow, which owes its present population size (1.3 billion in 1990) almost entirely to human livestock farming. Perhaps more significantly, there has during the past hundred years or so been a sustained increase in reproductive fitness. Not only does each generation produce a larger number of individuals who survive to contribute to the ancestry of future generations, but also a greater proportion of all those born do so. This in no way questions the moral issues raised by the existence of *any* degree of serious hunger, particularly when that could be avoided by greater equity without significant loss to anyone else. But it does suggest that if chronic hunger affects a large proportion of the world population, it is not severe or extensive enough to impair the biological *fitness* of the species as a whole. (As you saw in Chapter 5, fitness means to a biologist the successful transmission of genes to future generations; that is to say, the ability to survive long enough to reproduce and to protect that investment sufficiently to ensure that the offspring also have a chance to reproduce).

The most likely explanation of the apparent discrepancy between the biologist's view and that of the international agencies lies in the meaning they attach to the word 'hunger'. We need to be very careful to use this word and others like 'starvation' in a consistent way. The scientific definitions of these terms are not necessarily the same as when they are used colloquially, so we must spend a little time establishing the sense in which they will be used in the rest of this chapter.

That emotive word **hunger** has no scientific definition and there are no agreed methods for measuring it. Moreover, according to circumstance it has more than one common implication: for some people at some times it is a signal of desperation; for others it simply expresses a keen healthy appetite. Compare the likely implications of a complaint of 'hunger' by a child in an Ethiopian peasant family, with those of a similar plea made to almost any British parent!

Almost as problematic is **starvation.** The precise meaning is a sustained deficit of energy intake below energy expenditure. Because the first law of thermodynamics operates for people as well as for machines, this must mean a continuous loss of body weight. Although people do die from starvation caused by food shortages in some countries and some circumstances, prolonged starvation is probably quite rare except in the middle of famines, even in poor countries, and when death does occur it is more often due to disease than lack of available food.

Another term we must be clear about is **adaptation**, which refers to the physical attributes and capacities for responding to environmental stresses that a species displays in order to increase biological fitness. It may help you to understand this concept if you consider the extent to which a species can adapt to changes in the environment. The most adaptable individuals have the highest fitness because they are the most likely to survive and reproduce under the new environmental conditions. As you will see, one of the most important adaptations humans use in order to survive in situations with differing levels of food supply is to change average body size. But if we refer to the populations of poor countries, with their smaller average heights and weights, as being adapted to different (i.e. lower) food intakes than those of richer countries, we run the risk of being accused of excusing the continued existence of inequity.

To recap, not only are there problems in estimating the numbers of people who are affected by inadequate diets, there is also disagreement about what the numbers mean in terms of suffering. There are two ways of measuring the extent of malnutrition. We can try to measure what people are eating, and hence whether or not they are getting sufficient energy or nutrients to survive. Alternatively, we can try to measure the outcome, i.e. their *state of nutrition.*

Most of the statements about the extent of world hunger which have been made during the past fifty years (including Lord Boyd Orr's) have been based on attempts to measure the adequacy of food supplies reaching the populations of whole countries. In Chapter 7, we described the data, which is available from food balance sheets, of year-round per-capita food energy supplies, as well as some of the technical problems which limit the reliability of such data. Great efforts have been made to improve the reliability of this information and, through nutritional research, to establish the minimum levels of energy and nutrients that are needed in a country's food supply in order to avoid malnutrition. However, uncertainty about the reliability and interpretation of these assessments has, if anything, increased over time.

If it is difficult to establish the extent to which limitation of food supply has been a positive check to the health and growth of populations, can we perhaps find evidence of the converse? Have there been situations in the past in which populations have experienced *improvements* in health and survival which could be attributed to improved quantity or quality of available food? If so, it would be reasonable to conclude that they had previously been undernourished.

As you saw in Chapter 6, it was suggested by the medical historian Thomas McKeown that the improved food supplies available to the population of the United Kingdom from the beginning of the nineteenth century were the principal cause of the subsequent decline in mortality. However, you will also recall that the same data led the historical demographer Simon Szreter to challenge that hypothesis. The problem, of course, is that, unlike a controlled experiment under laboratory conditions in which only the food system of a whole community is changed while everything else is held constant, real-life changes in food supply are always associated with changes in economic and social factors which also have implications for people's behaviour, standards of living and hence of health.

Changes in body size: malnutrition or adaptation?

If it is so difficult to assess the adequacy or otherwise of the food available to past or present populations, can we simply observe the effects of food deprivation directly, i.e. assess people's **state of nutrition**? Only a few years ago, it was usual for international nutritionists to refer to measurements such as weight or height in children as indices of nutritional status. Individuals below certain critical size-for-age limits were classified as 'malnourished'. The implication was that body size in children could be used as a direct measure of the amount of food available to them as individuals, or to the households or communities in which they lived.

However, this view has changed over the past few years, to the extent that many health scientists now prefer to speak simply of assessing child growth or of 'anthropometry' ('human-measurement'), thus avoiding altogether the use of the terms 'nutritional status' or 'malnutrition' as the common direct cause of smallness.

How has this important change of views come about? First, studies from birth onwards of the patterns of growth of children living in economically and environmentally impoverished conditions have shown that certain **critical periods of growth** are of special importance. Growth is affected by any environmental stress (including a lack of nutrients), during the later stages of intra-uterine life and in the first two years or so after birth, in other words up to about the age when weaning is complete in pre-industrial societies. During this period, there is also a capacity to 'catch up' on any lost growth, provided the stress is reversed.

However, as the end of this critical period is approached, the ability to recover fully is reduced. The result is that a child who suffers repeated episodes of stress through and beyond the second year of life may end up with an accumulated short-fall—in both height and weight—which is permanent. Not only that, the deficit is 'carried over' into the next phase of life in the form of a modified set of 'instructions' for the mechanisms by which the body achieves its final adult size. These altered instructions, even in the absence of further stress, result in an adult who is shorter (and correspondingly lighter) than

he or she would have been without the stresses during infancy. It has been found that although this process of **stunting** can be reduced by improving the health environment of mothers and small children, relatively little further can be done to reverse its effects, even by intensive feeding treatments after the age of around two years.

The curve of growth in height shown in Figure 11.1 illustrates how this process might operate. A girl whose length as a baby follows the average of the normal range (the smooth curve labelled 50th centile), suffers a series of setbacks to growth. She catches up again at first, but after the age of two years further illness causes growth to fall away towards the lower end of the normal range (the dotted curve labelled '3rd centile'). Finally she becomes an adult whose height growth finishes at the lower end of the normal range.

Infectious diseases of early childhood, such as diarrhoeal or respiratory tract infections, not only affect growth directly, through the toxins they produce in the body, but also act indirectly through reduced appetite. If growth is severely affected, from whatever cause, there may also be damage to the immune system which defends the child from infections—increasing the likelihood of further severe illness. Thus, whatever the nature of the initiating event, disease or inadequate food, the outcome is likely to be the same: a self-reinforcing sequence of growth checks, with any remaining deficit in height after about two years being followed by a life-long pattern of smallness.

This means that we need to be very cautious of drawing conclusions about the adequacy of food supplies in a country on the basis of people's *current* body size. Adults are as likely to be the size they are because they were stressed in some way by their environment in the past, as because of their present situation. In addition, the source of that stress is just as likely to have been a series of infectious disease episodes as a simple lack of food.

Obviously, then, populations with large numbers of small adults are ones in which, *in the past*, many young children have suffered a good deal from infectious illness and perhaps also from a lack of care and attention (including parental care and other resources which might minimise the impact of illness). But can we say any more than that? For those that did survive and were not severely affected at the time, does being somewhat smaller than the average person in an industrialised society matter? Indeed, is it even some advantage?

To ask this question is not, of course, to imply that the process of illness and deprivation which results in children becoming permanently smaller might be regarded as acceptable. At the time it happens, it means that the children affected are living in an environment which is

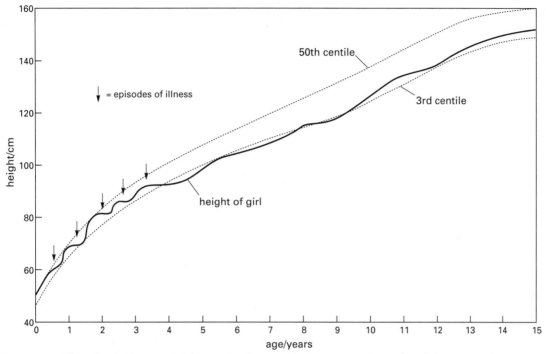

Figure 11.1 *Effect of early illness on height growth. The arrows indicate repeated episodes of illness. (Data from P. Payne, previously unpublished)*

socially and materially deficient. Moreover, if it is very severe, it carries a high risk of death at the time; and, even if the child does survive, there may be adverse effects on psychological development and on the capacity to withstand further illnesses. In addition, as you saw in the discussion in Chapter 10 of 'programming' and as you will see later, some epidemiologists believe that the impact of infectious diseases of very early childhood may pre-dispose the individual towards health problems, such as coronary heart disease in later life.

The point, however, is that there is little evidence that moderate shortness and lightness of the kind that distinguishes the average Asian adult from the average American or Briton carries any significant penalties *in itself*, in terms of physical, intellectual or social functioning (however, as noted in Chapter 10, above average height does tend to be *associated* with upward social class mobility). The Canadian nutritionist George Beaton has summarised all this as follows.

The primary conclusion that I have come to is that it is not *being* small that matters. Rather, it is *becoming* small that is critically important. It is that mix of environmental forces that leads to growth failure that also has consequences in

other aspects of development and may have long term sequelae for population development. The corollary to this conclusion is that the current emphasis on growth promotion, should be seen as an attack on *constraints to growth and development*. The real objective is not to make people bigger. (Beaton, 1989, p.37)

Of course, if programmes aimed at removing those constraints are effective and universally available, they will inevitably result in increases in the average body size of the populations of Third World countries. In the meantime, being small does quite usefully reduce overall food requirements. The upper part of Table 11.2 shows the body weight, from 6 months of age up to adulthood, of an average European girl. The lower part of the table shows that of a girl who is typical of many rural Asian populations.

☐ Comparing the weights, what pattern do you see?

■ They start to diverge sometime between 6 months and one year.

Below the values for weight for each girl, you will see those for the three components of **daily energy requirements**: *maintenance*, which is the energy cost of just

Table 11.2 The effect of reduced growth on energy needs

European girl age/years	0.5	1	5	10	25
weight/kg	7.2	9.5	17.7	35.2	57
energy needs/kcal					
maintenance	360	620	890	1140	1370
growth	80	50	25	70	0
activity	220	320	580	700	850
total per day/kcal	660	990	1495	1910	2220
lifetime total/kcal	**94 900**	**245 500**	**2 060 000**	**5 166 600**	**16 472 000**
Asian girl age/years	0.5	1	5	10	25
weight/kg	7.2	9	14	22.5	43
energy needs/kcal					
maintenance	360	590	700	790	1032
growth	80	20	20	30	0
activity	220	300	460	490	710
total per day/kcal	660	910	1180	1310	1742
lifetime total/kcal	**94 900**	**238 200**	**1 764 000**	**403 600**	**12 390 000**
Energy saved by smaller body size of Asian girl					
per day/kcal	0	80	315	600	488
lifetime/kcal	0	7300	296 000	1 130 600	4 082 000

Data from P. Payne, not previously published.

staying alive, with no energy used for physical activity or growth; *growth*, which is the energy needed to synthesise and store new tissue; and *activity*, the energy cost of moving the body and other objects around. The table shows the daily energy requirement of each girl, which is the sum of these three. The next row of values is for the total energy needed, added up for all the days these two girls have lived up to the particular ages at the top of each column.

The two rows at the bottom of the table show the amounts of energy 'saved' as a result of the smaller size of the Asian as compared with the European girl at each particular age. The daily savings are simply the differences between the daily rates. While the children are very young, the energy savings are relatively small amounts: at one year, the difference is 80 kcal a day. If you look back at the Bangladesh family profile in Chapter 4, you will see that the total needs of that family were between 7.8 (if resting) and 10 *thousand* kcal each day. Even that desperately poor family would hardly be likely to notice a saving of 80 kcal a day. However, the daily savings do become more significant as the girls become adult and, as the bottom row in the table shows, the cumulative differ-

ences (that is, the daily savings added up over the 25 years) are very substantial: by the time she reaches the age of 25, the Asian woman has used more than 4 million kcal less energy than the European. This would be sufficient to feed another younger sister up to the age of 10.

Changes in body size

Although the effect of an adverse environment on growth is more or less permanent in an individual if not corrected early in life, small size can be reversed gradually over successive generations. If the Asian woman described in Table 11.2 were to migrate to a better environment in which she had children, their growth would be along a faster track than their mother's. As adults, they would probably be taller and proportionally heavier than either of their parents. They would go on in their turn to have somewhat larger babies than they were themselves, and so on until an upper limit of size is reached. This explains the increases in adult size which have been seen in the offspring of Asian migrants to the United States and the slow upward trend in average height which occurred in Europe over three or more generations during the nineteenth and early twentieth centuries.

Conclusion

It seems that we can distinguish a number of food-related factors which have played a part in generating differences between human populations in lifespan, body size and, by implication, in general health. These differences have developed over time and between countries. However, food seems generally to have played an associated, as opposed to an initiating, role. The people of the industrialised world have become taller and heavier over the past two hundred years. As a result, their food requirements have increased. We can predict the same sequence of events for the peoples of the Third World as their physical stature undergoes the same trend, if there is a sustained improvement in their standards of living and general health provision.

As you saw in Chapter 7, world food supplies so far have kept pace with population growth. Evidence that food supply ever has been or is now a constraint to health and performance of the great majority of people in Third World countries is at best inconclusive. Certainly, it has not so far been sufficient to bring about a reduction in fertility to match the continuing decline in mortality.

Of course there have been and still are significant numbers of people who have to exist at the very margin of survival. For them, quite small adverse changes of circumstances may make the difference between bare adequacy and actual starvation—with death or permanent damage to health an inevitable outcome if the adversity is sustained. Because of the fragile nature of their food entitlement, they are often the first and the worst affected by domestic stresses, natural disasters, or famines—from whatever cause. Nevertheless, the *proportion* of people whose lives are threatened by disease and by the loss of food entitlement has declined, even if the growth in total numbers is sufficient to outweigh those gains.

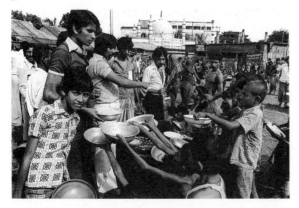

Feeding programme following floods in Bangladesh, 1980. Food queues are daily occurrences in Bangladesh, as in many other parts of the Third World. (Photo: Tom Learmonth)

Food supply and food entitlement: origins of the diet of industrialised countries

Dietary trends since the Industrial Revolution

Only some twenty years after Malthus published his first essay in 1800, William Cobbett, a journalist, political pamphleteer and enthusiast for all kinds of country pursuits, was writing his account of 'rural rides' around the English countryside. Cobbett was an enthusiastic agent of agricultural development, and he tells story after story of innovation and change, of new techniques and the adoption of new crop varieties and more varied patterns of production.

He also saw what he considered to be a complete refutation of Malthus' theory: namely, evidence of *depopulation* of the countryside at the same time that food production was expanding. On being told that the census figures showed a 40 per cent increase of the total population between 1801 and 1821 (see Figure 6.1), he wrote, 'A man that can suck that in, will believe, literally believe that the moon is made of green cheese.' What angered him was that relatively few of the peasants were receiving the benefit of expanding agricultural production. Writing about the food and wool produced in Somerset, he describes how:

> The infernal system causes it all to be carried away. Not a bit of good beef, or mutton, or veal and scarcely a bit of bacon is left for those who raise all this food and wool…and the canal that passes close by it…Devizes…is the great channel through which the produce of the country is carried away to be devoured by the idlers, the thieves and the prostitutes, who are all tax-eaters, in the Wens of Bath and London. (Cobbett, 1830, pp. 316–17)

Cobbett's detailed accounts of the economy of individual farms and cottage households give us a starting point for understanding what these changes must have meant for the nature of the food entitlement of working-class households. As far as rural life was concerned, Cobbett was obviously an idealist, but his description of what he called a 'fair share' of the produce of the labour of a family of five is probably a reasonable account of the largely self-sufficient food provisioning of labourers' households that he had known as a child:

> In order to come at the fact here, let us see what would be the consumption of one family; let it be a family of five persons; a man, wife, and three children, one child big enough to work, one big enough to eat heartily, and one a baby; …and this is a pretty fair average of the state of people in the country. (Cobbett, 1830, pp. 305–8)

If we make some 'guestimates' about what the body sizes, ages and work outputs of the members of this family are likely to have been, we can use the same method on which the values in Table 11.2 were based, to estimate that the family would have needed to expend something between 12–13 000 kcal per day.

You might remember from Chapter 4 that the peasant family of five in Bangladesh consumed and expended about 10 000 kcal per day. All but the youngest members of both families would have worked hard and long. The members of Cobbett's family, though not as large as contemporary Britons, would have been taller and heavier than the Bangladeshis, which largely accounts for their higher energy requirement.

Look at Table 11.3: the family would also have had some vegetables and fruit in season, which Cobbett does not mention. On this estimated diet, their week's food would indeed have provided the five of them with something over 13 000 kcal per day.

Table 11.3 Staple foods consumed over a week by a rural British family of five persons in around 1800

Food	Quantity	Energy/kcal
bread	35 lb (15.9 kg)	34 000
bacon	14 lb (6.4 kg)	41 000
mutton	7 lb (3.2 kg)	7 700
beer	10.5 gallons (47.7 litres)	8 000
total		**90 700**

Data from P. Payne, not previously published; based on Cobbett, W. (1830) *Rural Rides*, reprinted 1967 by Penguin English Library, Penguin, London.

To produce this weekly diet, the household would have needed basic grains for bread making, brewing and feeding to pigs, plus sheep for the mutton, all of which can be converted into contemporary cash equivalents as shown in Table 11.4.

Table 11.4 Quantities and costs of basic commodities needed for provisioning a British family of five for a year in around 1800.

Commodity	Quantity	Cost in 1800		
		Pounds	Shillings	Pence
wheat	3 quarters, 6 bushels	10	10	0
barley	22 quarters, 3 bushels	37	16	8
sheep	7 carcasses	14		
total		**£62**	**6**	**8**

Data from P. Payne, not previously published; based on Cobbett, W. (1830) *Rural Rides*, reprinted 1967 by Penguin English Library, Penguin, London.

Cobbett acknowledged that by the 1820s few labouring families could achieve even half of this cash income. How then did the rural labourers manage to live? His book, *Cottage Economy*, published in 1823, gives a vivid impression of the complex structure of food entitlement. A substantial part depended upon rights of access to land and forest, for producing their own food and fuel. That access might be wholly or in part through 'common' rights, or as land rented or in lieu of a portion of wages. Wages themselves would commonly be partly cash and partly in kind. Although small-scale rural industries still provided some cash income through employment of women and children, by 1820 these were already declining because of competition from the factories.

Entitlement to cash and resources, however, was only the starting point of provisioning. In addition to this, the labour component of preservation and preparation— salting, smoking, baking and brewing, to say nothing of growing vegetables and fruit, was of major importance for food security. The degree of self-sufficiency this gave was essential, not just as a way of minimising cash expenditure, but as a necessary hedge against widely fluctuating prices and wages from season to season and, because of weather, from year to year.

Some seventy years later, a survey of the food expenditure of 2 000 urban working-class families, representative of the whole country, was carried out by the Board of Trade. Table 11.5 shows the weekly purchases of those averaging 5 members, and earning just over £1 per week (the lowest of five income bands), 70 per cent of which was spent on food.

□ What do you think are the important differences between this list and Cobbett's peasant family's diet of the previous century?

■ First of all, the much greater variety of items; several of which (sugar, rice, tea, cocoa) were imported and many others were bought in a pre-prepared form (bread, bacon, cheese, currants, jam, etc.). Second, a much higher proportion of the energy comes from wheat flour and potatoes, but also sugar. Beer, which provided nearly 10 per cent of the cottager's energy, has been replaced by tea (although, quite possibly, drinking alcohol in any form was simply not regarded any more as a part of victualling, and anyway might not have been admitted to). Meat, and especially bacon, had become a secondary source. Bearing in mind also the likely trends in the *composition* of these meats, the proportion of energy from fat was probably much lower by 1900.

Table 11.5 Staple foods consumed over a week by a poor urban British family of five persons in around 1900.

Food	Quantity	Energy/kcal
bread and flour	28.4 lb (12.7 kg)	34 500
potatoes	14.1 lb (6.4 kg)	5 440
rice, oats	2.5 lb (1.1 kg)	3 960
sugar	3.9 lb (1.8 kg)	7 200
meat	4.4 lb (2.0 kg)	6 320
bacon	1.0 lb (0.5 kg)	3 250
milk	6.9 lb (3.1 kg)	2 015
cheese	0.7 lb (0.3 kg)	1 230
butter	1.1 lb (0.5 kg)	3 700
currants	0.4 lb (0.2 kg)	480
fruit and vegetables	not known	not known
tea, coffee, cocoa	0.6 lb (0.3 kg)	900
total		**68 995**

Data from P. Payne, not previously published; based on Burnett, J. (1966), *Plenty and Want*, Nelson, London.

The food energy supply per day of a little more than 10 400 kcal is much lower than that of Cobbett's cottagers, but this is consistent with the reduced energy demands of industrial as compared to agricultural labour, and the much lower energy cost of domestic food production and preparation.

What is interesting about the *entitlement* to this food, compared with the previous example, is its relatively simple pattern. By 1900, virtually everything to do with food acquisition depended upon a cash wage. Preparation would still have needed a lot of time, but much less than the time and labour needed to produce the cottager's food. The development of the urban supply system had already much reduced the need for the production, preservation and home processing of basic ingredients.

Ninety years further on, in the last decades of the twentieth century, the process of translocation of employment is almost total. Less than 1 per cent of the United Kingdom population now work *directly* in agricultural production, although a much greater proportion, perhaps as much as 30 per cent, are employed in some aspect of processing, packaging, promotion, distribution and sale of food. Table 11.6 and Figure 11.2 (overleaf) brings more up to date the sequence of family diets, with a weekly shopping list of a typical urban household of five people, living in the 1980s.

The daily energy intake works out at a little over 11 000 kcal, close to the estimated rate of expenditure of a British family having the same age and sex structure as the one we described as typical of rural Bangladesh—each British person being taller and heavier than their Bangladeshi counterpart, but leading a relatively much more sedentary urban life.

The point of Figure 11.2 is not so much to emphasise the *volume* of the 'modern' diet: a comparable photograph of a full year's food for the family in Cobbett's cottage would probably show it occupying an even

Table 11.6 Foods consumed over a week by an average British family of five persons, 1983

Food	Quantity oz	kg	Energy/kcal
white bread	110	3.12	7 270
brown bread	45	1.27	2 840
flour	30	0.85	2 704
cakes, biscuits, cereals	95	2.69	9 430
sugar and sweets	65	1.84	7 370
poultry	35	0.99	1 490
beef and veal	35	0.99	1 686
mutton and pork	40	1.13	2 490
bacon and ham	25	0.71	2 340
sausages	15	0.42	1 270
other meats	40	1.13	1 130
fish	25	0.71	710
cheese	20	0.57	1 700
milk	25	14.2	9 240
butter	20	0.57	4 190
margarine	20	0.57	4 140
fats and oils	15	0.43	3 820
eggs	20	1.40	2 060
vegetables: fresh	140	3.97	1 190
vegetables: frozen	85	2.41	1 080
potatoes	210	5.95	4 520
fruit: fresh	100	2.84	1 304
fruit: canned and frozen	40	1.13	290
tea and coffee	15	0.43	1 190
jams, pickles, sauces, spreads.	50	1.42	3 680
total			**79 170**

Data from P. Payne, not previously published, but based on calculations of the average food consumption per person in 1981, derived from the National Food Survey Committee (1983) *Household Food Consumption and Expenditure, 1981: Annual Report of the National Food Survey Committee*, HMSO, London.

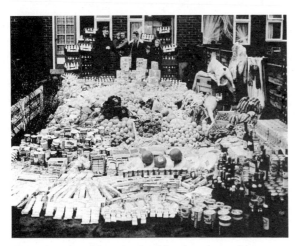

Figure 11.2 *Food for a family of five for a year—the 'average' diet in Britain in the 1980s. (Photo: Andrew Davidson, Camera Press)*

greater volume, because of the relative bulkiness of the staple foods of the time—but the greatly increased *variety* of the foods now available to the average family. What differs above all, however, is that most of the economic value added (and, as you will see later, the energy inputs) now take place during the stages *after* the agricultural production of the raw materials, and before the foods reach the larder.

You have now seen four contrasting examples of family energy budgets (three here and one in Chapter 4), selected from different locations, historical times and types of livelihood. The intention has been to illustrate households typical of their class: they were not chosen to present either the best or the very worst off but typical families, who on balance were surviving. That being so, they *must* have been able, over time, to balance the energy expended in pursuing their livelihoods against that obtained from the food they ate. Had those balances been struck at different levels, they would themselves have had to be different people—larger, or smaller, or leading different kinds of lives.

Dietary trends and health trends

Of course, there has been much speculation about the possible implications for health of the changes in the relative price and availability of foods in the United Kingdom over the past two centuries. Strictly comparable values for the availability of different foods and sources of energy and nutrients—in the form of national food balance sheets—are available only from 1939 onwards. This means that trends over longer periods of history rely on relatively anecdotal evidence. As the examples of family diets suggest, in Britain even the relatively poor

throughout the last century expected to eat quite a lot of meat. Already in 1880, at the national level, about 20 per cent of dietary energy was derived from animal sources. By 1910, at 25 per cent, the proportion was well on the way up to the 30 per cent of the 1980s.

Added to the uncertainty over the quantities of food eaten is doubt concerning their composition. For example, the average proportion of *fat* in meat has probably declined significantly since the nineteenth century, because of changes in animal husbandry. It is not necessarily correct therefore to think of previous generations as eating less animal fat than we do today. Indeed, Cobbett's cottagers may have been deriving some 42 per cent of their energy from fat—close to today's average. The pigs kept in 1820 would have been much older and bigger when they were slaughtered and would have been *very* much fatter. Cobbett's advice about fattening a pig, in his book *Cottage Economy,* was to keep it until it was well into its second year and to:

> make him *quite fat* by all means. The last bushel (of food) even if he sit as he eat, is the most profitable. If he can walk two hundred yards at a time, he is not well fatted. Lean bacon is the most wasteful thing that any family can use. The man who cannot live on *solid fat* bacon, well fed and well cured, wants the sweet sauce of labour, or is fit for the hospital. (Cobbett, 1823, pp. 121)

Evidently, the main purpose of keeping pigs at that time was not, as it is today, to produce lean meat as cheaply as possible, but was rather to store energy as fat and to preserve it throughout the year, by curing and smoking.

Another obvious change has been the increased consumption of *refined sugar*. It began with the introduction of cane sugar from the plantations of the West Indies around the middle of the eighteenth century, was later replaced by beet sugar and more recently has been complemented by glucose syrups made by breaking down starch extracted from cereals such as maize. The consumption of sugar has increased fivefold in little more than 200 years from about 20 grams per head per day around 1850 to its present 104 g (accounting for about 18 per cent of dietary energy).

Two changes that are not so obvious are in the levels of consumption of *salt* and of *vegetable fibre*. Throughout most of history, salt has been expensive. In addition to mining it, the manufacture of salt was an early component of industrial development. Since the process involves evaporation of large quantities of sea water, it is very energy demanding and salt production played a significant part in the deforestation of northern and eastern Europe in the seventeenth and eighteenth centuries

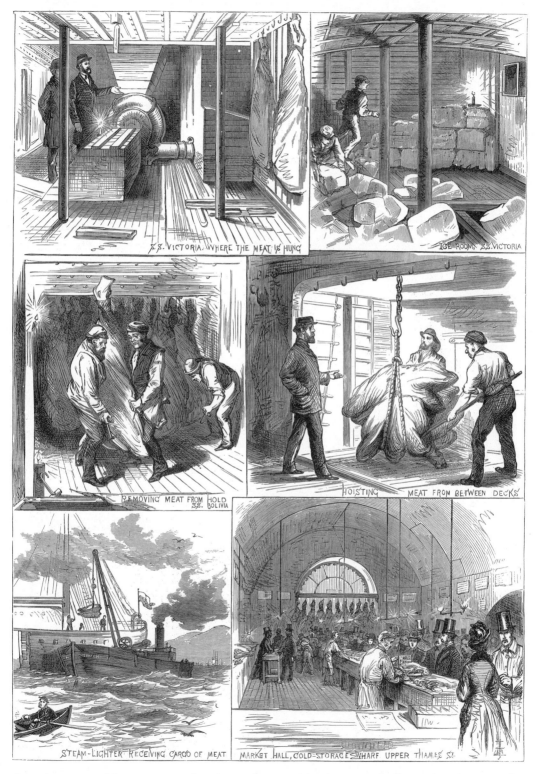

The trade in imported frozen meat was flourishing at the time of this drawing in the Illustrated London News *of 3 March 1877. (Source: The Mansell Collection)*

and was a major user of the peat whose excavation created the Norfolk Broads. With better technology and the introduction of cheap sources of fossil fuel, the price of salt has fallen considerably over the past 150 years in relative terms. It now takes only one-fifth of the time for the average worker to earn 1 kilogram of salt as it did in 1840. Not surprisingly, the consumption of salt has gone up and now averages about 12 grams per day, 5 g of which are added in cooking or at the table, with another 5 g consumed in traditional foods such as bread and 2 g in processed foods.

As for fibre, the greatly increased level of processing of foods prior to sale has resulted not only in the introduction of a wide variety of new substances—preservatives, stabilisers, flavourings and extenders—it has also removed from the diet much of the vegetable fibre contained in the original products.

All these changes in diet have had implications for the role of energy in food production. And more generally, the way the populations of the industrial countries now acquire their food has quite serious implications for the 'health' of the global ecology of which they are part. The next section takes a closer look at this issue.

Energy trends in food production

In his book *The Ecology of Agricultural Systems*, the geographer Timothy Bayliss-Smith gives an analysis of the amounts of energy needed for food production at different stages in the development of agriculture. Table 11.7 shows three examples, which you can relate to the three types of society, archaic, transitional and industrial, which were described earlier in this chapter. The last column in the table shows the ratio of food energy output to energy inputs.

The first row of values are for an example of a pre-industrial system, a tribe of people who cultivate food gardens in New Guinea. The next is for Fyfield Manor Farm in Wiltshire, for the year 1826, when it was visited by William Cobbett. You can also think of this as representing the transitional production systems upon which a major part of the world's population still depends. Finally, there are values derived from the energy budget for a mainly arable farm in the south of England in 1971.

☐ The differences between these systems are all quite dramatic, but which strike you as being the most significant?

■ The increase in productivity means that, by 1971, one man was able to produce enough food in each workday to feed 200 people for a day. The increase up to 1826 was achieved partly by using horses to supplement human effort. However, the really large increase has been achieved this century by using machines, which have now almost entirely replaced human and animal power. The increased productivity, however, has been bought at the cost of *much lower efficiency of energy conversion*. One unit of energy input in 1971 produced only 2.1 units of food energy, whereas in 1826 it produced 40.

For the twentieth-century farm, we have to count as part of the inputs not only the fuel used by machines, but also the energy for manufacturing and transporting fertilisers, herbicides and insecticides. In 1971, each full-time agricultural worker in the United Kingdom was backed by non-agricultural energy inputs equivalent to 11.2 tons of oil fuel per year.

The value of 2.1 units of food energy output for each unit of input on a contemporary farm applies only to grains. And high meat consumption has serious implications for energy use: systems of animal production, many of which depend on specially grown feed crops are even more inefficient than grain farming, returning energy ratios of nearer 1 : 1.

Table 11.7 Labour and energy productivity of agriculture

	Labour productivity Days of food per work day	Energy input/kcal from			Ratio energy output : energy input
		humans	animals	machines	
New Guinea, 1980	1	100	0	0	14 : 1
Wiltshire, 1826	7	77	21	2	40 : 1
South East England, 1971	200	0.2	0	99.8	2.1 : 1

Data from P. Payne, not previously published; based on Bayliss-Smith, T.P. (1982) *The Ecology of Agriculturral Systems*, Cambridge University Press, Cambridge.

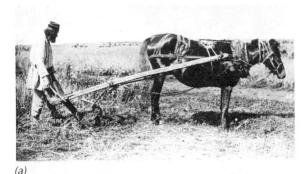

(a)

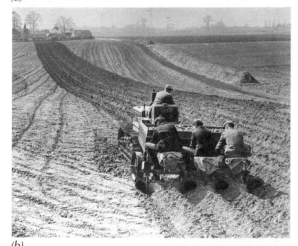

(b)

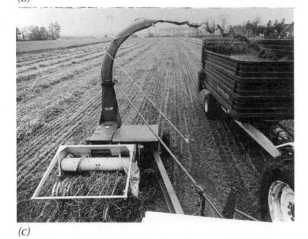

(c)

Rising labour productivity and falling energy productivity in agriculture. (a) Horse-drawn plough in Russia at the end of the nineteenth century. (b) Potato planting in England in the 1940s (c) Combine harvester in England in the 1960s (Sources: (a) Hulton-Deutsch Collection; (b) J. Topham Ltd.; (c) Sperry, New Holland)

□ Why do you think this is so?

■ If instead of eating plants ourselves, we first use an animal to convert plant material into meat, we are introducing an extra stage into the cycle.

Taking the animal production process as a whole, including the maintenance of breeding stock, the ratio of meat energy out to plant fodder energy in, is little better than $1 : 5$. This becomes even worse if the animal feed is itself purpose grown, using mechanised cultivation.

Even these values only include processes as far as the farm gate. Modern supermarket provisioning involves complex systems of factory processing, packaging and storage. Colossal supermarkets necessitate long-distance bulk transport, often followed by the use of personal car transport by individual purchasers. The energy costs of all of these are so variable as to be hard to represent meaningfully in a single value. However, one current estimate for the USA is that, whereas one farm worker can now produce the food needed by upwards of 1 000 other people, every kcal of food energy consumed requires on average a total expenditure of 9 kcal (including the cost of an average of 2 000 km of transport).

The food systems of industrial countries now account for nearly 20 per cent of their total energy use. This energy is mostly derived from coal and oil and is, of course, solar energy, which was trapped in plants millions of years ago. At first sight, this seems no different from the situation in 1826. This also involved trapping solar energy in fodder plants, feeding these to horses and using their muscle power to supplement human labour.

The difference, however, is in the recycling of *carbon*. The same amount of carbon was simply exchanged back and forth between horses and plants, whereas carbon released from burning fossil fuels leaves a *net increase* in atmospheric carbon dioxide. In addition to carbon dioxide, the huge populations of ruminants excrete carbon in the form of methane, a gas which has an even greater 'greenhouse' effect than carbon dioxide (in 1990 there were almost 29 million sheep in the United Kingdom, an increase of 35 per cent over the previous decade).

Food production in Third World countries also contributes to the greenhouse gases: the green algae which live in rice paddies and contribute to their fertility are also a major source of atmospheric methane. In this way, the food production and distribution systems of both the industrial countries and the developing countries are now substantial contributors to the problem of global warming.

In Chapters 5 and 8 you saw how the impact of humans on the environment and on natural resources has been contested for at least two centuries. The problem of greenhouse gases and global warming is no exception to this. However, Norman Meyers (1991) gives various estimates of the size of the global population that could be provided *equally* with an average diet similar in composition and volume to that currently eaten in the United Kingdom, without producing a continuous increase in the level of greenhouse gases and hence continued climatic change. The mid-range estimate works out to be around 2.5 billion. Barring a major catastrophe, the actual number alive in 2025 seems likely to reach nearer 8.5 billion (see Figure 5.2), even if the most effective population policies are universally adopted. Whether or not this figure turns out to be accurate, it does illustrate how human food production and human health are inextricably linked, not only directly, but also via the global environment.

Nutrition and health: the growth of scientific knowledge

We noted earlier that one aim of this chapter is to review the origins of the idea that a change in the pattern of food consumption would bring about a significant improvement in the general health of the United Kingdom population. To pursue this further, we need to consider in more detail the ways in which the quality of diets—that is, their chemical composition—may influence health and survival. We can do this by tracing the history of the growth of scientific knowledge of nutrition.

The origins of scientific knowledge of nutrition

In most branches of science, knowledge and more particularly the understanding and acceptance of knowledge seem to grow not just through the smooth progressive discovery and cataloguing of facts, but rather through sudden changes or even apparent reversals of accepted theories about how observations should be interpreted. Thomas Kuhn, in his book *The Structure of Scientific Revolutions* (1970), has described this as a process whereby existing theories, or *paradigms* as he calls sets of interconnected theories, gradually attract increasingly compelling criticism because of their failure to account for new facts. Finally, old theories are overthrown and are replaced by new ones. These then become for a while an accepted part of the culture of the time, only to be subjected in their turn to increasing attack and finally overthrow.[1] Occasionally, the proponent of a

'new' theory has to argue and struggle for a very long time before the conventional paradigm is discredited. Sometimes, like artists, they never live to see their ideas accepted. Something of this sort happened to delay the birth of nutritional science.

In 1753 the Scottish physician James Lind published his *Treatise on the Scurvy*. This showed that a disease which was frequently fatal for sailors on long voyages could be prevented simply by a daily ration of vegetables or lemon juice. The prescription was so effective that, whereas Anson in 1740 had failed to circumnavigate the globe largely because half his crew died of it, Cook in 1774 succeeded without the loss of a single man from scurvy. Despite this very practical success, Lind's theory was not popular. He believed that scurvy was caused by the *absence* of something in the diet—an idea that seems perfectly reasonable today, but which his contemporary medical scientists however found totally unacceptable. They 'knew' that diseases were caused by the *presence* of something bad—a poison, a miasma, or later a bacterium. Lind, who tried without success to produce scurvy in groups of volunteers by deliberate experiment, finally lost faith in his own idea and died disillusioned.

It was not until 1912 that the Polish-American biochemist Casimir Funk proposed the modern, general theory of essential nutrients and coined the term *vitamins* to describe the existence in foods of a collection of vital substances and a matching set of deficiency syndromes, which result from the absence of any one of them.

By the middle of the twentieth century, nutrition had become a quantitative experimental science. A very important feature of the development of nutritional science was the growth of research on farm animals. As you have seen, the industrial nature of agricultural development included increasingly intensive methods of meat production. The drive for increased economic efficiency of production, and the fast growth of the industry, generated a very high level of both public and private investment in research on agricultural animals, far greater than that which has ever flowed directly into research on human nutrition.

Although the cross-fertilisation between human and animal experimentation brought benefits to both sides, it is important to recognise that the objectives and hence the methods of the two are very different. Research on animal production is essentially aimed at maximising the rate of return on investment. The problem is how to feed the production 'units'—be they pigs, chickens or cattle—so as to generate the greatest value of meat (or milk or eggs) for each unit of value spent on food. The research programme is, roughly: (i) find out the chemical nature of as many as possible of the nutrients which are essential for *growth* in a particular species; (ii) of all these nutrients, find the relative proportions in the diet that give the

---

[1] Paradigm shifts in scientific knowledge and explanations are discussed in *Studying Health and Disease* (Open University Press, 1985; revised edition 1994).

maximum *rate* of growth; and (iii) get as close to that growth rate as possible, using the cheapest foodstuffs and chemical additives available.

The economics of commercial production are such that large-scale producers control virtually every aspect of the animal's environment and behaviour, and use genetic selection for maximum efficiency of energy conversion and minimum genetic variation between individuals.. In practice, this has meant concentrating research on the species, breeds and age ranges which have the greatest potential for fast growth. The nutrition research strategy adopted is essentially to try to measure the effects of changing the levels of single nutrients, one by one, while holding the influence of all the others as constant as possible. The number of different vitamins, minerals, fatty acids and amino acids (the building blocks in proteins) shown to be essential for some aspect of vital functions now stands at around 50, with some variation between species.

This animal research strategy implies the need for a level of detailed and precise quantitative knowledge about animal nutrition that is far beyond anything we could reasonably expect to acquire about humans: knowledge, moreover that would only be relevant to the performance of creatures living under the most rigidly controlled conditions. However, it did come to be widely accepted during the 1950s to 1970s that this kind of method could be used as a basis for assessing the diets eaten by people in poor countries, and hence estimating how many of them were suffering from hunger or malnutrition.

Nutrition research and Third World malnutrition

When this programme of nutrition research in the Third World got under way, there was a great deal of interest in **protein foods**, in part because the amounts of these eaten are so obviously different as between rich and poor people. During this period, the protein contents of a wide variety of the foods and diets from developing countries were measured, using tests based on animal growth—and found to be deficient in comparison with the amounts of protein then considered to be necessary for health.

At about the same time, physicians became very interested in *kwashiorkor*, an illness seen in small children in some poor countries. This is a condition in which the child, typically between the ages of 1 to 3 years, becomes listless and fretful, loses its appetite, develops a dry and flaking skin and a reddish tinge to its hair. Unlike the much more common problem of severe loss of weight, or prolonged failure to grow, these children look chubby and well covered, although in fact this is deceptive—the chubbiness is actually water, rather than normal flesh.

Although kwashiorkor occurs in a number of countries with differing traditional diets, it was first described in the Western medical literature by Cecely Williams, a doctor working in the Children's Hospital in Accra. Later, she used the Côte D'Ivoire word kwashiorkor, to describe the result of abrupt weaning onto maize gruel of a child whose mother has a new baby.

Cecely Williams herself never suggested that this disease was due to a lack of protein. However, maize flour does have a lower protein content than most weaning foods used in Europe and North America and these observations started off what came to be called the '**great protein fiasco**'. Beginning with the idea that the symptoms of kwashiorkor were the specific signs of protein deficiency, the theory rapidly became extended so that *all* the children of the Third World who were small and in poor health were believed to be suffering simply because their diets were deficient in protein.

In contrast to the reception of Lind's ideas about the cause of scurvy, the protein theory was eagerly embraced because it seemed to explain a lot of observations on both humans and animals. It was also attractive in other ways. Industrialised agriculture could produce protein-rich crops such as soy beans and protein-rich 'waste' products such as the residues after oil has been extracted from seeds like cotton. In addition, there were increasing surpluses and wastes from the meat, dairy and fish production industries of the industrialised countries. Finally, in those days of cheap mineral oil, there was even a prospect that yeasts or bacteria could be grown in bulk in continuous fermenters, using petroleum as a substrate, to form a cheap source of protein. Better still, since these protein concentrates could be added at low cost to existing staple foods, in the same way that vitamins and minerals are added to bread and breakfast foods in rich countries, there would be no need to wait for land or income to be redistributed. The poor could be cured of the physical symptoms of their poverty, without having first to make them richer.

The 'fiasco' came when, just as Kuhn describes such revolutions, contrary evidence built up to the point where more people rejected the theory than supported it. Further studies throughout the 1960s and early 1970s seemed to show two things: first, that kwashiorkor was not only caused by diets low in protein, and second, that the test animals (rats) used to measure the quality of the protein in the diets of poor countries did not have the same protein requirements as children. New committees of different 'experts' had in the meantime lowered the protein requirement figures appropriate for humans, so that by these new criteria most diets seemed to be adequate. Finally, the 'cure' did not seem to work: fortifying diets with additional protein either did not improve health and growth, or else children given extra dietary energy in the form of carbohydrates, and provided with better medical services, improved just as much.

There is still no agreement about what *does* cause kwashiorkor, although there are plenty of theories, including: psychological deprivation; the measles virus; dietary deficiencies of zinc or of essential fatty acids; and, most recently, toxic substances in foods produced by microscopic fungi. As to the causes of more widespread poor growth and health of children, you will remember from the discussion earlier in this chapter that the most recent view is that the primary cause may have as much to do with infectious disease in early life, as with diet.

Besides giving us a memorable example of a paradigm switch, this episode in the history of the growth of knowledge about human nutrition was an important demonstration of the way established power groups of professional scientist can determine—for a while at least—not only which ideas should be taken as the basis for policy, but also the priorities for ongoing research. From the beginning of the protein theory to its final abandonment—a period of some 15 to 20 years—a substantial diversion of resources for research and development took place. The beneficiaries were nutritionists, food scientists and plant breeders, rather than the people of the Third World.

In the field of international nutrition at least, the episode did have some lasting effect. Over the years, the reports of committees of experts on nutritional require-ments have steadily become longer and more packed with technical details about the scientific basis of the recommended values. However, since the protein fiasco, they have also become progressively more circumspect about what use can be made of them. Primarily, they seem to be telling us about the *minimum* quantities of energy and nutrients that groups of people are *likely* to be eating, *if they are healthy*. But they cannot with much confidence be used for determining to what extent exist-ing poor health in a population is the result of insufficient quantity or quality of food supply. Never again, it seems, is the world going to be switched from apparent adequacy to widespread malnutrition from lack of pro-tein or any other nutrient and back again, simply at the stroke of a pen in the report of a technical committee. The 'new' paradigm regards the problem of disease in human populations as inherently complex, variable and circum-stantial, and not likely to be solved simply by more accurate research on nutrient requirement levels.

Diet and health in the First World

Given this history of change and uncertainty about the role of food as a determinant of health, what confidence can we have that any of the ideas now current about eating and health are a valid basis for policy in the United Kingdom and other industrial countries? Are we likely to see a 'great fat fiasco'? Is there just something intrinsically difficult about human nutrition as a subject for research, so that we cannot expect anything other than constant changes of 'fashion'?

We have to remember that, although the human nutritionist can draw general conclusions about the nature of some fundamental processes from studies on other animals, he or she is working with a species which is inherently much more difficult to research.

☐ Can you suggest some reasons why this is so?

■ Humans are:

1   very slow growing: a farmer, faced with a piglet growing at the rate of a human baby, would very quickly dispose of it as a runt;

2   very long-lived: the pig goes to the slaughter house less than a year old (but already weighing more than an adult man);

3   very variable and unpredictable: humans are exposed intermittently to a large variety of physical and biological stresses, and because of their wide-ranging patterns of behaviour, some individuals have levels of food consumption twice as high as others of the same age, sex and size;

4   because of ethical or financial considerations, humans are not available for 'experiments' or for diet intervention trials except to a limited extent, and then only under conditions differing from those of normal life.

In addition to being difficult subjects to deal with, there is no single objective measurement of human nutrition, such as money output/money input, which can be max-imised. As a 1991 Department of Health Manual on Dietary Reference Values admits, 'there *is* no definition of optimum health'. Instead, there is a rather broad concern to identify the consequences for health or disease of deficiencies or surpluses of any of the thousands of single chemical entities or complex substances which occur in human diets. The overall objective of this venture is to extend the length and 'quality' of life.

For each individual human, the extent of the *interac-tions* between nutrients, between diet and infectious dis-eases and between diet and the genetic constitution may be so great that there simply is no ideal diet that would give the best possible outcome, regardless of circum-stances. It is even less likely that we shall ever be able to describe the perfect average diet for a *population*.

The consequences of all this are disappointing for some of the questions which excite the most popular interest—namely how can we avoid obesity, degenerative disease and premature death? In practice, most of the evidence about these questions still comes from epidemiological studies, which can by their nature only reveal *associations* between what we eat and our state of health.

The costs and benefits of prudent eating

There is no particular reason to suppose that today's paradigms will be much more resistant to attack than yesterday's. Indeed, since the growth of knowledge owes more to successful disproof of false ideas than to attempts to 'verify' the ones we happen to find attractive, we hope you will go away after reading this book and set about trying to prove us wrong. However, we need to describe those theories which are current among nutritionists and the health professions, in order to see the basis of present policy proposals and speculate about what might become options in the future.

Energy excess

First, what are believed to be the penalties of excess? The most obvious perhaps, is simply an excess of everything, i.e. too much food energy, i.e. **energy excess**. It is said that, at any one time, some 25 per cent of the United Kingdom population is trying some way of losing weight. Even if the motivation of many of these weight-conscious people is more related to cosmetic or psychological considerations than to any specific health problem, this is still a high level of popular concern. Moreover, some 45 per cent of all males and 36 per cent of females in the United Kingdom population are **obese**, i.e. above the upper levels of weight (taking account of their height) considered to be desirable by the Royal College of Physicians. This means that they *might* benefit from losing some weight, but probably need careful individual assessment and counselling to determine whether any practical benefit is likely. Also, there is an upwards trend in the proportion of theoretically overweight people in the United Kingdom population.

There is good evidence that people above the Royal College of Physicians definition suffer not only psychological trauma and social discrimination, but also from considerably increased risk of illness and death from a number of causes: heart disease, stroke, breast cancer, arthritis, diabetes and others. There is also evidence for some at least of these conditions that reaching *and sustaining* a lower weight reduces that risk. The problem lies in the word 'sustaining'.

As you might guess from the huge volume of both lay and professional writing on the subject, and the diverse nature of the methods used—from 'dieting', through surgery, wiring-up of jaws, to total starvation—weight loss can be and quite often is accomplished. Very often it is accomplished repeatedly by the same people: the difficulty lies in finding a way of *staying* lighter for life, or at least for a useful length of time. In practice, the success rate is poor. If we take as a reasonable criterion of a successful course of treatment an initial weight reduction followed by five years of stable and reduced weight, then, according to the clinical psychologist Kenneth Brownell, a person has a better change of being cured of most forms of cancer, than of obesity (Brownell, 1982). Simply suggesting to people that they should diet in order to avoid becoming overweight, or change to another diet if they do, is of little avail.

There is no convincing evidence that some kinds of food are *intrinsically* more 'fattening' than others, only that some—like fats and alcohol—pack a lot of calories into a small volume. Experiments have shown that subjects confronted with diets in which the energy was 'diluted' with water, indigestible gels or fibre, initially ate less than when the energy was more concentrated, even if they were not consciously aware of the difference. However, after a time they compensated, gradually increasing their intake of the diluted diet to the point where energy intake returned to its initial level. This means that low fat diets, or foods in which the energy has been diluted in some way, may be helpful in reducing weight, but like other treatments offer no special advantage in the long term.

As to the causes of obesity, it *has* to be the case that a person who is obese got that way because *at some time* in their development they had a greater excess of energy intake above expenditure than a non-obese person of the same age. However, it does not follow that they will go on continuously eating more than they expend when they have reached adulthood. Just as in the case of undernutrition we found it important to distinguish between the state of 'being small' and the process of 'becoming small', so it may be more helpful to study how some children get to be progressively more overweight for their age than others, than to study adults who are already obese.

One team of nutritionists from London University, which conducted serial measurements starting from the age of four years and repeated through adolescence, obtained some interesting results. First of all, the obese child's family is important. As compared to children whose parents are of average weight, children of obese parents are usually taller and heavier at all ages. They reach sexual maturity at an earlier age and often go on to become obese adults (Griffiths *et al*, 1990).

The chances of obesity happening are greatest if both parents are obese, somewhat less if only the mother, less still if only the father is. This looks very much like an inherited trait and although we cannot rule out some effect of the passing on of eating behaviour from parents to child, it has also been shown that identical twins, separated very soon after birth and reared apart, remain closely similar in weight and height throughout subsequent life. At least 25 per cent and perhaps as much as 80 per cent of the determinants of obesity are either genetic, or in some other way transmissible from parents at a very early age. A second and very important finding is that young children of obese parents eat *fewer* calories than those of average weight parents, despite their faster growth rate.

☐ How do you think they manage to do this?

■ Although they take in less energy, they also expend an even lower amount. In particular, they use less energy when they are at rest (the maintenance component of requirements in Table 11.2). It is the *difference* between intake and expenditure that decides the amount stored in the body, not the absolute amounts consumed.

It seems that what distinguishes obese people is that they are more *efficient* than the average person at storing energy. This might explain why the genes that predispose to obesity are so common in the population, despite the disadvantages to health. In the more distant past it could have been much more important—in order to cope with the uncertainties of hunting and scavenging—to have been able to store fat efficiently in times of food surplus and thus perhaps to survive a later hungry period.

As well as the difficulties of prevention or cure, there are costs involved in trying to deal with obesity by general advice to the public on diet and lifestyle. First, all we really know is that there are large numbers of people who are above a certain desirable *weight* for their height. Measuring body fat as such is too difficult and expensive outside the laboratory. But using this 'weight for height' definition means that, for example, a heavily muscled manual worker or a weightlifter might be classified as obese. Second, not all fat people will benefit to the same extent from slimming—it depends on *where* the fat is deposited. Abdominal fat seems to be associated with more of a health risk than peripheral fat. This means that quite a large proportion of overweight people would experience few health benefits even if they sustained a reduced weight. Most people would need access to

specialist help to find out whether or not they would be likely gainers. However, many overweight people do suffer considerably from the psychological stress which results from living in a society which has been encouraged to stigmatise fatness or heaviness not only as unhealthy, but as conditions which could perfectly well be avoided simply by less self-indulgence. Dieting can have beneficial psychological effects, but conversely there is also a growing problem of people suffering from weight obsession, obesity phobia and eating disorders such as anorexia nervosa.

Sugar

Obviously, anything such as sugar which has been consumed in such dramatically increasing amounts over the past 150 years is a prime suspect as a cause of any ills that have also seemed to be increasing over the same time. Nutritionists distinguish between 'intrinsic' and 'extrinsic' sugars: intrinsic sugars occur as part of the natural cellular structure of animal or plant tissues, whereas the extrinsic part comes as free sugar, which has been extracted from natural sources. Not surprisingly, extrinsic sugar has been accused of either initiating or exacerbating obesity, heart disease, diabetes and, of course, tooth decay. At the very least, its critics describe it as a source of 'empty' calories, meaning that apart from energy it brings nothing else with it to the diet in the way of nutrients or fibre.

Of all of these accusations, only that relating to tooth decay has seriously 'stuck'. Even then, the role of extrinsic sugar is once again better understood as a facilitator of a complex decay process, in which several other factors are involved—some environmental, but also behavioural. Tooth decay is caused by the action of bacteria in the mouth, which produce acid (hence dissolving away the enamel layer) and mineral deposits known as plaque, which gets in the way of the saliva that would otherwise protect the teeth. All forms of sugar in the diet are equally potent stimulators of this process. However, the critical factor is probably the length of time that sugar stays in the mouth. Obviously, this will tend to increase with greater intake, but just as (if not more) important, is the timing and the form in which it is eaten. Sweets between meals and sweetened drinks (which often also contain acids) are the main culprits, rather than total daily sugar intake per se. Even then, the impact is moderated by behaviour: oral hygiene, whether by direct cleaning, or subsequently eating other foods or taking drinks of the kinds which clean the mouth; and the application of fluoride, either on an individual or a community basis through water fluoridation.

Salt

There is a minimum physiological requirement for salt, but this appears to be no more than about 4 grams per adult per day. On average, an adult in the United Kingdom consumes about three times this amount per day. Salt is believed by many to be a prime candidate for causing hypertension (high blood pressure), specifically of the kind that increases with age and has no other obvious physical cause. Reducing salt intake does lower blood pressure in those people who already suffer from hypertension. However, in people whose blood pressure is within the normal range, only those who have a genetic sensitivity to salt respond in this way—about 10 per cent of the population. In addition, useful reductions of blood pressure require salt intakes to be reduced to less than one third of the population average (of about 12 grams per day), which, for many people is both inconvenient, because of the need to avoid very many of the common processed foods—and unpleasant.

Fat

Fat is certainly the most notorious example of a diet component which we are advised to avoid, particularly the kinds of fat which occur in meat, eggs and milk (the saturated fats, so called because of their low ability to combine with other molecules). Besides coronary heart disease (CHD), high levels of fat intake are suspected of causing cancers of the breast, colon and prostate, as well as having some association with overweight and hypertension. In all these cases, the suspicions started with the discovery of associations. Taking data from seven countries, the American epidemiologist Ancel Keys showed in 1980 that those with the highest average fat content in the national food supply were also the countries that experienced the highest mortality from CHD.

Figure 11.3a shows a scatter diagram of these data on CHD and fat content, and Figure 11.3b shows a similar plot for breast cancer.

However, attempts to conduct similar analyses between groups of people *within* single countries (for example, by grouping people by region, or by social class) have generally failed to show significant associations between degenerative diseases and fat intake.

□ Why do you suppose this is?

■ This may simply reflect the fact that the range of variation of fat intakes between such groups is usually a good deal smaller than that between the averages for different countries.

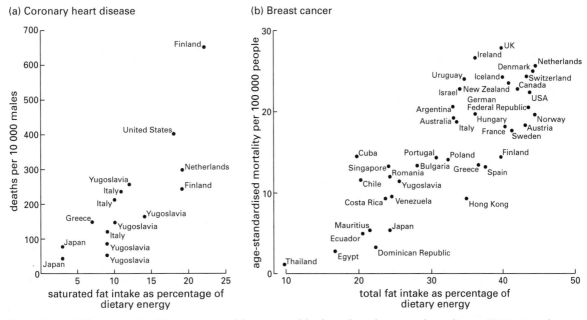

(a) Coronary heart disease

(b) Breast cancer

Figure 11.3 *(a) The association between saturated fat content of food supply and coronary heart disease (CHD). More than one data point is shown for some countries because data from more than one year has been used to construct this diagram. (b) The association between total food supply fat content and breast cancer. (Data from WHO, 1990,* Diet, Nutrition, and the Prevention of Chronic Diseases, *Report of a WHO Study Group, WHO Technical Report Series, No. 797, Geneva)*

Many of the industrial countries have collected longitudinal data which show a decline over time of CHD rates, paralleled (usually *after* a time-lag of ten years or more), by falling consumption of saturated fats. In the United Kingdom also, deaths of males from CHD have begun to decline quite rapidly, closely paralleling the decline in smoking, but with little evidence of diet change.

Cholesterol, a fatty component of all animal cells and hence of a good many foods, used to be regarded as the most dangerous of all dietary constituents. It is true that high concentrations of cholesterol in the blood of an individual are an indication of high risk of CHD: in fact measuring blood cholesterol is one of the best ways of predicting the likelihood of a person getting heart disease. This relationship also holds good at the national level. However, cholesterol in the *diet* is not now considered to be particularly important as a cause of CHD. This is because there is very little relationship between the amount of cholesterol a person eats and the level of cholesterol in the blood[2] for most of the population (although a minority show sensitivity to dietary cholesterol intake, as a result of their genetic constition).

Obviously, what started out as a fairly straightforward suggestion, that eating fats of animal origin is a specific cause of illness (rather like the idea that all malnutrition in Third World children is caused by lack of protein in their diets), seems to be getting more qualified and more complicated with further research. Partly, this is because epidemiological studies of any kind can only show *associations* : by themselves, they cannot identify *causes*. All that can be said so far is that various **risk factors** for CHD have been identified, i.e. factors that seem to be associated with different levels of heart disease in different countries.

☐ Can you think of some factors other than animal fat intake, which are said to be associated with CHD?

■ Smoking, excessive alcohol, levels in body tissues of free radicals (not a political party, but substances having a tendency to promote oxidation), low exercise levels, overweight, psychological stress, genetic susceptibility, and sex (in all populations, men seem to be much more at risk than women) have all been implicated as risk factors. More recently, early childhood diseases and (as you saw in Chapter 10) factors in infancy and even in fetal life have also attracted attention. Of all these, smoking in particular is

[2]This story is considered in more detail in *Dilemmas in Health Care* (Open University Press, 1993), Chapter 10.

widely regarded as having by far the greatest potential effect on the chances of dying from CHD.

Apart from the great range of possibilities, several things are interesting about this list. First, many of the risk factors *are associated with each other*. This could happen in different ways. For example, different risk factors such as smoking, high alcohol consumption and eating meat and cream might be *independent* causes of risk, but tend in practice to be associated statistically because all of them are related to something else—like income, or because they are all members of a set of behavioural traits in the culture or popular lifestyle of a country or a geographic region. Alternatively, some risk factors might turn out to be linked by a causal sequence—perhaps being overweight gives rise to hypertension, which is associated with high blood cholesterol, which is associated with CHD.

Finally, several factors might combine to have a more powerful effect on risk levels when they operate together, than singly: they might be 'synergistic' and augment each other. For example, it seems that with the exception of Japan (whose epidemiology always seems to stand on its own), all the countries in the lower half of the CHD scale are in the Mediterranean region. This is why many epidemiologists now seem to be interested in 'Mediterranean-type' diets. Characteristically, these include less animal fat, but more vegetable oil (especially olive oil), more fresh fruit, and more vegetables and wine than the United Kingdom diet. It might be wise however, before deciding to follow this prescription, to notice that there are also a good many cultural and climatic factors operating as well as diet. A comprehensive switch to a Mediterranean lifestyle might help the British population to postpone death from CHD but, as you will see shortly, it might simply make us die from something else instead.

In order to try to pin down the extent to which dietary fat is an independent *cause* of CHD, there have been a number of large-scale *intervention trials* in which people have been persuaded to reduce their intakes of total fat and especially of saturated fat for long periods (5–7 years). In all cases, there has been some reduction in coronary death rates. But reducing total fat intake has been worthwhile only when the subjects were pre-selected as being at high risk: for example, when they already had blood levels of cholesterol at the top end of the range (remember, that high cholesterol concentration in the blood is a reliable indication that a person is at risk). Intervention trials using *normal* members of the population have found either that reduced rates of death from CHD were offset by increased deaths from other causes such as cancer (or suicide!), so that there was no overall improvement in survival, or that the untreated control group improved to the same extent as those who changed their eating and smoking habits.

It has been a recurrent theme throughout this chapter that the health experience of adults may be influenced by adverse events or circumstances when they were very young—perhaps even while they were still in the uterus. This theme also occurred in Chapter 10, when we looked at the evidence for health 'programming'. This theory is still vigorously contested but, as the *British Medical Journal* remarked in an editorial in 1991, it is gaining ground and has all the hallmarks of a 'paradigm shift' in process.

☐ If this theory is correct, what would you expect to see happening to death rates from CHD over time?

■ They should decline, simply because of the progressive improvements in the health in early childhood of today's middle-aged people (because of better standards of living and child health care services).

Moreover, if the theory turns out to be correct, we would expect this to happen in addition to any changes due to *current* diet or to the *lifestyle* of those adults. The epidemiologists will probably still be arguing about what caused the apparent epidemic of CHD and what made it decline, long after it has done so!

Energy and physical activity

In contrast to the suggestion that some foods might be 'unhealthy', it is also said that people might gain from eating more of others, or of engaging in more exercise to 'burn off' excess calories.

Although overweight and obesity are seen to be a problem in industrial populations, there is also a theory that people are more sedentary than is good for them. This is because moderate levels of physical exercise have been shown to be a factor in reducing the risk of coronary and other circulatory diseases. There is therefore something of a paradox. At one and the same time, a large section of the population are considered to be overweight and hence feel themselves under social pressure to reduce their intakes of energy—which would reduce the national average consumption. At the same time, the 1991 report of the Committee on Medical Aspects of Food Policy, considers that, *for the population as a whole,* a higher level of physical activity would be desirable. However, if this was to be sustained in a long-term equilibrium, by implication it would entail *higher* average food intakes.

Dietary fibre

A proportion of what is left in the gut after a meal has been digested and absorbed is a mixture of carbohydrate materials, mainly coming from the walls of plant cells. This group of substances, generally known as *dietary fibre*, has over the years been credited with many health-protecting properties. Associations have been claimed between high fibre intakes and reduced incidence of heart disease, hypertension, bowel cancer, appendicitis, constipation, diverticular disease and haemorrhoids (piles).

However, the Department of Health Standing Committee on Medical Aspects of Food Policy said in 1991 about fibre (they call it 'non-starch polysaccharides', or NSP), that the methodological problems of most of the epidemiological studies are such 'that it is not currently possible to identify NSP as a major dietary factor in the aetiology of these diseases'. The committee also commented that '…NSP is not the major dietary determinant of blood lipid patterns', that is, cholesterol levels (although they do also suggest there may be something other than fibre which is good about oats and beans in this respect).

This is another nice example of an apparently simple idea which turns out to be complex. As with fat, the problem is one of multiple associations. High-fibre diets are by definition diets high in vegetables and fruit. Hence, they are nearly always also high in digestible starches and low in animal products. Like high intakes of fat, high intakes of fibre are better thought of as a *marker* of particular dietary (but therefore perhaps behavioural) patterns. The most convincing evidence of a causal role for fibre in protecting against illness is its value in reducing constipation. Both frequency and softness of stools increase with intake of fibre: but, don't forget, so does flatulence!

Alcohol

Considering their general enthusiasm for giving advice about personal behaviour, the health professions are remarkably coy about the fact that there is now quite good evidence (at least as good as that implicating fat in disease processes), that alcohol, *in moderate amounts,* exerts a protective effect against CHD and other circulatory diseases. Their problem, of course, stems from the fact that immoderate consumption results in a whole range of other health and social problems. High intakes cause liver disease, death and injury from accidents and personal violence, and have been associated with cancers of the alimentary tract. This is a case of what is called a 'J-shaped' risk relationship, namely one in which, starting from zero intake of alcohol, risks to health seem first to decline, passing through a minimum somewhere between 1 and 3 units[3] per day, and then increase again, rising steeply at more elevated levels of consumption. Taking all of this into account in trying to give advice on lifestyle presents formidable problems of communication.

Food and health policy: present and future

So far in this chapter, we have alternated between the more narrowly focused issues of how diet affects the health of individuals and broader concerns about the social, economic, resource and environmental factors which ultimately determine food entitlement. In addition, we have viewed these on a time-scale which includes individual lifespans as well as the prospects for global sustainability. In this last section, we need to try to integrate these aspects.

Present policy

First of all, in reviewing current opinions about the potential health benefits of following a 'prudent' diet, you have seen that initial observations that illness seemed to be associated with the intake of a number of the normal constituents of diets have, after more research, often given way to a more complex picture. Most degenerative diseases are the outcome of multiple causes—many of which are only indirectly related to diet and some of which are dependent on the constitution of the individual concerned. 'Constitution' is used here to mean partly the genetic endowment, but also characteristics engendered by events in the early life history of the person concerned. For example, variations in individual constitution determine the degree of sensitivity of response of blood pressure to reduced salt intake; the responsiveness of blood cholesterol levels to a diet with less saturated fat; and the extent to which the health risks of obesity are reduced by weight loss. Because of these interactions, the effectiveness of dietary prescriptions depends to some degree on *who* is following the advice and on their willingness to consider not just one, but probably a whole range of adjustments of consumption and of general lifestyle.

Second, implications of this for the *implementation* of food policy are quite profound. Until recently, dietary change was considered to be a promising area in which *mass control measures* (i.e. measures applied across the board to whole populations) to modify behaviour might lead to significant gains in the prevention of disease. Since the measures concerned would largely rely on

communication and persuasion, these would, it was believed, have the merit of cheapness, in comparison with the costs of long-term care or premature death.

Since dietary intakes vary widely between people, any attempt to persuade an entire population to eat less of something would, if successful, result in greater health benefits only for some—those whose previous intakes were highest. The proponents of mass control have argued that even those whose intakes were low would receive some benefit from following the advice. Moreover, since low-risk people form the largest proportion of the population, even a small reduction of individual risk would result in a socially valuable saving of lives.

The ethical as well as the practical validity of this argument depends on the assumption that most individuals, if only they were possessed of all the 'facts', would consider that the benefits of a reduced likelihood of suffering or dying from a diet-related disease outweighed the costs (loss of pleasure, inconvenience, or economic costs, etc.) associated with a permanent change of diet. Or, that even if the cost was perceived by them to be greater than the benefits, they would still be willing to change for the sake of contributing to the *collective* benefit of a reduction in the social burden of illness.

However, there have always been disputes among members of the health professions about the effectiveness of this kind of mass intervention approach.

☐ Can you suggest an alternative basis for policy?

■ Another way would be to identify individuals whose constitution, habitual diet, and other patterns of habitual behaviour puts them at high risk. Having 'screened' them out, such people could be offered treatment or counselling appropriate to their specific needs. Everyone else would be left to their own devices.

Those who wished to persuade the United Kingdom government to make mass control the basis of its food and health policy have encountered strong resistance. In part, this has been because the 'facts' have continued to be in dispute. For example, in a report in 1983, the National Advisory Committee on Nutrition Education (NACNE) made repeated claims that the professional consensus about the causal role of dietary fat was so strong that it was unnecessary to wait for further research before implementing policies designed to bring about reduced consumption (Health Education Council, 1983). In fact, individual academics have continued to challenge publicly both the causal nature of the associations and the

[3]A unit of alcohol is the equivalent of 1 glass of wine, or a measure of spirits.

extent of the benefits likely to accrue to the average individual. For its part, government has been reluctant to endorse one particular set of scientific opinions over another. This lack of professional consensus, and the changes over time in professional dietary advice, have combined to reinforce public scepticism. According to a survey of attitudes towards diet conducted by the polling organisation MORI in 1992, although 95 per cent of the British public believed that eating healthy food was important for a healthy life, over 70 per cent thought that messages from health professionals on healthy eating were inconsistent. Over 40 per cent ignored food and diet advice and ate what they liked. (National Dairy Council, 1992)

The decade of the 1980s has also seen a fundamental shift of political ideas in virtually all the industrialised countries away from the responsibility of the state and towards individual behaviour and choice. In the 1970s, it was quite commonly assumed that governments ought to accept the responsibility of intervention, so as to regulate individual consumption on the grounds of health—if necessary through price policy. For example, in 1976 the government of Norway adopted a combination of mass education and macro-economic strategy to encourage a trend away from the consumption of dairy foods. Since the 1980s, the emphasis in most of the industrialised countries has swung even further away from detailed government economic management, public expenditure and provision, and welfare, and towards 'free-market' strategies. At the same time, social policy has placed greater emphasis on individual choice, as well as individual responsibility, for health.

The future: a speculative account

This shift of outlook is likely to have profound implications in the future for many aspects of health raised in this book. In the former USSR and other ex-communist countries, a move towards a functioning market economy, if successfully accomplished, may lead to health gains as gross industrial pollution and other health-damaging features of these societies are reduced. But it may also have detrimental health consequences if the government-promoted routes to low mortality pioneered in a number of Third World countries via concerted public action (discussed in Chapter 8) encounter increasing ideological hostility to any form of government intervention.

Some particular questions concerning food policy and dietary advice are also raised by this shift in outlook. If people living in a 'free-choice' society are to be enabled to make responsible decisions between the enjoyment of

present consumption and the likely future consequences of that for their health, what kind of information do they need to have? What should be the role of government and the health professions in meeting that need? Given that freedom of choice is to be regarded as something to be valued in its own right, provided no harm is done to others in exercising it, what principles should govern communication with consumers? Remember that dietary advice comes not only as advice from government, or other institutions, but also from commerce through promotion of products and as advocacy from the health professions.

It is evident that people need to know, through labelling, something about the content of the foods they buy. The problem is that the information has to be in a useable form. The average British family purchases more than a hundred different food items a week and chooses each of these from a wide range of alternatives, so the more detailed the description of the contents of each item, the more severe the demands made on the time and motivation of the consumer.

☐ Would such labelling be enough to enable the consumer to choose a health-promoting diet?

■ No. Each individual would also need to have a personal profile, summarising their own constitutional and behavioral risk factors, together with an evaluation of the implications these might have for food choice.

This profile might, in theory, be made available from the medical practitioners of the future as part of a system of periodic health checks or 'well-patient' clinics, so that there could be an entitlement to regular updating. Personal profiles would have to be linked in some practical way to the system of labelling of food items and this would require access to advice either from human or machine- based 'expert' systems.

Clearly, as in other areas of environmental health, prevention of diet-related diseases will require *more* rather than *less* government intervention on behalf of the consumer if it is attempted on the basis of our current rather limited understanding of causes, and is as likely to *increase* as to *reduce* the total cost of health provision.

There are, however, reasons other than those connected directly with health for expecting to see significant changes in diet over the next few decades. Health promotion is only one of a number of popular ideas and trends which are together having a cumulative impact on what people choose to eat. Many of these ideas spring from concerns which are apparently unconnected, except that in different ways they all represent a widespread feeling that our industrialised food procurement system fails to deal sensitively with the environment, or to give people a sense of integration with nature. Fears about the dangers of pollution and contamination link up with desires for more conservation-oriented production, causing continued growth of demand for 'organic' and 'whole' foods. Concern for conservation and for better animal welfare has not only brought a demand for less intensive (and more expensive) methods of production, but has given a new momentum to vegetarianism. Coincidentally, this has become much more scientifically respectable. The same research which precipitated the protein 'fiasco' of the 1960s showed not only that human needs for protein were much less than previously thought, but that there was *no* specific need for animal as opposed to vegetable protein in the diet.

Alongside these informal movements, we can already envisage the likely effect of government responses to national and global environmental issues on food prices, particularly animal products. For example, we might anticipate tighter regulations regarding the environmental impact of food production, covering animal waste disposal, the pollution of water sources, and so on. These will likely be followed by taxes on the emission of carbon dioxide and probably methane, as part of international agreements to contain the build-up of 'greenhouse' gases. Alongside these developments, the large subsidies paid to farmers in industrialised countries which were noted in Chapter 8 are likely to come under increasing pressure. And many Third World countries will be arguing for the realisation in practice of the free trade in goods and services, and not least in foodstuffs, which the industrialised countries proclaim in theory.

The effects of these developments on aggregate demand, whether through preference or price, are uncertain, but there may be some interesting prospects of convergence. The 'prudent' diet described in this chapter is moving in the same direction as that selected by those who favour 'whole foods' or one of the many degrees of vegetarianism; it is also convergent with the diet of all but the poorest people in many parts of the Third World. Perhaps the important question for nutritional science to answer is not so much 'what is the composition of a diet which is optimal for health?' but rather, 'what will be the health implications of a diet which is sustainable around the globe in the long run, assuming also an acceptable degree of equity?'

And perhaps this prompts a concluding question for all of us: what will be the health implications of some way of *living* which is sustainable around the globe in the long run, assuming an acceptable degree of equity? For the prevailing patterns of world health and disease as set out in this book would be regarded by few people as acceptably equitable, while increasingly urgent questions of equity and sustainability are raised by the present trajectory of world population growth and development.

OBJECTIVES FOR CHAPTER 11

When you have studied this chapter, you should be able to:

11.1 Make a critical assessment of the evidence for the role of food availability and food consumption in accounting for the differences in health between the industrialised and Third World countries.

11.2 Describe how the growth of children and the body size of adults are determined by the interaction of the effects of nutrition and infectious diseases.

11.3 Describe the main changes that have taken place during the past century in the patterns of food entitlement and consumption of typical households in the United Kingdom.

11.4 Discuss the changes that have taken place in the relationship between human work inputs and the energy outputs of food production systems, from prehistoric times to the present day, and identify the significance of these changes for the future sustainability of global food supplies.

11.5 Describe the problems involved in using (i) epidemiological techniques, and (ii) laboratory measurements, to find the relative importance of nutrition, genetic constitution and other environmental factors in determining human health.

11.6 Discuss the implications for the state and for the individual consumer, of different proposals for implementing a food and health policy.

QUESTIONS FOR CHAPTER 11

Question 1 (*Objective 11.1*)

What kind of evidence would be needed to show that the health of a population was limited by its supply of food?

Question 2 (*Objective 11.2*)

Contrast the significance for food and health policies in a developing country, of (a) small average stature of adults, (b) interrupted growth of children of less than two years.

Question 3 (*Objective 11.3*)

If a typical family of today were transported back two hundred years in time to become agricultural workers, in what ways would their energy consumption and energy output change?

Question 4 (*Objective 11.4*)

How has the increased productivity of farm workers been achieved during the past century? What kind of changes in the food systems of the industrial countries will be needed in future, to limit their adverse effects on the environment?

Question 5 (*Objective 11.5*)

Why is it so difficult to interpret 'standardised' laboratory tests on human subjects so as to understand more about how the food we eat determines our health?

Question 6 (*Objective 11.6*)

Why do some people object to the proposal that policies should be designed to change the diet of the entire population of the United Kingdom?

References and
further reading

References

Abdullah, M. and Wheeler, E. (1985) Seasonal variations and the intrahousehold distribution of food in a Bangladeshi village, *American Journal of Clinical Nutrition*, **41**, pp. 1305–13.

Bairoch, P. (1982) International industrialization levels from 1750 to 1980, *Journal of European Economic History*, **11** (2), pp. 269–333.

Barker, D. J. P., Osmond, C., Golding, J. *et al.* (1989) Growth in utero, blood pressure in childhood and adult life, and mortality from cardiovascular disease, *British Medical Journal*, **298**, pp. 564–7.

Bayliss-Smith, T. P. (1982) *The Ecology of Agricultural Systems*, Cambridge University Press, Cambridge.

Beaton, G. H. (1989) Small but healthy? Are we asking the right question? *Human Organisation*, **48** (1), pp. 31–7.

Bebbington, A. C. (1991) The expectation of life without disability in England and Wales: 1976–88, *Population Trends*, **66** (Winter), pp. 26–9.

Behm, H. (1979) Socioeconomic determinants of mortality in Latin America, *Proceedings of the Meeting on Socioeconomic Determinants and the Consequences of Mortality*, UN/WHO, Mexico.

Benjamin, B. (1989) Review article: Demographic aspects of ageing, *Annals of Human Biology*, **16** (3), pp. 185–235.

Berthoud, R. (1986) *Selective Social Security*, Policy Studies Institute, London.

Braudel, F. (1981) *The Structures of Everyday Life: the Limits of the Possible*, Collins, London.

Brownell, K. D. (1982) Obesity: understanding and treating a serious, prevalent and refractory disorder, *Journal of Consultant Clinical Psychology*, **50**, pp. 820–40.

Burnett, J. (1966) *Plenty and Want*, Nelson, London.

Caldwell, J. C. (1986) Routes to low mortality in poor countries, *Population and Development Review*, **12** (2), pp.171–220.

Central Statistical Office (1989) *Regional Trends No. 24*, HMSO, London.

Central Statistical Office (1991) *Regional Trends No. 26*, HMSO, London.

Central Statistical Office (1992) *Family Spending: a Report on the 1990 Family Expenditure Survey*, HMSO, London.

Central Statistical Office, Zimbabwe (1990) *Zimbabwe Demographic and Health Survey Report*, CSO, Harare.

Centre for Urban Studies, Dhaka (1989) *Report of the Centre for Urban Studies*, University of Dhaka, Dhaka.

Chambers, I. D. (1972) *Population, Economy and Society in Pre-industrial England*, Oxford University Press, Oxford.

Chen, L. C. (1986) Primary health care in developing countries: overcoming operational, technical and social barriers, *Lancet*, **ii**, pp. 1260–5.

Cipolla, C. (1974) *The Economic History of World Population*, 6th revised edn, Pelican, London.

Coale, A. J. (1991) Excess female mortality and the balance of the sexes in the population: an estimate of the number of 'missing females', *Population and Development Review*, **17** (3), pp. 514–24.

Cobbett, W. (1823) *Cottage Economy*, reprinted in 1974 by Landsman's Bookshop, Bromyard, Herefordshire.

Cobbett, W. (1830) *Rural Rides*, reprinted in 1967 by Penguin English Library, Penguin, London.

Crimmins, E. M., Saito, Y. and Ingegneri, D. (1989) Changes in life expectancy and disability-free life expectancy in the United States, *Population and Development Review*, **15**, pp. 235–67.

Davies, J. M. (1982) The prevention of industrial cancer, in Alderson, M. R. (ed.), *The Prevention of Cancer*, Edward Arnold, London.

Dawkins, R. (1976) *The Selfish Gene*, Oxford University Press, New York.

Department of the Environment (1988) *English House Condition Survey 1986*, HMSO, London.

Department of Health and Social Security (1980), *Inequalities in Health*, Report of a Working Group (the 'Black Report'), DHSS, London.

Diamond, J. (1991) *The Rise and Fall of the Third Chimpanzee*, Vintage, London.

Drèze, J. and Sen, A. (1989) *Hunger and Public Action*, Clarendon Press, Oxford.

Dubos, R. (1979) *Mirage of Health*, Harper and Row, New York.

Ehrlich, P., Ehrlich, A. and Holdren, J. (1970) *Ecoscience: Population, Resources and Environment*, Freeman, New York.

Flinn, M. W. (1965) *An Economic and Social History of Britain 1066–1939*, Macmillan, London.

Food and Agriculture Organisation (1991) *The State of Food and Agriculture 1990*, FAO, Rome.

Forbes, T. R. (1979) By what disease or casualty: the changing face of death in London, in Webster, C. (ed.) *Health, Medicine and Mortality in the Sixteenth Century*, Cambridge University Press, Cambridge.

Fox, J. and Adelstein, A. M. (1978) Occupational mortality: work or way of life? *Journal of Epidemiology and Community Health*, **33**, pp. 73–8.

Fox, J. and Goldblatt, P. (1982) *OPCS Longitudinal Study, 1971–5, Socio-Demographic Mortality Differentials*, Series LS, No. 1, HMSO, London.

Fox, J., Goldblatt, P. and Jones, D. (1990) Social class mortality differentials: artifact, selection or life circumstances? in OPCS (1990) *Longitudinal Study: Mortality and Social Organisation*, HMSO, London, pp. 99–108.

Frenk, J., Bobadilla, J. L. and Stern, C. (1991) Elements for a theory of the health transition, *Health Transition Review*, **1** (1), pp. 21–38.

Fries, J. F. (1989) Compression of morbidity: near or far? *Milbank Quarterly*, **67**, pp. 208–32.

Fry, J. (1983) *Common Diseases*, 3rd edn, M.T.P. Press, Lancaster.

Gardner, M. J., Snee, M. P., Hall, A. J. *et al.* (1990) Results of case-control study of leukaemia and lymphoma among young people near Sellafield nuclear plant in West Cumbria, *British Medical Journal*, **300** (6722), pp. 423–9.

Ghana Health Assessment Project Team (1981) A quantitative method of assessing the health impact of different diseases in less developed countries, *International Journal of Epidemiology*, **10** (1), pp. 73–80.

Gillespie, S. and McNeil, G. (1992) *Food, Health and Survival*, Oxford University Press, London.

Goldblatt, P. (1989) Mortality by social class, 1971–85, *Population Trends*, **56** (Summer), pp. 6–15.

Goldblatt, P. (1990) Mortality and alternative social classifications, in OPCS (1990) *1971–1981 Longitudinal Study: Mortality and Social Organisation*, HMSO, London, pp. 163–92.

Griffiths, M., Payne, P. R., Stunkard, A. K., Rivers, J. P. W. and Cox, M. (1990) Metabolic rate and physical development in children at risk of obesity, *Lancet*, **ii**, pp. 76–8.

Halstead, S. B., Walsh, J. A. and Warren, K. S. (1985) *Good Health at Low Cost: Proceedings of a Conference held at the Bellagio Center, Bellagio, Italy*, 29 April–2 May 1985, Rockefeller Foundation, New York.

Harrison, P. (1979) *Inside the Third World*, Penguin, London.

Hartmann, B. and Boyce, J. K. (1983) *A Quiet Violence*, Zed Press, London.

Health and Safety Commission (1991) *Annual Report 1989/90*, HMSO, London.

Health Education Council (1983) *Report of the National Advisory Committee on Nutrition Education (NACNE)*, HEC, London.

HMSO (1989) *Health and Personal Social Services Statistics for England, 1989*, HMSO, London.

HMSO (1992) *Social Trends 22:1991*, HMSO, London.

Hobsbawm, E. (1969) *Industry and Empire*, Weidenfeld and Nicolson, London.

Institute of Nutrition, Dhaka (1971 and 1981) *Bangladesh National Nutrition Surveys*, Institute of Nutrition, Dhaka.

James, W. P. T. and Schofield, C. (1990) *Human Energy Requirements: a Manual for Planners and Nutritionists*, Oxford Medical Publications, Oxford.

Johnson, P. and Webb, S. (1990) *Poverty in Official Statistics: Two Reports*, Institute for Fiscal Studies Commentary No. 24, IFS, London.

Johnson, P. and Webb, S. (1991) *UK Poverty Statistics: a Comparative Study*, IFS Commentary No. 27, IFS, London.

Jones, D. R. (1987) Heart disease mortality following widowhood: some results from the OPCS Longitudinal Study, *Journal of Psychosomatic Research*, **31** (3), pp. 325–33.

Kelly, A. C. (1988) Economic consequences of population change in the Third World, *Journal of Economic Literature*, **XXVI**, pp. 1685–728.

Keys, A. (1980) *Seven Countries: a Multivariate Analysis of Death and Coronary Heart Disease*, Harvard University Press, London.

Kinnersley, P. (1974) *The Hazards of Work: How to Fight Them*, Pluto Press, London.

Kreitman, N., Carstairs, V. and Duffy, J. (1991) Association of age and social class with suicide among men in Great Britain, *Journal of Epidemiology and Community Health*, **45** (3), pp. 195–202.

Kuhn, T. S. (1970) *The Structure of Scientific Revolutions*, University of Chicago Press, Chicago.

Laslett, P. (1971) *The World We Have Lost*, 2nd edn, Methuen, London.

Littlewood, R. and Lipsedge, M. (1982) *Aliens and Alienists: Ethnic Minorities and The Psychiatrist*, Penguin, Harmondsworth.

Lopez, A. D. (1993) Causes of death in the industrialized and the developing countries: estimates for 1985, in Jamison, D. T. and Mosley, H. (eds) *Disease Control Priorities in Developing Countries*, Oxford University Press, New York.

Malcolm, L. A. (1974) Ecological factors relating to child growth and nutritional status, in Roche, A. F. and Falkner, F. (eds) *Nutrition and Malnutrition*, Plenum, New York.

Malthus, T. R. (1798) *An Essay on the Principles of Population*, reprinted in 1970 by Penguin, London.

Marmot, M. G. (1986) Social inequalities in mortality: the social environment, in Wilkinson, R. G. (ed.) *Class and Health: Research and Longitudinal Data*, Tavistock, London, pp. 21–33.

Marmot, M. G., Adelstein, A. M. and Bulusu, L. (1984) *Immigrant Mortality in England and Wales 1970–78*, OPCS Studies on Medical and Population Subjects No. 47, HMSO, London.

Marmot, M. G., Smith, G. D., Stansfield, S. *et al.* (1991) Health inequalities among British civil servants: the Whitehall II study, *Lancet*, **i**, pp.1387–93.

McEvedy, C. and Jones, R. (1978) *Atlas of World Population History*, Penguin, London.

McKeigue, P. M., Marmot, M. G., Adelstein, A. M. *et al.* (1985) Diet and risk factors for coronary heart disease in Asians in northwest London, *Lancet*, **ii**, pp. 1086–90.

McKeown, T. (1976) *The Modern Rise of Population*, Edward Arnold, London.

McNeill, W. (1976) *Plagues and People*, Basil Blackwell, Oxford.

Meyers, N. (1991) Mass extinctions, in Sharpton, V. L. and Ward, P. D. (eds) *Global Catastrophes in Earth History: Impacts, Volcanism and Mass Mortality*, Special Paper No. 247, Geological Society of America, Boulder, Colorado.

Morgan, M. (1980) Marital status, health, illness and service use, *Social Science and Medicine*, **14A**, pp. 633–43.

Moser, K., Goldblatt, P. and Jones, D. (1990) Unemployment and mortality, in *OPCS Longitudinal Study 1971–81: Mortality and Social Organisation*, HMSO, London, Chapter 5.

Moss, R., Watson, A. and Ollason, J. (1982) *Animal Population Dynamics*, Chapman & Hall, London and New York.

National Dairy Council (1992) *Food and Health: What Does Britain Think?* National Dairy Council and MORI, London.

National Food Survey Committee (1983) *Household Food Consumption and Expenditure, 1981: Annual Report of the National Food Survey Committee*, HMSO, London.

OPCS (1984) *Census 1981: Economic Activity in Great Britain*, CEN 81 EA, HMSO, London.

OPCS (1986a) *Registrar General's Decennial Supplement on Occupational Mortality 1979–83*, HMSO, London.

OPCS (1986b) *Mortality Statistics, Perinatal and Infant: Social and Biological Factors for 1984*, Series DH3, No. 17, HMSO, London.

OPCS (1988a) *Occupational Mortality:Childhood Supplement*, OPCS Series DS, No. 8, HMSO, London.

OPCS (1988b) *The Prevalence of Disability among Adults*, OPCS Report No. 1, HMSO, London.

OPCS (1989) *General Household Survey 1986*, HMSO, London.

OPCS (1990a) *General Household Survey 1988*, HMSO, London.

OPCS (1990b) *Longitudinal Study 1971–81 England and Wales: Mortality and Social Organisation*, OPCS Series LS, No. 6, HMSO, London.

OPCS (1990c) *Mortality and Geography: a Review in the mid-1980s; England and Wales*, OPCS Series DS, No. 9, HMSO, London.

OPCS (1991a) *General Household Survey 1989*, OPCS Series GHS, No. 20, HMSO, London.

OPCS (1991b) *Mortality Statistics: Cause 1990*, OPCS Series DH2, No. 17, HMSO, London.

OPCS (1991c) *National Population Projections, 1989-based*, OPCS Series PP2, No. 17, HMSO, London.

OPCS (1991d) *OPCS Monitor*, No. ss91/3, HMSO, London.

Open University (1982) D301 *Historical Data and the Social Sciences*, Units 5–8 *Historical Demography: Problems and Projects*, The Open University, Milton Keynes.

Pamuk, E. R. (1985) Social class inequality in mortality from 1921 to 1971 in England and Wales, *Population Studies*, **39**, pp. 17–31.

Parkes, C. M., Benjamin, B. and Fitzgerald, R. G. (1969) Broken heart: a statistical study of increased mortality among widowers, *British Medical Journal*, **1**, pp. 740–43.

Phelps Brown, E. H. and Hopkins, S. V. (1956) Seven centuries of the prices of consumables compared with builders' wage-rates, *Economica*, **23**, pp. 296–314.

Phillimore, P. and Morris, D. (1991) Discrepant legacies: premature mortality in two industrial towns, *Social Science and Medicine*, **33** (2), pp. 139–52.

Platt, S. D. and Dyer, J. A. (1987) Psychological correlates of unemployment among male parasuicides in Edinburgh, *British Journal of Psychiatry*, **151**, pp. 27–32.

Polo, Marco (1968 edn) *The Travels of Marco Polo*, translated by Latham, R. E., Penguin, London.

Powles, J. (1973) On the limitations of modern medicine, *Science, Medicine and Man*, **1** (1), pp. 1–30.

Pryer, J. (1990) Socioeconomic and environmental aspects of undernutrition and ill health in an urban slum in Bangladesh, PhD thesis, London.

Rappoport, R. A. (1968) *Pigs for the Ancestors: Ritual in the Ecology of a New Guinea People*, Yale University Press, New Haven.

Razzell, P. (1977) *The Conquest of Smallpox: the Impact of Inoculation on Smallpox Mortality in Eighteenth Century Britain*, Caliban Books, Firle, Sussex.

Registrar-General (various years) *Annual Abstract of Statistics*, HMSO, London.

Rockney, B. P. (1991) *Soviet Statistics since 1950*, Dartmouth, Aldershot, UK.

Royal College of General Practitioners/OPCS/DHSS (1986) *Morbidity Statistics from General Practice: Third National Study*, OPCS Series MB5, No. 1, HMSO, London.

Royal College of General Practitioners/OPCS/DHSS (1986) *Morbidity Statistics from General Practice: Third National Study: Socio-economic Analysis*, OPCS Series MB5, No. 2, HMSO, London.

Sahlins, M. (1974) *Stone Age Economics*, Tavistock, London.

Simon, J. (1981) *The Ultimate Resource*, Princeton University Press, Princeton.

Sivard, R. L. (1989) *World Military and Social Expenditures 1989*, World Priorities, Washington, DC.

Swerdlow, A. J. (1979) Incidence of malignant melanoma of the skin in England and Wales and its relationship to sunshine, *British Medical Journal*, **179**(2), pp. 1324–7.

Szreter, S. (1988) The importance of social intervention in Britain's mortality decline c. 1850–1914: a re-interpretation of the role of public health, *Social History of Medicine*, **1**, pp. 1–37.

Thompson, E. P. (1967) Time, work-discipline and industrial capitalism, *Past and Present*, **38**, pp. 56–97.

Townsend, P. (1979) *Poverty in the United Kingdom*, Penguin, London.

Townsend, P., Davidson, N. and Whitehead, M. (1990) *Inequalities in Health*, Penguin, London.

United Nations (1986) *Determinants of Mortality Change and Differentials in Developing Countries: a 5-country Case Study Project*, Population Studies No. 94, UN, New York.

United Nations (1989) *World Population Prospects 1988*, Population Studies No. 106, UN, New York.

United Nations (1990) *World Population Monitoring 1989: Special Report: the Population Situation of the Least Developed Countries*, Population Studies No. 113, UN, New York.

United Nations (1991) *United Nations Demographic Yearbook 1989*, UN, New York.

United Nations Development Programme (1991) *Human Development Report 1991*, Oxford University Press, Oxford and New York.

United Nations Development Programme (1992) *Human Development Report 1992*, Oxford University Press, Oxford and New York.

United Nations Population Division (1992) *Long-range World Population Projections: Two Centuries of Population Growth 1990–2150*, UN, New York

US Department of Health and Human Services (1991) *Health US 1990*, National Center for Health Statistics, Maryland.

Velazquez, A. and Bourges, H. (eds) (1984) *Genetic Factors in Nutrition*, Academic Press, London and New York.

Walsh, J. A. (1988) *Establishing Health Priorities in the Developing World*, United Nations Development Programme, New York.

Warr, P. (1987) *Work, Unemployment and Mental Health,* Clarendon Press, Oxford.

Webb, P. (1981) Health problems of London's Asians and Afro-Caribbeans, *Health Visitor*, **54** (April), pp. 141–7.

Westoff, C. F. (1974) The populations of the developed countries, *Scientific American*, **231** (3), September, pp. 108–22.

Wilkinson, R. G. (1986a) Socio-economic differences in mortality: interpreting the data on their size and trends, in Wilkinson, R. G. (ed.) *Class and Health: Research and Longitudinal Data*, Tavistock, London.

Wilkinson, R. G. (1986b) Income and mortality, in Wilkinson, R. G. (ed.) *Class and Health: Research and Longitudinal Data*, Tavistock, London.

Winter, J. M. (1982) The decline of mortality in Britain, 1870–1950, in Barker, T. and Drake, M. (eds) *Population and Society in Britain, 1850–1950*, Batsford Academic and Educational, London.

Woodhouse, P., Keatinge, W. R. and Coleshaw, S. R. K. (1989) Factors associated with hypothermia in patients admitted to a group of inner city hospitals, *Lancet*, **ii**, pp. 1201–4.

World Bank (1982) *World Development Report 1982,* Oxford University Press, Oxford and New York.

World Bank (1991) *World Development Report 1991,* Oxford University Press, Oxford and New York.

World Bank (1992) *Global Economic Prospects and the Developing Countries,* World Bank, Washington.

World Health Organisation (1958) *Constitution of the World Health Organisation,* WHO, Geneva.

World Health Organisation (1990) *Diet, Nutrition, and the Prevention of Chronic Diseases,* Report of a WHO Study Group, WHO Technical Report Series, No. 797, Geneva.

World Resources Institute (1992) *World Resources 1992–93,* Oxford University Press, Oxford and New York.

Wrigley, E. A. and Schofield, R. S. (1989) *The Population History of England 1541–1871: a Reconstruction*, paperback edn, Cambridge University Press, Cambridge.

Further reading

Disease Control Priorities in Developing Countries, edited by D. T. Jamison and H. Mosley (1993, Oxford University Press, New York) contains a number of very valuable contributions on world patterns of mortality and morbidity; one such is *Causes of Death in the Industrialized and the Developing Countries: Estimates for 1985*, by A. D. Lopez.

A very entertaining and accessible speculation on palaeopathology, the hunter-gatherers and the influence of our evolutionary past is *The Rise and Fall of the Third Chimpanzee*, by Jared Diamond (1992, Vintage, London). In *Changing the Face of the Earth: Culture, Environment, History* (1989, Blackwell, Oxford and Cambridge, Mass.) I. G. Simmons gives a most enjoyable and wide ranging account of how the human species, throughout its evolution, has continuously modified its own environment. *The Atlas of World Population History* by C. McEvedy and R. Jones (1978, Penguin, London) gives a compact and fairly up-to-date summary of research on the history of the world's human population by major region.

For those interested in world health, population, development and environment, the following annual publications are always worth referring to, for information, commentary, analysis and references to other research: *Human Development Report* (United Nations Development Programme, Oxford University Press, Oxford and New York) gives an overview of social and economic development around the world during the past few decades and of the prospects for the next; *World Development Report* (World Bank, Oxford University Press, Oxford and New York) concentrates more on economic development. It is an essential source of economic, demographic and health-related data, with annual features on topics such as environment, debt or population; and *World Resources: A Guide to the Global Environment* (World Resources Institute, Oxford University Press, Oxford and New York) provides a wealth of information on conditions and trends in the global environment.

An authoritative study of England's historical experience of mortality, fertility, population, famine, marriage and related topics is *The Population History of England 1541–1871: a Reconstruction* by E. A. Wrigley and R. S. Schofield (1989, Cambridge University Press, Cambridge). A scholarly, readable and well-referenced examination of causes of hunger in today's world and what could be done to eradicate it is provided by Jean Drèze and Amartya Sen in *Hunger and Public Action* (1989, Clarendon Press, Oxford).

The Nation's Health: a Strategy for the 1990s, a report from an independent multidisciplinary committee edited by Alwyn Smith and Bobbie Jackson (1988, Oxford University Press for the King's Fund, London), provides a good introduction to changes in Britain's health during the 1970s and 1980s, with an accessible and well-referenced commentary.

Nutrition, Diet and Health by Michael J. Gibney (1986, Cambridge University Press, Cambridge and New York) gives a good exposition of the broad scientific principles of the general subject of human nutrition, and is an entertaining guide to the controversies surrounding their implications for public policy. Finally, the relationship between the food needs of populations and the agricultural and energy resource bases from which food is produced is explored in *The Food Resource* by John T. Pierce (1990, Longman Scientific and Technical, Harlow).

Answers to self-assessment questions

Chapter 2

1   Your answers should be as follows.

(a)   This is a straightforward calculation. All that is required is to add the percentages of the female population in the age bands from 65 upwards. Obviously this can only be done roughly from Figure 2.2 but the percentages in the age groups above 65 add up to between 2 and 3 per cent. This is a much smaller figure than for, say, Sweden, where there is a similar percentage in the 65–69 group alone. Such profound differences have serious implications for patterns of disease, as you will see in Chapter 3, and for the organisation of health care.

(b)   From Figure 2.9:

(i)   The pyramid in Figure 2.9a indicates a population in transition from Third World to industrialised. The narrowness at the top of the pyramid suggests there has been high mortality and fertility in the past. However, the shape at the bottom suggests that child and infant mortality rates have been falling, and the indentation right at the bottom suggests a decline in fertility, perhaps as a result of a family planning programme. Taken together, these features suggest a Third World country that is industrialising fairly rapidly. The country is the Republic of Korea in 1987. The pyramid in Figure 2.9b indicates a population in which birth and death rates have been low for many years, and in which the proportion in older age-groups—particularly females—is high. These features suggest a country that has been industrialised for a long time. The country is the United Kingdom in 1988.

(ii)   Because of the relatively large number of older people in the United Kingdom we might reasonably expect the crude death rate there to be fairly high, but the age-standardised death rates to be low. This is typical for industrialised countries. In contrast, the reverse would be expected in the Republic of Korea in 1987. With its young population it would be expected to have a low crude death rate but higher age-standardised rates. In fact, the crude death figures for the United Kingdom and the Republic of

Korea were respectively 12 and 6 per 1 000. If the Republic of Korea had the same age–sex structure as the United Kingdom but the present age- and sex-specific death rates, its crude death rate would have risen to 22 per 1 000.

(c)   This would only be possible if the conditions in the country were to remain constant over the lifetime of the child. For many countries this is not so. A population pyramid is a snapshot of the population at a given time—it is based on cross-sectional data. The predictions it makes about the evolution of a system over time must be treated with great scepticism.

2   The crude death rate is useful in that it covers deaths occurring in the entire population, whereas the infant mortality rate only measures deaths in a very narrow age-band. However, because the crude death rate covers the entire population, it is influenced by the age- and sex-structure of the population; consequently it may be misleading to compare the crude death rates in two different countries if their populations do not have a similar structure. Because the infant mortality rate only covers those aged up to 1 year old, it does not have this problem. A country's infant mortality rate may not be an accurate guide to more general levels of mortality in that country, but normally it provides a rough indication.

3   The absolute difference between the IMR in India and the average for the more developed world has narrowed, from around 134 to 84 per 1 000 live births. However, the *relative* difference has widened substantially, from 3.4 times higher in 1950–55 to 6.6 times higher in 1985–90. In other words, the IMR in the more developed world has been falling at a faster rate than it has in India.

Chapter 3

1   In general, the chapter showed that the so-called 'tropical' diseases are not in fact the major cause of death in Third World countries, and that the major causes of death in the Third World also occur in industrialised countries—good examples are the respiratory diseases such as pneumonia, influenza, measles, bronchitis and whooping cough. The mortality differences between

Third World and industrialised countries arise in part from the very different impact these diseases have. In addition, the different age structure of the populations in industrialised countries, with a much higher proportion of older people, means that the degenerative diseases contribute a higher proportion of deaths there than in the Third World.

2   This method weights deaths according to the age at which they occur. Infant and childhood deaths are very much more common in Third World countries than in industrialised countries, and the 'years of potential life lost' measure is very good at emphasising this difference.

3   All of the following are important in terms of mortality in the Third World but less important in terms of disease prevalence: circulatory and degenerative diseases, malaria, measles, injuries, cancers and meningitis and tetanus. The main diseases that are more important in terms of disease prevalence than of mortality are diarrhoeas and respiratory tract infectious diseases. However, both diarrhoeas and respiratory diseases are also very important causes of death in the Third World: annual deaths from diarrhoeas are more than 4 million, while respiratory tract infectious diseases together account for almost half of Third World mortality.

4   Zoonotic diseases are shared by humans and other species and are transmissable to humans from the disease reservoir in these species, either directly or by a disease vector (an intermediary insect or animal). Examples of zoonotic diseases include brucellosis, rabies, plague, tuberculosis, gastroenteritis and typhus. Rabies is an example of a directly transmitted disease, and yellow fever is a vector-borne disease, transmitted from monkeys and rodents to a human by certain kinds of mosquito. Zoonotic diseases may be difficult to control because reservoirs of infection exist in other species and these may be hard to detect and eliminate.

5   You may have used data from Table 2.3 from the previous chapter alongside Table 3.6 in this chapter.

(a)   Expectation of life at birth in Bangladesh is greater for males (56.9 years) than for females (56 years). In the United Kingdom the females have the longer life expectancy at birth—77.6 years compared with 71.9 years for males.

(b)   In Bangladesh the male advantage persists for at least the first 30 years. However, by the age of 50 the difference is reversed and females have a longer remaining life expectancy than males. In the United Kingdom the female advantage in life expectancy at birth persists at all ages.

(c)   Bangladesh has a population structure in which the actual ratio of males to females is higher than might be predicted from the demography of African, Latin American or European countries, and this is equivalent to 1.6 million 'missing' women.

6   It is very likely that education will be linked to higher incomes, better social conditions and better access to health care, all of which will be associated to some extent with childhood mortality. However, studies have been able to demonstrate that childhood mortality and parents' education are associated, even after allowing for the effect of income. One interpretation of this is that better education encourages awareness and use of good health practice.

Chapter 4

1   Case studies are a way of combining the features of particular situations and especially sequences of events over time, into a narrative description of processes, and relating the outcome to quantitative data on populations. In this respect, qualitative material provides a complement to statistical data, which on its own may have the limitation that it reduces everything to a 'snapshot' of averages. The difficulty and potential danger of case studies is of striking a balance between the particular and the general. Descriptive material on particular situations or people or groups must be selected which conveys information about their lives and is also a valid description of processes which apply more generally.

2   There are two direct problems that relate to the transmission of disease:

(a)   The growth of resistance to chemical control, by both disease organisms and the insect vectors which form part of the cycle of transmission, as in the case of the malarial parasites and the mosquitoes that transmit infection.

(b)   The existence of reservoirs of infection outside the borders (and hence out of reach of control programmes) of Bangladesh.

The underlying problem, which makes both of these more intractable, is widespread poverty and continued population growth—in Bangladesh itself and in the neighbouring countries of the region. Increasing numbers of people are forced to leave the land and migrate to cities, where they live in situations in which the control of water-associated diseases is difficult, resources for public control are limited and people are too poor to afford private means (e.g. antimalarial drugs, mosquito nets, insecticides). Poverty and the violence that goes with it is generating increasing numbers of political and economic refugees, who carry disease across national boundaries.

For a small farming family in Bangladesh:

(a) Improved access to basic health services would have an impact on child survival (e.g. through better immunisation programmes) and this could be expected to increase the survival of girls to levels comparable with that of boys. It would also reduce the risk of maternal mortality through the provision of contraceptive services and ante- and post-natal care. Easier availability of essential drugs, especially antibiotics, would benefit all age groups and might especially reduce the risk of loss of production or employment through illness at critical times of the year.

(b) Improved food security would mean not only the ability to avoid seasonal hunger and reduce the impact of infectious diseases by improving resistance, but it would also reduce indebtedness and even perhaps allow families to build some reserves of cash or credit against the risk of natural disasters. It might make investment possible—in more education for a child perhaps.

These two kinds of improvements are not mutually exclusive, but to have any meaning, both have to be treated as investments in a future. The 'twist' to the question of course is that the food security of such households could only be improved in a sustained way by structural changes in the security of land tenure and the availability of secure employment and reasonable credit—in other words by laying the foundations of a future.

Chapter 5

1 Infectious diseases such as measles cannot remain endemic in very small and scattered populations. The Agricultural Revolution raised food production and so populations increased and agricultural areas became more densely populated. This provided the conditions under which many new types of infectious diseases could have a fairly constant presence (for example, food stores attract vermin).

2 This is a broadly accurate statement in relation to human population in total, which was probably remarkably stable over long periods with a very low growth rate. However, the 'punctuation marks' of sudden changes in death rates were very frequent: data from France indicates up to 13 general famines in the course of a century. And at the local level there may well have been substantial rise and fall.

3 Population and real wages are linked in two different ways in the Malthusian model. Changes in real wages can affect mortality rates, thus changing population size. But real-wage changes also alter *nuptiality*, and this affects

the fertility rate and thus population size. In Figure 5.3 these two different links were represented by different loops.

4 The Industrial Revolution was effecting changes in the social structure of people's lives that greatly increased the importance of coordinated routines and time-keeping. Technological change was also cheapening certain goods such as watches, making them available to a mass market. Finally, many industrial towns were accumulating sufficient wealth to erect public buildings as symbols of civic pride and opulence.

5 Many people were being forced to leave rural areas as a result of landlessness due to enclosures or unemployment, and had nowhere to go but to the cities. Also, although conditions were appalling in the cities, they may have been no better in many rural areas because of the changes the Industrial Revolution was making to the country as a whole.

Chapter 6

1 The most likely cause is autonomous infectious disease—the evidence in the chapter indicates that crises of subsistence only increased the mortality rate by three or four times, whereas the mortality crises listed in the question are six to ten times greater than the underlying mortality rate.

2 You may have thought of the following: (i) changes in definition and terminology since 1550; (ii) changes in medical knowledge and science; (iii) the lack of qualified persons to make the diagnosis (few people had access to a physician in 1550); (iv) the lack of adequate and reliable records from the sixteenth century.

3 A rise in fertility and a decline in mortality both contributed to the expansion in population between 1680 and 1850. The evidence in the chapter suggests that the rise in the birth rate contributed two and a half times as much to the increase in population as did the decline in the death rate.

4 According to Szreter, McKeown's thesis runs as follows: declines in the air-borne diseases were the main factor in reducing mortality during the nineteenth century; there is no evidence of effective public health measures to contain or combat them during this period; therefore the population must have become more resistant to them, and the most likely way this happened was by improved nutrition. However, Szreter argues that McKeown has over-emphasised the decline in air-borne diseases and under-estimated the decline in water-borne diseases during the nineteenth century. This allows him to

suggest that public health measures against water-borne disease in the nineteenth century and against air-borne diseases in the twentieth century were of great importance, and that the role of nutrition as an isolated factor is less clear than McKeown concluded.

As Figure 6.2 shows, the period from 1541 to the start of the eighteenth century was one in which birth rates and death rates both oscillated, but broadly birth rates were falling while the death rate was static or rising. This pattern does not fit precisely any of the stages of the model of demographic transition: stage 1 of the model is characterised by a high death rate and a high birth rate. However, almost by definition, models are simplifications of reality and often put erratic and irregular events to one side. And this particular model does fit the broad pattern of events in England from the eighteenth century onwards.

Chapter 7

1 In 1800 manufacturing production in the United Kingdom was only a small fraction of manufacturing production in the Third World. Even in 1850 United Kingdom production was half that in the Third World. In this sense it was not 'the workshop of the world'. However, the phrase is more accurate in conveying the notion of a great concentration of manufacturing production in one not very populous country. And, as the table shows, by 1880 the United Kingdom was producing more manufactured goods than the whole Third World, and continued to do so until the late 1950s.

2 It is true that a country's level of GNP per person is not always a reliable guide to standards of health, education or other aspects of human development. This is partly due to the fact that a nation's wealth may be unequally distributed across the population or may be directed to other policy objectives and areas of spending, such as military expenditure or industrial expansion. The Human Development Index does go some way to take account of health, education and income distribution, and so does move away from means towards ends. However, it does not take account of important issues such as civil liberties. There is in fact a broad association between the GNP and HDI measures. On a different point, some people may consider that education and health are not 'ultimate ends', but are themselves means to attaining an end, such as prosperity or security.

3 The Third World does have a much larger population than the industrialised countries: in fact over 80 per cent of the world's population are in low-income or middle-income countries. But these countries are so much poorer that their share of world GNP is very small indeed: as the text noted and Table 7.2 showed, the 60 per cent of the world's population in the poorest (low-income) countries accounts for just 5 per cent of world GNP.

4 The two most important common difficulties are:

(a) that production may go unrecorded because it is in the subsistence sector, or within the family, or is bartered or exchanged unofficially; and

(b) that in both cases the average per person is likely to disguise inequalities in distribution, so that many people may not in fact get the average or anything like it.

5 No. Sen and Drèze stress that food availability must be one of the factors that determine entitlement. They list four ways in which the two may be linked: subsistence farming can be thought of as 'direct entitlement'; entitlement is influenced by the price of food, which is influenced by food availability; food production can be a major source of employment; and a stock of available food in a public distribution system can be an important instrument to combat starvation and improve entitlement. However, their central point is that a range of other factors also influence the command over food which different sections of the population can exercise.

Chapter 8

1 It is true that population change is subject to many factors and uncertainties, some of which are poorly understood. And projections frequently have turned out to be inaccurate and have had to be revised substantially. However, most population projections include a range of different assumptions (for example, high, middle or low projections given different rates of fertility decline). Moreover, populations have a fair degree of momentum built into them, so that short-term projections are unlikely to be very wide of the mark. Finally, projections are not always intended as predictions, but rather as illustrations of what might happen if present trends continue. Their merit is in illustrating a possible outcome against which informed public debate can take place.

2 Three main factors have been identified: first, the overall level of development, and in particular education levels and rates of child survival; second, the cultural setting, including the influence of particular religions; and third, government population policies, including family planning programmes. Education levels (particularly female literacy) and child survival seem to be particularly important, followed by family planning programmes.

3   It is true that the objective of most Third World countries is low mortality in absolute terms. But as Table 8.2 showed, the countries that have achieved a lower *relative* mortality rate than might have been predicted on the basis of their income level have also achieved lower mortality and longer life expectancy in *absolute* terms than the group of countries doing particularly badly in relation to their income level. The relevance of the countries that are superior health achievers is in demonstrating that low mortality is not an automatic spin-off from rising levels of income.

Chapter 9

1   Although skin diseases are not mentioned in the chapter among the important causes of death, and are not a common reason for admission to hospital (Figure 9.5), they do cause considerable morbidity. They are one of the commonest reasons for consultations in general practice (Tables 9.1 and 9.4). Skin diseases do not appear to cause much physical impairment (Figure 9.7), though people who suffer severe skin conditions may well experience considerable social handicap.

2   Almost certainly not. The younger cohort are unlikely to experience the same rate of dental decay suffered by the older cohort. For instance, the younger groups may have benefited from using fluoride toothpaste, eating less refined sugar and receiving better dental care, so a higher proportion may retain their teeth than was true for the older cohort who were born around 1910 and have not enjoyed these benefits. Figure 9.6 contains some evidence of such cohort effects: for example, 64 per cent of the group who were aged 55–64 in 1968 had already lost all their teeth, but ten years later, when they were aged 65–74, this had increased a further 10 per cent to 74 per cent. In comparison, 48 per cent of the group aged 55–64 in 1978 had lost all their teeth, but ten years later, when they were aged 65–75, this percentage had barely increased at all. So at the same stage of the life cycle, the groups born more recently were more likely to have some of their own teeth and were losing them at a much slower rate.

3   No. The consultation ratio for all conditions combined for divorced (actually divorced and widowed) women is the same as for men. For some specific conditions, such as diseases of the musculo-skeletal system or accidents, poisonings and violence, divorced women do have higher consultation rates, but the reverse is true for mental disorders, in which the ratio for men is higher than that for women.

4   First, it should be noted that minority ethnic groups are not a homogeneous group, and that there are difficulties of definition and measurement. In general, migrants to England and Wales experience excess mortality in comparison with the population as a whole (Table 9.3). Overall, GP consultation ratios amongst minority ethnic groups are not very different from those for the population as a whole (Figure 9.13), but they are much higher for serious complaints and conditions. The limited information available on reasons for consulting a GP suggests that minority ethnic groups differ from the general population mainly in the degree to which they consult rather than in the kind of conditions they bring.

5   For a biological explanation (a), you may have suggested the influence on the human body of climatic or geological factors, such as hours of sunshine or water hardness; for a social explanation (b), variations in housing standards or in income or occupation; and for a life-history explanation (c) alcohol or tobacco consumption (although this is also a social explanation as levels of consumption may be affected by income).

6   The only exception mentioned in the chapter was that of breast cancer mortality (Figure 9.18), which is highest in social class I and lowest in social class V. Although this pattern is true for a few other conditions, the vast majority of diseases either show no social class gradient or are commoner in lower social classes. This is true whether mortality, morbidity, or disability is being measured.

7   Low-back pain is likely to increase with age due to biological 'wear and tear' on the backbone and its musculature, but the increase will be greatest in those regularly engaged in occupational or domestic heavy lifting, i.e. those in the lower social classes. Thus the *combined* influence of age and social class needs to be taken into account, and an analysis of either factor alone will distort the apparent distribution of back pain in the population.

Chapter 10

1   Data to answer this question are contained primarily in Table 10.1 and Figure 10.1. Figure 10.1, which shows trends in mortality among men by social class, from 1931 to 1981, suggests that health inequalities have widened substantially over this period. It has been suggested that these data, which are based on Decennial Supplements on Occupational Mortality, might be prone to various measurement errors. However, the OPCS Longitudinal Study, which avoids most of these, also shows that betwen 1971–5 and 1981–5 there was a widening of health inequalities across social classes (Table 10.1).

2   The proportion of the population in the lowest social classes (classes IV and V) fell from 38 per cent in 1931 to 30 per cent by 1961 and 26 per cent by 1981. These are the social classes with poorest health experience. However, there are at least two reasons why this does not necessarily imply that health inequalities must have declined also. First, there are inequalities within social classes as well as between them, and when the population is stratified using some other form of social classification, as in Table 10.3, much larger percentages of the population are revealed to have a relatively poor health experience. Second, most measures of inequality do not simply count the proportions at the lowest end of the distribution, but attempt to assess the degree of inequality above as well as below the average. The highest social classes with the best health experience have grown substantially in size, and so, on most measures, inequality in health has not diminished.

3   Patterns of smoking do vary substantially by social class (Table 10.5), and, as smoking is a major cause of death (Chapter 9), this is likely to be reflected in mortality differences between social classes, although it may take many years for current patterns of smoking to be reflected in mortality. The influence of drinking is less certain: as Figure 10.4 shows, there are no consistent differences in heavy alcohol consumption by social class among men, and among women the differences run in the opposite direction to most health differences: drinking appears to be more prevalent in the higher social classes.

4   Occupations do have different health consequences, and injury and death rates are much more common in manual occupations such as construction work. However, it is possible to standardise death rates between occupations for the social classes of the people in the occupation, and doing this removes around 80 per cent of the differences between occupation. In other words, occupation itself may account for up to 20 per cent of the health differences between social classes, but most of the differences are due to more indirect effects. Occupation remains a useful way to classify people by social class because it contributes to these indirect effects through income and hence housing tenure, and so on.

Chapter 11

1   A sustained deficit of energy, affecting a significant proportion of the population, would imply the existence of famine—continuing loss of body weight and a rising death rate from starvation. If the situation then stabilised, with a fixed, but reduced supply, there would be many very thin people and deaths from starvation would reduce population growth to zero.

If there were none of these signs of energy deficit, then some other nutrient in the food supply might be limiting health. The information needed would be the prevalence of some deficiency disease.

2   (a)   Small average stature of the adult population by itself has few implications for health policy, since nothing can be done to correct it. It may simply be a reflection of adverse factors or circumstances when those adults were very young.

(b)   Frequent faltering of growth of children under two years old is evidence of impoverished home environments, leading to high risk of infections and/or low levels of care, including inadequate feeding. The policy implications are for better access to basic preventive health services, better housing and sanitation, better employment conditions and education, especially for women. More food in the house would help, but it would probably be more effective to raise household income and hence free more time and resources for child care, rather than to provide more food. The real problem would be deciding which of all these to concentrate on first.

3   They would all have to engage in work that was *physically* much harder—probably the man at labouring and the children and wife at growing, preserving and preparing whatever food the wages would not cover. Probably they would lose some body weight and because of that, would reduce their maintenance needs for energy, hence raising their work efficiency. If Cobbett's figures are correct, after these adjustments, they would be eating about 30 per cent more food than before their time trip.

4   The increased productivity has been achieved partly by improved farming practice—better crops and the use of fertilizers (dung and later chemicals); partly by more efficient management of human labour—leading to economies of scale; and mainly by a large increase of energy inputs (lately in the form of fuel oil), hence the large net production of carbon dioxide. Changing this will entail improving energy efficiency, by using lower energy techniques—less working of soils, using high energy chemical inputs more sparingly and (as part of a general response to the need to reduce carbon emissions) using more renewable energy sources. Also, a lot less meat and dairy production—i.e. much higher prices for these foods!

5   Most of the things we would like to know more about involve tests and measurements over long periods—ideally, over an appreciable fraction of the human

lifespan. Since everything interacts with everything else, we need to try to keep as many factors of the environment and of behaviour as constant as possible. People either end up living in a way which bears almost no resemblance to real-life, or start cheating. Poor James Lind's subjects, after months on a diet without fruit or vegetables, probably got their relatives to pass them a few things through the window.

6   The problem with changing the diet of the whole population so as, for example, to reduce average consumption of fats, is that only those at the highest risk (of early death) would experience sufficient benefit to make it seem worthwhile to them as *individuals*. Most of the population would not get a perceived benefit, since their reduction of risk would be so small in comparison with other causes of death. They would get only the knowledge that the community as a whole would have reduced costs to bear (the economic loss of early death of productive members, health care costs, etc.). They might perhaps appreciate the better position of the United Kingdom in the European league tables of percentage of the population dying of CHD—or the smiles on the faces of public health nutritionists. But perhaps not! The objection is essentially the ethical position that people should be able to make their own free choice about these matters, on the basis of information which is *relevant to their own quality of life.*

Acknowledgements

Grateful acknowledgement is made to the following sources for permission to reproduce material in this book.

Figures

Figure 3.2 adapted from Walsh, J. A. and Warren, K. S. (1979) Selective primary health care, *New England Journal of Medicine*, Vol. 301, p. 968, reprinted by permission of the New England Journal of Medicine; *Figure 3.4* Science Photo Library, London; *Figure 3.5* Werner, D. (1979) *When There Is No Doctor*, Hesperian Foundation © David Werner; *Figures 4.1, 4.2, 4.5* OXFAM/Philip Jackson; *Figure 4.3* OXFAM/Walter Holt; *Figure 4.4* OXFAM/Sheena Grossett; *Figure 4.6* OXFAM; *Figure 5.2* adapted from McEvedy, C. and Jones, R. (1978) *Atlas of World Population History*, Penguin Books, Copyright Colin McEvedy and Richard Jones 1978, reproduced by permission of Curtis Brown Ltd, London; *Figure 5.4* from Wrigley, E.A. and Schofield, R. S. (1981) *The Population History of England 1541–1871: A Reconstruction*, Edward Arnold; *Figures 6.3, 6.4* Forbes, T. R. (1979) By what disease or casualty: the changing face of death in London, in Webster, C. (ed.) *Health, Medicine and Mortality in the Sixteenth Century*, Cambridge University Press; *Figure 6.5* Bodleian Library, MS Ashmole 216, Folio 116ʳ; *Figure 6.7 (bottom)* Registrar-General (1992), *Annual Abstract of Statistics*, reproduced with the permission of the Controller of Her Majesty's Stationery Office; *Figure 10.7* From the *Health and Safety Commission Annual Report 1989/90*, reproduced with the permission of the Controller of Her Majesty's Stationery Office; *Figure 11.2* Photo: Andrew Davidson, Camera Press; *Figure 11.3a* Reprinted by permission of the publishers from *Seven Countries: A Multivariate Analysis of Death and Coronary Disease* by Ancel Keys, Cambridge, Mass., Harvard University Press, Copyright © 1980 by the President and Fellows of Harvard College.

Tables

Table 3.6 Coale, A. J. (1991) Excess female mortality and the balance of the sexes in the population: an estimate of the number of 'missing females', *Population and Development Review*, **17**(3), pp. 514–24, The Population Council; *Table 3.8* adapted from the *Zimbabwe Demographic & Health Survey Report* (1990), Central Statistical Office, Zimbabwe; *Table 6.1* Forbes, T. (1979) By what disease or casualty: the changing face of death in London, in Webster, C. (ed.) *Health, Medicine and Mortality in the 16th Century*, Cambridge University Press; *Table 6.2* adapted from Szreter, S. (1988) The importance of social intervention in Britain's mortality decline, c. 1850–1914: a reinterpretation of the role of public health, *Journal of the Social History of Medicine*, Oxford University Press; *Table 7.7* Drèze, J. and Sen, A. (1989), *Hunger and Public Action*, Oxford University Press; *Table 9.1* adapted from Fry, J. (1979) *Common Diseases*, reprinted by permission of Kluwer Academic Publishers; *Table 10.1* OPCS (1989) Goldblatt, P., Mortality by social class 1971–85, *Population Trends 56*, Summer, reproduced with the permission of the Controller of Her Majesty's Stationery Office; *Table 10.3* adapted from OPCS (1990) *Longitudinal Study: Mortality and Social Organisation*, reproduced with the permission of the Controller of Her Majesty's Stationery Office; *Table 10.4* Wilkinson, R. G. (1986) *Class and Health: Research and Longitudinal Data*, Tavistock Publications; *Table 10.6* From the *Health and Safety Commission Annual Report 1989/90*, reproduced with the permission of the Controller of Her Majesty's Stationery Office; *Table 10.7* Johnson, P. and Webb, S. (1990) *Poverty in Official Statistics (Two Reports)*, Institute for Fiscal Studies.

Un-numbered photographs/illustrations

p. 3 Walter Holt/Oxfam; *pp. 14, 27, 96, 171* Tom Learmonth; *p. 16* Photos courtesy of Teaching Aids at Low Cost (TALC), P. O. Box 49, St Albans; *pp. 30, 67* C. J. Webb, London School of Hygiene and Tropical Medicine; *pp. 31, 34* Tom Learmonth/Christian Aid; *p. 33* Hutchison/Crispin Hughes; *p. 36* Popperfoto; *pp. 52, 56, 61, 81, 175* The Mansell Collection; *p. 57* Institute of Agricultural History, Reading; *p. 59* Punch; *p. 60* Wood, R. from Shellard, P. (1970) *Factory Life In 1774–1885*, Evans Bros; *p. 72* Royal Collection; *p. 75* Punch; *p. 78* Oxford University Press; *p. 83 (bottom)* Illustrated London News, 21 November 1896; *p. 86* Terry Fincher, Camera Press; *p. 93* Gerald Scarfe; *p. 95* From a drawing by Mr H. Smith, Cork; Illustrated London News,

30 January 1847; *p. 102* OXFAM/Mark Edwards; *p. 105* Panos Pictures/Paul Harrison; *p 106* Sally and Richard Greenhill; *p. 117* Maclean Hunter Ltd, Medical Division; *p. 122* White and Reed, Reading; *p. 123* Imperial War Museum; *pp. 157, 159* Shelter Photographic Library: Nigel Dickinson; *p. 166* Papua New Guinea Church Partnership; *p. 177a* Hulton–Deutsch Collection; *b* J. Topham Ltd; *c* Sperry, New Holland.

Index

Entries and page numbers in **bold type** refer to key words which are printed in **bold** in the text. Indexed information on pages indicated by *italics* is carried mainly or wholly in a figure or table.